89-1475

RC
607
.A26
R23
1988

# Radiology of AIDS

# Radiology of AIDS

### Editors

**Michael P. Federle, M.D.**
*Professor of Radiology*
*University of California, San Francisco*
*Chief, Department of Radiology*
*San Francisco General Hospital*
*San Francisco, California*

**Alec J. Megibow, M.D.**
*Associate Professor of Radiology*
*Director of Body Computed Tomography*
*University Hospital*
*New York University Medical Center*
*New York, New York*

**David P. Naidich, M.D.**
*Associate Professor of Radiology*
*Director of Body Computed Tomography*
*Bellevue Hospital*
*New York University Medical Center*
*New York, New York*

RAVEN PRESS ❧ NEW YORK

Raven Press, 1185 Avenue of the Americas, New York, New York 10036

© 1988 by Raven Press, Ltd. All rights reserved. This book is protected by copyright. No part of it may be reproduced, stored in a retrieval system, or transmitted, in any form or by any means, electronical, mechanical, photocopying, or recording, or otherwise, without the prior written permission of the publisher.

Made in the United States of America

**Library of Congress Cataloging-in-Publication Data**
Radiology of AIDS.

Includes bibliographies and index.
1. AIDS (Disease)—Diagnosis. 2. Diagnosis, Radioscopic. I. Federle, Michael P. II. Megibow, Alec J. III. Naidich, David P. [DNLM: 1. Acquired Immunodeficiency Syndrome—radiography. WD 308 R129]
RC607.A26R23    1988    616.97′920757    87-45366
ISBN 0-88167-406-0

The material contained in this volume was submitted as previously unpublished material, except in the instances in which credit has been given to the source from which some of the illustrative material was derived.

Great care has been taken to maintain the accuracy of the information contained in the volume. However, neither Raven Press nor the editors can be held responsible for errors or for any consequences arising from the use of the information contained herein.

Materials appearing in this book prepared by individuals as part of their official duties as U.S. Government employees are not covered by the above-mentioned copyright.

9 8 7 6 5 4 3 2 1

*To our families—Lynne, Andrew, and Tim; Marilyn, Matilda, David, and Louie; Jocelyn and Zachary—and to those physicians, surgeons, housestaff officers, and nurses who continue to provide care and comfort*

# Preface

Initial reports of the acquired immunodeficiency syndrome (AIDS) were first made to the Centers for Disease Control in 1981. Since then an epidemic of world-wide proportions has been documented. Unfortunately, despite the tremendous strides that have been made to date in elucidating the clinical syndromes which characterize this disease, as well as the discovery of its causative agent, the human immunodeficiency virus (HIV), effective therapy, and prophylaxis are lacking. The number of reported cases continues to grow at an alarming rate, making recognition of the diverse manifestations of this syndrome increasingly important.

This volume is an outgrowth of an extensive interchange of experience and ideas between members of the Departments of Radiology at the San Francisco General Hospital, and the New York University-Bellevue Hospital Centers. Situated as we are in large, diversely populated urban settings, each of us has developed considerable experience in the radiologic diagnosis and management of patients with this syndrome. Based on collaboration with our respective Departments of Clinical Medicine and Pathology, our goal is to provide the most comprehensive overview possible of the enormous spectrum of radiographic manifestations of AIDS.

Rather than present an atlas of images, we have attempted to integrate important radiologic findings and appropriate imaging strategies as they apply in day-to-day clinical practice. An introductory chapter details basic virology, epidemiology, and therapeutics. The following chapters describe the most important radiologic findings utilizing an organ system approach. Included are the central nervous system; the thorax; and the gastrointestinal tract. Separate chapters are devoted to imaging in neoplastic disease, including a discussion of lymphadenopathy, and pediatric manifestations. A final chapter is devoted to the handling of AIDS patients specifically within Departments of Radiology.

It is hoped that this volume will prove valuable not only to radiologists who are as yet unfamiliar with this syndrome, but to all physicians involved in the day-to-day care of patients with AIDS. With time and increasing experience significant changes in the diagnosis and especially the treatment of AIDS will occur. We expect these changes will be reflected in changes in the radiographic appearances of this syndrome and an increasing role of radiologic imaging to monitor treatment responses. We hope that this volume may serve as a stimulus towards continued collaboration between those responsible for the care of AIDS patients.

*Michael P. Federle*
*Alec J. Megibow*
*David P. Naidich*

# Contents

1. **Human Immunodeficiency Virus: Epidemiology, Biology, and Spectrum of Clinical Syndromes** .................................................. 1
   *Laura J. Bessen, Kenneth B. Hymes, and Jeffrey B. Greene*

2. **Neuroradiology of AIDS** .................................................. 21
   *Walter L. Olsen and Wendy Cohen*

3. **Pulmonary Manifestations of AIDS** .................................................. 47
   *David P. Naidich, Stuart M. Garay, Philip C. Goodman, Benito J. Rybak, and Elissa L. Kramer*

4. **Gastrointestinal Radiology in AIDS Patients** .................................................. 77
   *Alec J. Megibow, Susan D. Wall, Emil J. Balthazar, and Benito J. Rybak*

5. **Malignant Neoplasms: Kaposi's Sarcoma, Lymphoma, and Other Diseases with Similar Radiographic Features** .................................................. 107
   *Michael P. Federle, David A. Nyberg, Donald H. Hulnick, and R. Brooke Jeffrey, Jr.*

6. **Pediatric AIDS** .................................................. 131
   *Nancy Branom Genieser, Marta Hernanz-Schulman, Keith Krasinski, M. Alba Greco, and William Borkowsky*

7. **Handling AIDS Patients in the Radiology Department** .................................................. 143
   *Mary Anne G. Johnson*

**Appendix A** .................................................. 147

**Subject Index** .................................................. 159

# Contributors

**Emil J. Balthazar, M.D.**
*Professor of Radiology
Director, Gastrointestinal Radiology
New York University Medical Center
560 First Avenue
New York, New York 10016*

**Laura J. Bessen, M.D.**
*New York University Medical Center
560 First Avenue
New York, New York 10016*

**William Borkowsky, M.D.**
*Associate Professor of Pediatrics
New York University Medical Center
550 First Avenue
New York, New York 10016*

**Wendy Cohen, M.D.**
*Assistant Professor
Department of Radiology
University of Washington
Seattle, Washington 98195*

**Michael P. Federle, M.D.**
*Professor of Radiology
University of California, San Francisco
Chief, Department of Radiology
San Francisco General Hospital
San Francisco, California 94110*

**Stuart M. Garay, M.D.**
*Assistant Professor of Clinical
  Medicine
New York University Medical Center
560 First Avenue
New York, New York 10016*

**Nancy Branom Genieser, M.D.**
*Professor of Radiology
Director, Pediatric Radiology
New York University Medical Center
560 First Avenue
New York, New York 10016*

**Philip C. Goodman, M.D.**
*Chief, Chest Imaging
Clinical Associate Professor of
  Radiology
San Francisco General Hospital
San Francisco, California 94110*

**M. Alba Greco, M.D.**
*Associate Professor of Pediatric
  Pathology
New York University Medical Center
560 First Avenue
New York, New York 10016*

**Jeffrey B. Greene, M.D.**
*Clinical Associate Professor of
  Medicine
New York University Medical Center
560 First Avenue
New York, New York 10016*

**Donald H. Hulnick, M.D.**
*Assistant Professor of Radiology
New York University Medical Center
560 First Avenue
New York, New York 10016*

**Kenneth B. Hymes, M.D.**
*Assistant Professor of Medicine
Division of Hematology
New York University Medical Center
560 First Avenue
New York, New York 10016*

**R. Brooke Jeffrey, Jr., M.D.**
*Professor of Radiology
University of California, San Francisco
San Francisco General Hospital
San Francisco, California 94110*

**Mary Anne G. Johnson, M.D.**
*Assistant Clinical Professor of
  Medicine
University of California San Francisco
Medical Director/Laguna-Honda
  Hospital
San Francisco, California 94110*

**Elissa L. Kramer, M.D.**
*Assistant Professor of Clinical
  Radiology
New York University Medical Center
560 First Avenue
New York, New York 10016*

**Keith Krasinski, M.D.**
*Associate Professor of Pediatrics
New York University Medical Center
560 First Avenue
New York, New York 10016*

**Alec J. Megibow, M.D.**
*Associate Professor of Radiology
Director of Body Computed
  Tomography
University Hospital
New York University Medical Center
560 First Avenue
New York, New York 10016*

**David P. Naidich, M.D.**
*Associate Professor of Radiology
Director of Body Computed
  Tomography
Bellevue Hospital
New York University Medical Center
560 First Avenue
New York, New York 10016*

**David A. Nyberg, M.D.**
*Associate Professor of Clinical
  Radiology
University of Washington
Department of Radiology
Swedish Hospital
747 Summit Avenue
Seattle, Washington 98104*

**Walter L. Olsen, M.D.**
*Chief, Neuroradiology
Assistant Professor of Radiology
San Francisco General Hospital
San Francisco, California 94110*

**Benito J. Rybak, M.D.**
*Assistant Professor of Pathology
Mount Sinai Medical School
City University of New York
New York, New York 10016*

**Marta Hernanz-Schulman, M.D.**
*Assistant Professor of Radiology
New York University Medical Center
560 First Avenue
New York, New York 10016*

**Susan D. Wall, M.D.**
*Assistant Professor of Radiology
Chief, Abdominal Imaging
San Francisco Veterans
  Administration Hospital
San Francisco, California 94110*

# Radiology of AIDS

CHAPTER 1

# Human Immunodeficiency Virus: Epidemiology, Biology, and Spectrum of Clinical Syndromes

Laura J. Bessen, Kenneth B. Hymes, and Jeffrey B. Greene

Since the first description in 1981, more than 35,000 persons in the United States and as many as 1 million persons worldwide have contracted the acquired immune deficiency syndrome (AIDS). It is estimated that between 1 and 2 million persons in the United States already have been infected with the causative agent of AIDS, the human immunodeficiency virus (HIV). Many of these individuals will develop clinical disease within the next decade. AIDS was described initially in a limited number of high-risk groups defined alternatively by male homosexual practices, parenteral drug use, or prior blood product infusion (whole or packed red blood cells or coagulation factor concentrates). As the scope of the epidemic broadens, some of the newly reported cases of AIDS fall outside the originally recognized risk groups, and include female sexual partners of bisexual men and intravenous (i.v.) drug users, and infants born to HIV-infected women. The diagnosis of AIDS in the first 3 to 4 years of the epidemic usually was made on clinical grounds and rested on the recognition of an opportunistic infection or Kaposi's sarcoma in a patient with no other identifiable cause of immune dysfunction. In the past 3 years a firmer understanding of the etiology of AIDS and the spectrum of HIV infection has allowed for a more elaborate classification of HIV-associated diseases (Table 1).

As the incidence of AIDS continues to rise, the care of patients with this illness will no longer be restricted to research centers or municipal hospitals of large urban areas. Every health care establishment in the nation and physicians from every subspeciality will be called upon to familiarize themselves with the pathophysiology and clinical manifestations of AIDS.

## EPIDEMIOLOGY

The earliest reports of what would later be termed AIDS appeared in 1981 with the recognition of Pneumocystis carinii pneumonia (PCP) and Kaposi's sarcoma (KS) in homosexual men and i.v. drug users (1–3). Although these two rare diseases were known to occur in the setting of severe immune depression, no clearly definable cause of immune deficiency was apparent in these individuals. During the next 12 months, more than 500 cases of unexplained life-threatening opportunistic infections and neoplasms were reported, raising the awareness of a new epidemic of acquired immune deficiency. As of August 1987, more than 40,000 cases in the United States were reported to the Centers for Disease Control (CDC), and more than 50% of these have ended in death (4).

In the United States, 95% of the adult AIDS cases occur in persons belonging to one of several risk groups (Table 2). The nature of these risk groups is consistent with the theory that AIDS is horizontally transmitted by intimate contact with blood or body fluids. Despite the growing number of cases over the past 6 years, the relative percentages of cases within each risk group has remained virtually constant. Most reassuring is that today only 3 to 4% of cases occur in persons not reporting any risk factors, similar to the percentage in the period prior to 1983 (see Table 2). This implies that the epidemic has been limited in extent because of the inability to transmit AIDS by casual contact.

While the number of AIDS cases continues to increase each year, the time to double the number of cases has lengthened from 5 months in 1982 to 11 months in

**TABLE 1.** *CDC classification of HIV infection*

Group I: Acute HIV infection
  Mononucleosis-like syndrome associated with seroconversion
Group II: Asymptomatic infection
  Positive HIV antibody assay or viral culture (may have abnormal CBC, platelet counts, T-cell subsets, etc. . .)
Group III: Persistent generalized lymphadenopathy
  Palpable lymphadenopathy (at least 1 cm) at two or more extrainguinal sites for more than 3 months in the absence of concurrent illness to explain the findings
Group IV: Other HIV-associated disease
  Subgroup A: Constitutional disease
    Fever, diarrhea for more than 1 month, involuntary weight loss of 10% of baseline weight in the absence of concurrent illness to explain symptoms
  Subgroup B: Neurologic disease
    Dementia, myelopathy, or peripheral neuropathy in the absence of a concurrent illness or condition
  Subgroup C: Secondary infectious diseases
    Category C-1: Symptomatic or invasive disease due to 1 of 12 specified diseases listed in the surveillance definition of AIDS: Pneumocystis carinii pneumonia, chronic intestinal cryptosporidiosis, isosporiasis, toxoplasmosis, extraintestinal strongyloidiasis, cryptococcosis, histoplasmosis, invasive candidiasis, atypical mycobacterial infection (M. avium complex, M. kansasii), cytomegalovirus infection, chronic mucocutaneous or disseminated H. simplex infection, progressive multifocal leukoencephalopathy
    Category C-2: Symptomatic disease due to one of six other specified diseases: oral hairy leukoplakia, multidermatomal varicella-zoster, recurrent salmonella bacteremia, nocardiosis, tuberculosis, and oral candidiasis (thrush)
  Subgroup D: Secondary cancers
    Kaposi's sarcoma, non-Hodgkin's lymphoma (small, noncleaved lymphoma or immunoblastic lymphoma), Burkitt's lymphoma, primary brain lymphoma
  Subgroup E: Other symptomatic conditions in HIV infection
    Chronic lymphoid interstitial pneumonia, secondary infectious diseases, and neoplasms not listed above

From CDC: Classification system for HIV infections. *M. M. W. R.*, 35:334, 1986.

1985 (5). The rate of increase in homosexual/bisexual cases has fallen significantly, due to intensive educational efforts and changes in sexual practices. The numbers of cases among female sexual partners of HIV-infected men have the most rapid percentage growth. The epidemiology of AIDS is somewhat different in New York City (Table 3): This geographic area contributes almost 30% of the nationally reported cases. Intravenous drug use is implicated in 27% of the reported cases, and Blacks and Hispanics account for a disproportionately high number of those diagnosed (6).

Soon after AIDS was reported in the United States, several countries in Europe and Central Africa as well as Haiti also began recognizing cases (7–9). The availability of a reliable serologic test for HIV provided the means of establishing the presence of this virus in Africa as early as the 1960s (10). Forty countries have now reported AIDS and this disease has become a major focus for the World Health Organization. In Africa, the distribution of cases of AIDS is equal among men and women, reflecting the predominantly heterosexual mode of transmission in that region (8). In Central Africa, the virus is more widely prevalent in the general population than it is in the United States or Europe.

In the United States, the rate of HIV seropositivity among healthy blood donors ranges between 0.02 and 0.04% (11). In civilian recruits for military service who were systematically subjected to mandatory HIV testing, a seroprevalence of 1.5/100 was reported (12). In contrast, the prevalence of HIV infection in members of the various risk groups is significantly higher. Cohort studies of homosexual men in San Francisco have identified an HIV-seroprevalence approaching 70% (13). Similarly, the rate of positive HIV antibodies among i.v. drug users approximates 50% (14). Hemophiliacs receiving Factor VIII concentrates have an HIV seroprevalence of 64 to 72% (15).

The natural history of HIV infection is better understood by a recent study of 6,700 homosexual men reported at the Third International Conference on AIDS (16). The risks of developing AIDS following HIV infection were 15% at 60 months and 36% at 88 months of followup.

There is strong epidemiologic evidence to support the contention that AIDS is not easily transmitted by casual or occupational exposure to infected individuals. Only one of the 40,000 cases of AIDS reported to the CDC

**TABLE 2.** *Cases of HIV infection in U.S. adults by risk group*

| Risk group | Before 1983 (%) | 8/83–8/84 (%) | 8/84–8/85 (%) | 8/85–8/86 (%) | 8/86–8/87 (%) | Total (%) |
|---|---|---|---|---|---|---|
| Homosexual/bisexual | 1,430 (72) | 2,512 (73) | 5,062 (75) | 8,140 (73) | 11,924 (73) | 29,068 (74) |
| I.V. drug abuser | 330 (17) | 628 (18) | 1,155 (17) | 1,920 (17) | 2,473 (15) | 6,506 (16) |
| Hemophiliac | 15 (<1) | 26 (<1) | 33 (<1) | 113 (1) | 169 (1) | 356 (1) |
| Heterosexual | 127 (6) | 146 (4) | 230 (3) | 383 (3) | 646 (4) | 1,532 (4) |
| Transfusion recipient | 20 (1) | 41 (1) | 117 (2) | 231 (2) | 430 (3) | 839 (2) |
| Undetermined | 56 (3) | 100 (3) | 151 (2) | 278 (2) | 599 (4) | 1,184 (3) |
| Total | 1,978 (100) | 3,453 (100) | 6,752 (100) | 11,067 (100) | 16,243 (100) | 39,493 (100) |

TABLE 3. *Adult AIDS in New York City (5/87)*

| Risk group | % of cases |
|---|---|
| Homosexual/bisexual | 63 |
| Homosexual/bisexual i.v. user | 5 |
| i.v. drug user | 27 |
| Sex partner of at-risk group | <1 |
| Blood product associated | <1 |
| No identified risk | <1 |
| Other/under investigation | <5 |
| Race/ethnicity (cumulative) | |
| White | 45 |
| Black | 31 |
| Hispanic | 23 |
| Unknown | 1 |

Adapted from ref. 6.

was in a nonsexual household contact of another patient with AIDS (17). This was the mother of a hemophiliac child who failed to observe infection control precautions despite frequent blood and fecal soiling. A formal study of 350 household contacts of AIDS patients demonstrated the absence of acquisition of HIV serologic and virologic methods (18).

The risk of HIV infection to health care workers has been studied. Among 1,500 health care providers (half of whom reported needle-stick injury or mucosal exposure to infected material), 26 were seropositive but only three of these persons had no other risk factors (19). Three other health care employees were found to have acquired HIV infection by unusual exposure to infected blood, presumably by the transcutaneous or transmucosal route (20). Therefore, the occupational risk of HIV infection for the health care worker is extraordinarily low and can be reduced further by adherence to recommended infection control practices.

## IMMUNE ABNORMALITIES AND IMMUNOPATHOGENESIS

The earliest clinical observations in patients with AIDS centered on the secondary infectious diseases they incurred. Because most of the etiologic agents of these infections were ubiquitous intracellular pathogens, AIDS was felt to be due to a profound defect in cell-mediated immunity (CMI). Current knowledge of the immune defects in AIDS implicates a much wider range of abnormalities involving the humoral, cellular, and monocytic arms of the immune system (Table 4).

Absolute lymphopenia is a common finding in HIV-infected individuals, usually due to a depletion of circulating T-helper lymphocytes ($CD_{4+}$). This may be preceded by an increase in the number of T-suppressor cells ($CD_{8+}$). Thus, the $CD_4/CD_8$ ratio is inverted and tends to decline with disease progression due to further decreases in the $CD_4$ cell population (21).

Functional T-lymphocyte abnormalities are widely apparent in HIV-infected persons. The wide sweeping immune defects caused by HIV infection in large part may be understood by the central regulatory role played by the T-helper lymphocytes (22). This cell is involved with B-lymphocyte maturation, $CD_{4+}$ cell proliferation, plasma cell antibody production, and induction of cytotoxic lymphocytes. The delayed-type hypersensitivity (DTH) reaction often is absent with cutaneous anergy to multiple recall antigens. T-lymphocyte dependent proliferative responses to mitogens and antigens are severely depressed. Similarly, alloreactivity in mixed lymphocyte culture is abnormally low or absent. Antibody-dependent cytotoxic cellular response (ADCC), natural killer cell (NK) activity, and decreased function of T-helper cells in stimulating B-cell immunoglobulin production are all observed (22,23).

The B-lymphocyte defects are manifested by polyclonal hyperimmunoglobulinemia. Excessive immunoglobulin production usually is associated with circulating immune complexes and antilymphocyte antibodies (23,24). Despite excessive spontaneous synthesis of immunoglobulin, *de novo* production of specific antibody is impaired. Serologic response to neoantigens such as keyhole limpet hemocyanin is poor, and serologic responses to reactivation of latent infectious agents (e.g., Toxoplasma gondii) may be less than expected. T-lymphocyte dependent pokeweed mitogen B-cell responses also are depressed (23,24).

Altered monocyte function is marked by decreased chemotaxis, decreased cytotoxicity, and decreased interleukin-1 production. Other immunologic epipheno-

TABLE 4. *Immune defects in HIV-infected individuals*

Humoral
  Hyperimmunoglobulinemia (polyclonal)
  Decreased antibody response to neoantigens
  Circulating immune complexes

Cellular
  Absolute lymphopenia
  Decreased $CD_{4+}$ population ⎫
  Increased $CD_{8+}$ population ⎬ Inverted $CD_4/CD_8$ ratio
  Diminished delayed-type hypersensitivity to cutaneous antigens
  Decreased lymphoproliferative response *in vitro* to mitogens and allogeneic cells
  Decreased natural killer cell activity
  Decreased interleukin-2 production

Monocytic
  Decreased chemotaxis
  Decreased intracellular killing

Miscellaneous
  Elevated acid-labile alpha interferon
  Elevated beta-2 microglobulins

mena include high levels of acid-labile alpha-interferon (formerly described in autoimmune diseases), serum suppressor factors of interleukin-2 production by T-helper cells, and increased levels of beta-2 microglobulins (25,26).

The clinical implications of such generalized immune defects can be recognized easily. The severely depressed T lymphocyte and monocyte function might explain the high incidence of opportunistic intracellular pathogens, such as cytomegalovirus (CMV), Toxoplasma gondii, and mycobacteria, and probably the secondary neoplasms. Abnormal B-lymphocyte function may impair defense against bacterial pathogens and limit the utility of serologic diagnostic tests. Excessive antibody production may cause immune complex-mediated diseases such as immune thrombocytopenic purpura (27).

The immunopathogenesis of the HIV retrovirus is beginning to be unravelled. The virus surface glycoprotein (gp-120) binds directly to the $CD_4$ molecule on the T-helper lymphocyte cell membrane (28). This observation explains the preferential infection of T-helper cells by HIV. The viral cytopathic effect is directly related to the concentration of the $CD_4$ molecule on the cell surface (29). Many T-helper cells will be killed osmotically during initial infection by HIV due to increased membrane permeability. Alternatively, T-helper cell surface-bound HIV may induce syncytial cell formation and cell-to-cell infection (30). While these two mechanisms clearly reduce T-helper number, other indirect and as yet obscure factors may be involved to explain the marked decrease in this cell population.

Monocytes have a lower density of $CD_4$ molecules on the cell surface, which allows for limited HIV cellular penetration. While cell death does not occur, the direct infection may be the cause of abnormal monocyte function. In addition, it is believed that the circulating monocytes may bring the HIV to such extravascular sites as the central nervous system (10).

Measurable immune abnormalities tend to be irreversible in HIV-infected individuals and the absolute $CD_4$ counts tend to fall in parallel with progressive clinical disease.

## ETIOLOGIC AGENT OF AIDS

Four years have elapsed since the reporting of convincing evidence that a human retrovirus was the etiologic agent of AIDS. During this period, a great deal of knowledge has accrued concerning the basic biology and molecular genetics of this newly described organism.

The previously described human retroviruses, human T-lymphotropic viruses I and II (HTLV-I,II), were discovered in 1978 and 1982, respectively, and were linked to human leukemia (31). In view of the fact that these viruses have long latency periods, have the potential to cause neoplasms and immune deficiency, and spread epidemiologically within well-defined populations (e.g., islands off Japan's coast), the possibility of a new retrovirus causing AIDS was considered. In 1983, Montagnier et al. at the Pasteur Institute reported a new retrovirus isolated from patients with the lymphadenopathy syndrome and termed this virus lymphadenopathy virus (LAV) (32). Soon thereafter, Gallo et al. at the National Institutes of Health isolated a similar retrovirus from individuals with AIDS-related complex (ARC) and AIDS (33). They named the isolates human T-lymphotropic virus-III (HTLV-III). It was later determined that these retroviruses were the same organism, now known as human immunodeficiency virus (HIV).

The HIV is a ribonucleic acid (RNA) retrovirus, so named because it uses its RNA template to produce deoxyribonucleic acid (DNA) via the action of the enzyme reverse transcriptase. The virus is composed of a glycoprotein envelope that has two structural subunits (gp41 and gp120) (10). There is a small eccentric ribonucleoprotein core that is seen as a dense crescenteric structure by electron microscopy (34). The provirus is more complex than previously described retroviruses. There are three structural genes and at least five regulatory genes critical to the expression of either viral latency or active replication. The tat-III transactivating gene is the major up-regulator of viral replication. Another regulatory gene, 3'-orf, has negative control modulation of replication (35). The five regulatory gene products are all immunogenic. The structural proteins include two envelope proteins (gp41 and gp120) and the core antigen (p24) (35).

The HIV lacks extensive nucleotide homology with members of the oncovirinae, such as HTLV-I and HTLV-II. It is more closely related to the Lentivirnae, such as Visna (sheep), Caprine encephalitis virus, and Equine infectious anemia virus (36). Viral isolates from West Africans have yielded an organism related to but distinct from HIV. This new retrovirus has been termed HIV-2 (or HTLV-IV, LAV-2) (37). This virus is prevalent in African green monkeys and humans in western African nations.

The body of evidence that HIV is the cause of AIDS is extensive. The biologic properties of HIV, such as cytopathic effect in human cell lines, T-helper cell tropism, syncytia formation, and long latency periods, explain many of the clinically observed features of AIDS. Furthermore, HIV can be isolated from a majority of persons with ARC or AIDS (38). Serologic studies using highly specific antibodies to HIV document a correlation between seropositivity and acquisition of clinical disease (39). Simian-AIDS is induced by the simian T-lymphotropic virus (STIV-III) a retrovirus related to HIV (40). This lends further support of the disease-causing potential of this class of virus.

While few investigators question the role of HIV in

AIDS, many have considered cofactors to be important in determining the degree of clinical illness. Such cofactors may include genetic determinants, concomitant viral infections (e.g., CMV, Epstein-Barr virus [EBV]), or coinfection with other retroviruses (e.g., HTLV-I) (41,42). Dual retrovirus infection is now being uncovered in i.v. drug abusers in the United States (42).

HIV is highly susceptible to inactivation by a variety of physiochemical conditions. Wet heat at 56°C for 30 min, 0.01% sodium hypochlorite, 0.125% glutaraldehyde, 0.1% formaldehyde, 25% ethanol, and 3% hydrogen peroxide all inactivate the virus effectively (43).

## CLASSIFICATION

The earliest case definitions of AIDS used by the CDC for surveillance purposes required the diagnosis of a rare opportunistic infection in a person without an identified cause of immunodeficiency. These infections were caused by Pneumocystis carinii, Cryptococcus neoformans, Toxoplasma gondii, and Mycobacterium-avium intracellulare (44). With the development of accurate serological assays for HIV exposure, it became clear that some persons with AIDS developed infections with more common pathogens such as Histoplasma capsulatum. In 1985, a revision of the original case definition of AIDS added other infections to the list of "indicator diseases" if there was concomitant serological proof of HIV infection (45). The most recent revision of the CDC's case definition was published in August 1987 and expands the definition of AIDS to include clinical syndromes attributable to HIV infections (e.g., wasting syndrome and dementia) in the absence of secondary pathogens (46) (see Appendix A). In addition to this change, the new case definition of AIDS allows for the presumptive diagnosis of indicator diseases (e.g., the diagnosis of KS based on gross appearance, or the diagnosis of PCP based on clinical and radiographic findings) without confirmatory laboratory evidence. The goal of these changes is to enable public health departments to track HIV-related morbidity and simplify reporting of AIDS cases. Application of this classification schema will increase the number of reported cases and improve the understanding of the natural history of this disease.

## OPPORTUNISTIC INFECTIONS COMPLICATING AIDS

The recognition and treatment of opportunistic infections in patients with AIDS poses a real challenge to clinicians. The usual manifestations of infection may be altered significantly by the host's profound immune depression and lack of inflammatory response. As such, a cryptococcal meningitis might not be associated with meningeal symptoms, abnormal cerebrospinal fluid chemistries, or pleiocytosis. Similarly, disseminated mycobacterioses may not display tissue granulomatous responses or systemic symptoms until very late in the course of infection. Certain laboratory diagnostic measures cannot be relied upon in the setting of AIDS. For example, the serologic response to infection by Toxoplasma gondii often is less than anticipated, thus making the titer of antibody an unreliable diagnostic indicator. The treatment of opportunistic infections also is particularly difficult in the AIDS patient. Some newly recognized pathogens (e.g., Mycobacterium avium-intracellulare [MAI], cryptosporidium) have no standard therapies. The frequent lack of clinical or laboratory signs of infection may make following a response to therapy quite difficult. Finally, the profound immunologic defects encountered in AIDS places the antimicrobial agent in a central role without the assistance of a host-immune response. This undoubtedly accounts for the high failure and relapse rates seen in this population.

It is convenient to consider the various opportunistic infections complicating AIDS in terms of the symptom complexes they cause (Table 5). The most frequently encountered symptom complex is pulmonary. The patient usually will report a nonproductive cough, dyspnea on exertion, shortness of breath, vague chest pain, and fever to 101 to 102° F. These symptoms often are present for weeks or months before diagnosis. The most

**TABLE 5.** *Presentations of opportunistic infections in AIDS*

| Symptom complex | Likely pathogens |
|---|---|
| Pulmonary | Pneumocystis carinii<br>Cytomegalovirus<br>Mycobacteriae<br>Cryptococcus neoformans |
| Central nervous system | |
|   Chronic meningitis | Cryptococcus neoformans<br>Mycobacteriae<br>Toxoplasma gondii<br>Histoplasma capsulatum |
|   Diffuse encephalitis | Human immunodeficiency virus<br>Toxoplasma gondii<br>Progressive multifocal leukoencephalopathy<br>Mycobacteriae |
| Gastrointestinal | |
|   Stomatitis esophagitis | Cytomegalovirus<br>Herpes simplex<br>Candida albicans |
|   Dysentery-like | Cryptosporidia<br>Isospora belli |
|   Colitis | Cytomegalovirus<br>Mycobacteriae<br>Clostridium difficile |
| Fever of unknown origin | Mycobacteria avium-intracellulare<br>Other mycobacterium |

likely pathogen in this setting is Pneumocystis carinii. Other possibilities include CMV, mycobacteria, histoplasma, or pulmonary cryptococcus.

Alternatively, patients may present with a neurologic syndrome, which may take the form of chronic meningitis with photophobia, headache, nucchal, and lumbar tenderness. This is usually caused by Cryptococcus neoformans. Meningitis caused by mycobacteria, histoplasmosis, or toxoplasmosis is far less frequently encountered. Patients also may present with diffuse encephalitis. The most common cause of this syndrome is HIV-induced subacute encephalopathy. It is marked by a slow onset of vague neurologic symptoms including memory deficit, change in personality, difficulty with conversation and reading, attenuation of fine motor skills, and occasionally a severe manic psychosis. Other causes of encephalopathy in AIDS include Toxoplasma gondii, progressive multifocal leukoencephalopathy (PML), and mycobacterial brain abscesses. Toxoplasmosis and PML usually present with focal neurologic signs and symptoms.

Gastrointestinal presentations of opportunistic infections in AIDS patients usually involve diarrhea. This may be a voluminous dysentery-like syndrome usually without fever and associated with cachexia and dehydration. Cryptosporidiosis should be anticipated in this setting, as well as isosporiasis. More commonly, colitis associated with tenesmus, hematochezia, mucousy stools, and fever is encountered and caused by CMV or MAI.

Finally, a presentation of unexplained fevers without localizing symptoms may be seen. These individuals often exhibit weight loss, hepatosplenomegaly, lymphadenopathy, severe anemia, and abnormally elevated cholestatic liver enzymes. Generally the workup will reveal disseminated mycobacterial infection.

The following discussion focuses on the clinical manifestations of the most common AIDS-related disorders affecting the lungs, central nervous system, and gastrointestinal tract.

### Pneumocystis Carinii Pneumonia

Pneumocystis carinii pneumonia (PCP) is the most frequently diagnosed opportunistic infection in patients with AIDS, accounting for more than 60% of all infectious episodes (5). Pneumocystis carinii is a parasite that normally resides in the lungs of rodents, small domestic mammals, and man. In immunosuppressed patients, the dormant cystic forms may multiply, resulting in a life-threatening interstitial pneumonia (47).

Individuals with AIDS may present with a fulminant pneumonia within days of the onset of symptoms. More often, however, symptoms may persist for weeks or even months before the diagnosis is established (3). Significant fever ($\geq 101.5°$ F) usually is the earliest sign, followed by vague nonpleuritic chest discomfort, nonproductive cough, dyspnea on exertion, and shortness of breath. More than one-half of patients will report a mild diarrhea.

The physical examination usually reveals few signs. In the more ill patient, air hunger, cyanosis, and bibasilar rales can be demonstrated. However, the pulmonary exam typically will be normal and the remainder of the findings nonspecific.

The chest roentgenogram usually reveals a bilateral, diffuse interstitial pneumonitis most prominent in the perihilar and basilar regions. Many other patterns of chest x-ray (CXR) findings have been described in patients with PCP (see Chapter 3). In as many as 10% of patients with PCP, the initial CXR may be normal. These individuals usually will have abnormal Gallium$^{67}$ ($Ga^{67}$)-citrate pulmonary scans with diffuse parenchymal uptake persistent at 72 to 96 hours (48). This abnormal pattern of $Ga^{67}$ uptake is highly sensitive and moderately specific for PCP.

Other abnormal laboratory findings include hypoxemia, a widened arterial-alveolar $O_2$ gradient, and an elevated serum lactate dehydrogenase (LDH) in the absence of elevations of other liver chemistries. In our experience, the degree of LDH elevation correlates roughly with the severity of illness and is one of the earliest parameters to begin to normalize with successful therapy (49).

The definitive diagnosis of PCP requires the histologic demonstration of the organisms. Transbronchial lung biopsy can be performed with a low complication rate and high yield, exceeding 95% (50). This diagnostic modality also allows diagnosis of concomitant or other pulmonary processes. Some centers have reported an acceptably high yield using bronchial alveolar lavage without transbronchial biopsy (50). The polychrome stains (e.g., Gram-Weigert, Giemsa) highlight the trophozites and the silver stains (e.g., modified Grocott's) reveal the cyst wall. This histopathology of pneumocystis pneumonia is notable for an exuberant intralveolar proteinaceous exudate with little interstitial inflammation.

The treatment of first episode PCP is generally successful, with a "cure rate" of about 85% (51). Patients presenting with respiratory failure or extremely high serum LDH levels, or patients with recurrent PCP have a worse prognosis. The treatments of choice are trimethoprim/sulfamethoxazole (tmp/smx) and pentamidine isoethionate. Tmp/smx has a rapid onset of action, can be given orally, and is relatively inexpensive. The use of tmp/smx is complicated by an extraordinarily high rate of allergy in patients with HIV infection. Approximately 55% of patients with AIDS will develop fever, rash, cholestatic hepatopathy, or neutropenia by the second week of therapy (52). The reasons for this observed rate of adverse reactions is unknown but is peculiar to persons with HIV-induced immune suppresson. Pentamidine is a parenterally administered drug with a wide range of possible side-effects. These include azotemia, sterile abscess formation, severe orthostatic hypotension, granulocytopenia, hypoglycemia, and diabetes mellitus (permanent) (53). Effective levels may not be reached in pulmonary tissue for 4 to 5 days.

The dose of tmp/smx is 15 to 20 mg/kg/day of tmp and 75 to 100 mg/kg/day of smx in four divided doses for 14 to 21 days. Pentamidine is given slowly at 4 mg/kg/day in a single daily intramuscular or i.v. dose for 14 to 21 days. Although the patient may have a good clinical response, follow-up bronchoscopic studies may demonstrate persistence of pneumocystic organisms weeks after completion of therapy (54).

The attendant toxicities of tmp/smx and pentamidine in treating PCP have prompted a search for other effective therapies. Dapsone with trimethoprim, dapsone alone, deoxyfluoromethoxyornithine (DFMO), and trimetrexate (a methorexate analog) have shown acceptable cure rates in the treatment of PCP (55).

Antimicrobial prophylaxis of PCP is an important consideration in any patient who has had this pneumonia, in view of its high recurrence rate. Oral tmp/smx in low doses is effective in preventing PCP in those patients who tolerate this drug (56). Dapsone 100 mg. p.o. daily may be an effective alternative regimen, although some cross-sensitivity should be anticipated (57). Fansidar (sulfadoxine/pyrimethamine) given once weekly also may be efficacious (58). Aerosolized pentamidine administered biweekly currently is under study as a means of PCP prophylaxis, with promising initial results (59).

While Pneumocystis carinii is most commonly implicated as a cause of pneumonia in patients with AIDS, extrapulmonary infections rarely have been seen. Involvement of the skin, otic structures, and retina have been reported (60–62).

**Cerebral Toxoplasmosis**

Toxoplasma gondii is a prevalent infection in the general population (40–50%) (63). In patients with AIDS, reactivation of central nervous system toxoplasmosis is a common cause of encephalitis. The illness presents as a focal neurologic illness sometimes with seizures. Computed tomography (CT) performed with i.v. contrast reveals multiple ring-enhancing abscesses with surrounding edema favoring the basal ganglia and the periventricular region (64; see Chapter 2). It is important to consider this diagnostic possibility so that a CT scan may be performed to rule out mass effect prior to performing lumbar puncture. Recent evidence for local cerebrospinal fluid production of immunoglobulin G antitoxoplasma antibodies provides a basis for future development of a diagnostic test for cerebral toxoplasmosis (65). Currently, the therapy for this disease is begun empirically.

The antimicrobial regimen employed is a combination of pyrimethamine and sulfadiazine (63). Additionally, anticonvulsants and corticosteroids may be needed for seizure control and cerebral edema, respectively. Clindamycin has not shown convincing usefulness in the therapy of cerebral toxoplasmosis despite its *in vitro* activity against T. gondii (66). Other antimicrobial agents, such as trimetrexate, are being evaluated for effectiveness and safety (67).

Neurologic and radiographic improvement may be anticipated to occur within two weeks of initiating therapy. Failure to demonstrate improvement should raise other diagnostic possibilities, including mycobacterial brain abscess or a primary central nervous system lymphoma. In such cases a brain biopsy is needed to make a definitive diagnosis.

The duration of treatment should probably be for the patient's lifetime. There is a high rate of relapse within 4 to 6 months of withdrawing antitoxoplasma therapy.

**Cryptococcus Neoformans**

Cryptococcus neoformans, a yeastlike fungus, is the most common cause of meningitis in patients with AIDS. In this population there frequently is evidence of concurrent cryptococcal sepsis (positive blood cultures or serum cryptococcal antigen) with visceral involvement of the lungs, bone marrow, skin, pleura, lymph nodes, or adrenal glands (68). The meningitis may be extremely insidious in onset because of the diminished inflammatory response seen in the cerebrospinal fluid (CSF). It is not unusual to detect CSF cryptococcal antigen at levels exceeding 1:10,000 with normal CSF chemistries and absence of pleiocytosis. In some patients diagnosed late in the course of cryptococcal infection, cryptococcoma of the brain has been observed.

The treatment of cryptococcus requires the prolonged use of amphotericin-B, at a dose of 0.4 mg/kg/day. The addition of 5-fluorocytosine may potentiate the effectiveness of amphotericin-B therapy, but bone marrow suppression may limit the usefulness of this drug (69). The proper duration of therapy is unknown. Cessation of amphotericin, even after substantial duration of therapy, is associated with a high relapse rate (68). Lifetime amphotericin-B treatment is made difficult by the cumulative toxicities of the drug and the need for permanent central venous access. A new approach to the treatment of cryptococcosis in AIDS has been afforded by the development of a new imidazole drug, fluconazole. This antifungal agent may be administered orally and penetrates the blood-brain barrier well. It shows excellent *in vitro* activity against cryptococcus neoformans and clinical studies currently are underway (70).

## Cryptosporidiosis

Cryptosporidiosis is an intestinal protozoan infection that presents with a self-limited diarrheal illness in immunocompetent persons (71). When cryptosporidiosis occurs in the setting of AIDS, a severe dysentery-like illness ensues (72). There is typically no fever, little abdominal cramping, and no tenesmus or hematochezia. The infection usually is not remitting, although the diarrhea may wax and wane. The organism tends to inhabit the brush border of the small bowel although it is also found in the colon. Ectasia of the common bile duct with obstruction and cholecystitis have been associated with cryptosporidiosis (73). Isolation of cryptosporidia from the lower respiratory tract also has been described (74).

The cryptosporidial oocysts may be demonstrated easily in stool by the sugar flotation method (75). They are acid-fast and also stain by the auramin-rhodamine immunofluorescent technique (76).

The treatment of intestinal cryptosporidiosis is often supportive. Total parenteral nutrition, antidiarrheal agents, and hydration are important adjuncts. A variety of antimicrobials have been tried with little success in this illness. Early reports of response to spiramycin (Rovamycin) have not been substantiated (77). Recently at New York University several patients were treated with bovine transfer factor prepared from cryptosporidia-infected cows. Preliminary results appear promising, with a decrease in the volume of diarrhea and a decrease in the numbers of organisms shed in the stool (78).

## Cytomegalovirus

Cytomegalovirus (CMV) is a DNA herpes virus. Cytomegalovirus has a prevalence of 40 to 60% in the general population and greater than 98% in homosexual men (79). In the patient with AIDS, CMV may cause severe clinical syndromes including CMV retinitis, colitis, and pneumonia. At postmortem examination, CMV is uniformly demonstrated in many tissues.

CMV retinitis may be unilateral, bilateral, or sequential over time. The patient usually presents with symptoms of vitreal floaters, blind spots, or a decrease in visual acuity. When lesions are peripheral in location they may be incidentally discovered in the course of a routine ophthalmologic examination. CMV retinitis lesions are hemorrhagic, necrotic, and occasionally are associated with significant vitritis. The lesions may progress to new retinal areas by direct extension. CMV retinitis must be distinguished from nonspecific cotton-wool spots, retinal toxoplasmosis, fungal enophthalmitis, and herpes retinitis. CMV retinitis is rapidly progressive and nonremitting (80).

The treatment of CMV retinitis is with ganciclovir, 9-(1,3-dihydroxy-2-propoxymethyl) guanine, or DHPG (81). This drug currently is available on an investigational basis from Syntex Laboratories. Consolidation therapy with 10 mg/kg/day in two divided doses for 2 weeks results in arrest of spread of retinal lesions, resolution of retinal edema, and a decrease in hemorrhage. A high rate of early relapse mitigates in favor of lifetime maintenance therapy with 6 mg/kg/day for 5 to 7 doses weekly. The major toxicity of ganciclovir is neutropenia. An unusual occurrence of rhegmatogenous retinal detachment following treatment has been reported (82).

Colitis due to CMV in patients with AIDS is a common cause of fever and diarrhea. Colonoscopic examination reveals submucosal hemorrhage and occasional ulcerations that reveal CMV inclusion cells on biopsy. This entity usually is seen in patients who have had AIDS diagnosed previously and is rarely its first manifestation. Colonic perforation, obstruction due to involvement of the ileocecal region, and significant colonic bleeding have been observed. CMV gastric or esophageal ulcers also are found.

The treatment of CMV colitis is identical to CMV retinitis. A 74% response rate to ganciclovir therapy was reported for CMV colitis with similar results in other extracolonic gastrointestinal sites of involvement (83). There is a similarly high rate of clinical relapse if maintanence therapy is not employed.

## Disseminated Mycobacterium Avium-Intracellulare

MAI is an acid-fast bacilli belonging to Runyon's Group III. This slow-growing, nonphotochromogen is ubiquitous and free living in the environment (84). Clinical isolation of MAI is far more common than M. tuberculosis in homosexual men with AIDS and mycobacterial infection. In AIDS patients with a high premorbid exposure to M. tuberculosis, (e.g., Haitians and i.v. drug abusers), the recovery rate of this organism may approximate MAI (85). The illness may be variable in the presentation, but fever, pancytopenia, elevations of alkaline phosphatase and 5' nucleotidase, and lymphadenopathy with splenomegaly are common. Cavitary lung disease is rare, although the organism may be cultured from sputum or bronchial secretions. Clinical infection by MAI may follow by many months the recovery of the organism from the stool. A persistent mycobacteremia may be documented using a commercially available blood culture system (86). Bone marrow and liver biopsies have a high diagnostic yield, as do lymph node biopsies. In patients with AIDS, the histopathology may reveal a paucity of poorly formed granulomata, but acid-fast stains may disclose huge numbers of mycobacteria (87).

The treatment of disseminated MAI infection is difficult because of the high grade *in vitro* antimicrobial resistance patterns of this organism. Certain groups have published uniformly poor clinical outcomes despite treatment (88). Like others, we have adopted a combination of two conventional antituberculous agents (isoniazid and ethambutol) with ansamycin and clofazimine (89). Ansamycin (LM-427) is a rifamycin-s derivative that, unlike rifampin, can penetrate the MAI cell wall. The drug may be obtained through the CDC. Clofazimine (Lamprene®, Ciba-Geigy) is an antileprosy drug that also inhibits many isolates of MAI *in vitro* at clinically achievable concentrations. In our experience this regimen usually results in a clinical response in more than half of the treated patients. Defervescence, decreased transfusion requirements, reduction of adenopathy, and splenomegaly are seen. Infection by MAI usually is a late manifestation of AIDS, and even when there has been a therapeutic response, survival for more than 6 to 8 months after diagnosis is unusual.

### HIV-Dementia

Dementia induced by HIV (subacute encephalitis) is marked by a triad of cognitive, motor, and behavioral dysfunction. This clinical entity is now accepted as criteria for the diagnosis of AIDS by the CDC (Appendix A). In some patients, HIV-dementia may be the first AIDS-associated illness. The clinical course is variable. In some individuals the onset is abrupt and in others may span months. The most frequent symptoms include difficulty in concentrating, short-term memory impairment, poor verbal skills with strained word finding, gait unsteadiness, changes in fine motor skills (e.g., handwriting), and personality alterations (90).

Neurologic evaluation reveals cerebral atrophy in virtually all symptomatic patients. Magnetic resonance imaging demonstrates patchy white matter abnormalities (90). Lumbar puncture reveals mild mononuclear pleiocytosis and modest elevations of the CSF protein. The HIV has been isolated from spinal fluid (91). There is a distinct neuropathology noted in HIV-dementia. Reactive hyperplasia and degeneration of oligodendrocytes and astroglial cells occur with subsequent demyelination. Electron microscopic studies have revealed HIV particles in these two cell types as well as in the endothelium of brain capillaries (92).

Recent studies have suggested that early in the course of HIV-dementia, treatment with Zidovudine (Retrovir, AZT) may reverse some of the symptoms of this illness (93). It should be kept in mind that patients with HIV-dementia are particularly susceptible to the extrapyramidal toxicity of anticholinergic drugs used to treat nausea or psychosis. This may be in part due to the decreased levels of cholinergic neurotransmitters in persons with HIV-dementia.

### Kaposi's Sarcoma and AIDS-Associated Neoplasms

AIDS is associated with a variety of neoplastic diseases. The incidence of KS exceeds all the other tumors combined and represents the initial manifestation of AIDS in almost 30% of the reported cases.

Before 1979, KS typically was diagnosed in elderly men of Ashkenazi Jewish or Mediterranean extraction. The disease in this setting was extremely indolent, favored the skin of the lower extremities, and rarely was the primary cause of death. The usual survival duration following diagnosis was 8 to 10 years. When treatment was indicated, local radiation therapy or single-agent chemotherapy was employed (94).

In addition to the aforementioned classic form of KS, two other clinical variants of this disease were known to occur in subSaharan Africa. Adult men in that region developed indolent tumors similar to the classic variety except that they were more locally invasive. Life expectancy after diagnosis was 5 to 8 years (95). Another form of KS seen in Africa is the so-called lymphadenopathic type. This variant affects children between the ages of 2 and 15 years and extensively involves lymph nodes and viscera early in the course of the disease. This form of KS is fatal within 2 to 3 years after diagnosis (96).

In the United States before the AIDS epidemic, KS was reported to occur *de novo* in the setting of iatrogenic immunosuppression employed during organ transplantation (97). While lesions favored the classical distribution, namely the lower extremities, tumor spread to regional nodes and viscera were reported. Some patients had complete regression of the tumors upon the discontinuation of immunosuppressive therapy (98).

Kaposi's sarcoma in the setting of AIDS has a clinical course that closely resembles the African lymphadenopathic form of the disease. The recent, sudden appearance of this form of KS in large numbers of patients in the western hemisphere justifies the term of epidemic Kaposi's sarcoma (EKS).

The etiology of KS is unknown. Among AIDS patients with this tumor, 95% are homosexual men, and only rare cases are seen in members of other risk groups. As AIDS becomes more widespread among i.v. drug users and transfusion recipients, the incidence of KS as a presenting symptom has decreased overall but remains highest in homosexual men (5). This implies that there may be one or more necessary cofactors operating in the development of KS. Hypothetical cofactors include genetic components, the influence of recreational drugs (such as inhaled amyl nitrites) and coincidental DNA viral infection (e.g., HSV, CMV, EBV) (99–101).

KS in the setting of AIDS is histologically identical to the lesions found in the classical, African, and transplantation-associated forms of the disease. Biopsies of the lesions show fascicles of spindle-cells surrounding cleftlike spaces containing extravasated erythrocytes. Other areas of the lesions show hemosiderin deposition, plasma cell and polymorphonuclear cell clusters, and dilated lymphatic and capillary channels. These changes can be identified in biopsies of skin lesions in organ parenchyma (see Fig. 30, Chapter 3) (102).

The origin of the malignant cell in KS remains a topic of some controversy. Factor VIII antigen has been identified in the spindle-cell of KS lesions by immunoperoxidase staining, suggesting that these cells arise from the vascular endothelium (103). Similar studies performed by other investigators were unable to identify this antigen by either immunoperoxidase or enzyme histochemical techniques on fresh frozen or paraffin-embedded tissue. This latter data would implicate the lymphatic rather than the blood vessel endothelium as the origin of the malignant cell in KS (104).

The cutaneous lesions of EKS are pigmented and appear pink, violaceous, or even brown in dark-skinned individuals. There may be a single lesion at the onset of EKS or multiple areas of involvement. The early lesions usually are macules, and later progress to raised, palpable masses that are fixed subcutaneously. The lesions are ovoid in shape and their long axis is oriented parallel to the cleavage lines of the skin. The disease may present in any area of the body, without the predilection for the lower extremities as seen in classical KS. Mucous membranes of the oral cavity often are involved.

Gastrointestinal lesions are demonstrable in 40 to 50% of all patients with EKS, and rarely (<5%) the gastrointestinal tract may be the only site of involvement at presentation (105). Endoscopically the tumors appear as cherry red, raised, nonulcerated, smooth masses covered by intact mucosa. These lesions, even when extensive, rarely cause symptoms or bleeding. In an autopsy series, liver involvement was seen in 35% of cases, but significant hepatic EKS is rare (106).

Pulmonary involvement with KS is present at some point in the disease in 30 to 40% of all cases (107). These lesions often are symptomatic, with chronic cough, hemoptysis, exertional dyspnea, and shortness of breath. The chest roentgenographic findings are nonspecific and frequently may be mistaken for opportunistic infections. Pleural effusions are common findings (see Chapter 3). The histologic demonstration of KS is difficult by transbronchial biopsy, with a diagnostic yield of only 15 to 20% (108). This technique is effective in ruling out opportunistic infections; in the setting of aggressive KS this technique leads to a presumptive diagnosis of pulmonary KS. In patients with no or few skin lesions and abnormal CXR, an open lung biopsy may be indicated.

Pleural effusion secondary to progressive KS is a problem that deserves special mention. Thirty to 50% of the patients with pulmonary KS pleural fluid can be detected by physical examination, plain chest radiograph, or CT scans (109). With successful systemic treatment there usually is dramatic reduction or complete disappearance of the fluid. However, it has been the author's experience that large pleural effusions do not respond well to local measures such as repeated thoracenteses or chest tube placement with or without instillation of sclerosing agents. These effusions respond best to systemic chemotherapy, and failure of the tumor to respond to treatment in this setting carries a poor prognosis. The majority of patients with AIDS who actually die of KS usually do so in the setting of progressive pulmonary compromise due to recurrent pleural effusions.

Lymphadenopathy is commonly seen in patients with KS, although the presence of enlarged lymph nodes does not insure that there will be histopathologic evidence of KS. Many other AIDS-associated conditions also may cause lymphadenopathy, including infections with MAI, mycobacterium tuberculosis, and malignant lymphomas or progressive generalized lymphadenopathy (PGL). Conversely, biopsy of enlarged lymph nodes in patients with ARC may reveal foci of KS in the absence of evident cutaneous or mucosal tumors. These observations need to be considered when assessing the response of patients with KS to antineoplastic treatment. Failure of a lymph node mass to regress may reflect the presence of an infection or another opportunistic neoplasm rather than failure of the treatment to control the KS.

In none of the earliest studies of either classical or African KS was there any attempt to stage patients systematically according to extent of disease or to correlate a staging system with prognosis. After the recognition of the AIDS-related epidemic of KS, a staging system based on a large, clinical experience was developed at New York University Medical Center (Table 6) (110). This system staged the anatomic extent of disease and tumor-associated symptoms (e.g., fever and weight loss). It did not include the presence or absence of concurrent or prior opportunistic infections (OI) as a variable in determining the survival of EKS patients.

Current or previous OI subsequently has been shown to have a powerful effect on survival of patients with EKS as indicated by subsequent data. Patients with all stages of KS but without OI had a survival rate of 80% at 39 months (median survival not reached), while those with any stage of KS and OI have a median survival of only 16 months. If only patients with no history of OI are considered, survival correlates well with the anatomic extent of disease (111).

To define prognostic features further in EKS, studies of immunologic parameters in patients with this dis-

**TABLE 6.** *Staging system for epidemic Kaposi's Sarcoma*

| Stage I | Cutaneous, locally indolent |
|---|---|
| Stage II | Cutaneous, locally aggressive with or without involvement of lymph nodes |
| Stage III | Generalized mucocutaneous or lymph node involvement |
| Stage IV | Visceral |
| A | No systemic signs or symptoms |
| B | Systemic signs: > 10% weight loss or fever > 100°F orally lasting two weeks without identifiable source |

order were performed (111,112). Reduction in the number of $CD_{4+}$ lymphocytes correlated with a poor prognosis, a finding that seemed to be independent of tumor stage or the presence or absence of constitutional tumor symptoms. Those patients with absolute $CD_{4+}$ counts of 300 and a $CD_4/CD_8$ ratio of 0.5 had an 85 to 95% one-year survival while those with 200 $CD_{4+}$ cells and a $CD_4/CD_8$ ratio of 0.2 had a 25% one-year survival. These data strongly suggest that simple clinical staging of patients is inadequate to predict prognosis both for purposes of clinical management and for planning clinical trials. A combination of extent of tumor, evidence for OI, and laboratory assessment of immune function need to be integrated in order to select and statify patients accurately.

There is no definitive treatment of KS. The mainstay of therapy generally has been the use of radiation therapy for localized disease and chemotherapy for disseminated KS. The drugs most commonly used for treatment include vinblastine, vincristine, and etoposide (VP-16). Other single-drug regimens undergoing investigation are adriamycin (doxorubicin), mitoxatrone, bleomycin, and recombinant alpha-interferon.

Vinblastine has been shown to be active in both AIDS and nonAIDS related KS. This treatment has resulted in an objective response rate of 25% and stabilization of the extent of disease in an additional 50%. This agent is convenient to use, relatively nontoxic, and only minimally immunosuppressive. Because vinblastine is slow on onset of action, 6 to 8 weeks should be allowed before assuming a nonresponse and reverting to an alternative regimen (113).

Vincristine, like vinblastine, is also active as a single agent against KS. It has been noted to cause severe peripheral neuropathy and should be used with caution in patients with AIDS-related neuropathies. However, vincristine may be more appropriate for patients with severe neutropenia or thrombocytopenia (114).

Etoposide (VP-16) may be more effective in treating EKS than the vinca alkaloids. One study reported a 76% response rate to etoposide as a single agent. Subjective side-effects were minimal and objective toxicity was acceptable (115).

Trials with combination chemotherapy were employed for patients with more aggressive forms of EKS. Initial trials of adriamycin, bleomycin, and vinblastine resulted in a response rate approximating that of VP-16. The opportunistic infection rate, however, was higher with the three-drug regimen (115).

Presently, alpha-interferon is being tested as an alternative to the traditional chemotherapeutic agents (116). Objective response rates comparable to single-agent chemotherapy with vinblastine or VP-16 has been demonstrated. Side-effects tend to be minimal and opportunistic infections were less commonly encountered in the patients who responded to this treatment.

## AIDS-RELATED LYMPHOMA

Non-Hodgkin's lymphoma (NHL) and Hodgkin's disease (HD) were identified as part of the spectrum of AIDS-related diseases shortly after its description (117). Although these tumors are histologically identical to the commonly described lymphomas, they have a unique biological behavior that distinguishes them from sporadically occurring lymphoproliferative diseases.

The appearance of NHL and HD in AIDS is far less frequent than the infectious complications of this disease, and certainly far rarer than KS (118). While less than 10% of patients with AIDS will develop either NHL or HD, it is common for these malignancies to coexist with a variety of infectious diseases. In such cases, the infection is as likely as the neoplasm to be the cause of death (118). Unlike KS, the incidence of NHL and HD is proportionally distributed among the classical risk groups and their clinical presentation is similar among homosexual men, i.v. drug users, and transfusion recipients.

The mechanisms that induce NHL or HD in AIDS patients is unknown. There is indirect evidence that EBV may be responsible for some of the Burkitt's lymphomas (BL) seen in AIDS patients (119).

Non-Hodgkin's lymphomas in persons with AIDS are almost exclusively high or intermediate grade as classified by the Working Formulation (120). In a review of patients from two studies, 40% had diffuse large cell, noncleaved lymphomas, 35% had diffuse small cell noncleaved lymphoblastic lymphomas (BL), and 20% had immunoblastic sarcomas. Only 1% of the patients had nodular histology and 4% had low-grade diffuse lymphomas (118,121). These lymphomas usually have the pre-B cell or B cell immunopathologic markers of surface immunoglobulin and B1 antigen, although a rare T-cell malignancy may be seen. Leukemic transformation of these lymphomas are exceedingly uncommon.

Patients with AIDS and HD have been described with all histologies, including lymphocyte predominance, nodular sclerosis, mixed cellularity, and lymphocyte depletion, although the number of patients with mixed cellularity and nodularity sclerosis is somewhat overrepresented (122). The histopathology of the lymph nodes or bone marrow is often typical with Reed-Sternberg cells on a background of eosinophils, plasma cells, and lymphocytes. Occasionally, the Reed-Sternberg cells will be mononuclear and atypical in appearance but these patients cannot be distinguished clinically.

The clinical hallmark of NHL and HD in AIDS is the high incidence of stage IV disease and the unusual sites of extranodal involvement. In NHL, the central nervous system, small and large bowel, perirectal area, gingiva, tonsil, and skin are sometimes involved clinically. In two large studies of patients with AIDS and NHL, only 18% had stage I or II disease, while the remaining 82% had advanced stages (118,121). Constitutional symptoms (fevers, chills, night sweats, and weight loss) are so common in patients with AIDS and no neoplasia that is difficult to ascribe them to a coexistent lymphoma. Nonetheless, more than 80% of the patients had one or more of the "B" symptoms (118,121).

There is a high incidence of extranodal disease in patients with NHL or HD, and as such one should anticipate a wide variation in the presentation of patients with these disorders. Further complicating the evaluation of these patients is the possibility that symptoms associated with the lymphoma can be directly due to HIV infection, concurrent OIs, or KS. Thus, the diagnosis of lymphoma must be made only on examination of adequate biopsy specimens and not on the pattern of clinical signs and symptoms.

Almost all patients with AIDS associate NHL or HD present with either peripheral, retroperitoneal or mesenteric adenopathy, and/or splenomegaly. In the few patients with HD and no lymph node or splenic involvement, isolated bone marrow infiltration has been described. Between 10 and 15% of cases of NHL in AIDS patients with primary central nervous system involvement. It is far more common to find brain involvement when other sites of disease are present (118).

The risk of developing NHL in HIV-infected persons may be as much as 1,000 times the risk of the general population (123). No meaningful data is available to guide the physician on when it is appropriate to pursue lymph node biopsies in patients with persistent generalized lymphadenopathy (PGL; 124). A decision tree that has proven helpful has been to biopsy any palpable node that is greater than 3 cm, doubles in size over a period of 1 month, or occurs in a patient with unexplained elevation of serum lactate dehydrogenase.

Although other authors have reported that the diagnosis of lymphoid malignancy in AIDS patients may be made by using fine-needle aspiration, we have found this technique to have limited utility. In our experience cytopathologists may be capable of identifying malignant lymphoid cells from needle aspirate specimens. However, it may be impossible to differentiate between Burkitt's lymphoma, large cell noncleaved lymphoma, or atypical variants of Hodgkin's disease with cytologic preparations, and since the treatment of these entities may vary, adequate surgical biopsy is required to differentiate the histologies of these lymphomas.

Patients with HD demonstrate a 70 to 90% response rate to aggressive combination chemotherapy (125). In contrast to the patients with NHL, some patients with HD respond well to treatment, with median survival rates exceeding 2 years in some small series. As in the case of treating KS, patients may have their malignancy controlled successfully only to succumb to an OI.

Non-AIDS patients with stage III or IV diffuse large cell NHL usually respond well to combination chemotherapy. Complete response rates in these individuals to such regimens as PrOMACE-MOPP, m-BACOD, and MACOP-B range from 70 to 90%, with as many as 40 to 60% of all patients achieving long-term unmaintained disease-free remissions and possibly cures (126–128). In contrast, the AIDS patient with NHL does not demonstrate favorable responses to treatment. Although these lymphomas have impressive initial sensitivity to treatment with these types of regimens (with up to 97% of evaluable patients achieving a complete or partial remission) it is common for these lymphomas to recur rapidly and often during brief interruptions in treatment (121). This is especially problematic in the AIDS population where interruptions in chemotherapy for cytopenias and intercurrent infections are common. Despite the high initial response rate the median survival for patients with diffuse noncleaved NHL was only 5 months, while that for patients with BL was 3 months (121,129).

A small number of reports have described the appearance of several solid tumors in patients suffering from AIDS. These tumors include anorectal squamous cell carcinoma and testicular carcinoma.

Squamous cell of the anorectal region has been reported. This tumor is locally invasive and usually presents as a mass, a nonhealing ulcer, or with rectal pain or discharge (130). At diagnosis, most lesions are invasive but not metastatic and have responded to local treatments including surgical excision, radiation therapy, and electrocurettage. Although the etiology of these tumors remains unknown, some evidence implicating condyloma virus is available. Dysplastic and frankly carcinomatous changes in the rectal epithelium adjacent to lesions of condyloma accuminata have been reported (131). Furthermore, the incidence of antipapilloma antibodies is higher in patients with squamous cell carcinoma of the anorectal region than in healthy homosexual male controls (132).

Other solid tumors, including nonseminomatous germ cell tumors, malignant melanoma, and adenocarcinoma of the lung have been observed in HIV-seropositive patients. Although there is a suspicion that the appearance of those tumors may be related to the patient's underlying immunosuppression, there is inadequate data to identify these malignancies as "AIDS-related".

## AIDS-Related Complex

Soon after the first descriptions of AIDS appeared in the literature, physicians began seeing patients in defined risk groups for the disease who were ill but who did not satisfy the criteria for diagnosis outlined by the CDC. This group of individuals exceed the number of AIDS patients by 10-fold and their conditions were alternatively termed "preAIDS," "lesser AIDS," or "AIDS-related complex" (ARC). For this chapter we will use the term ARC to refer to those HIV-associated illnesses or conditions that are not accepted by the CDC as criteria for the diagnosis of AIDS (Table 7).

ARC is a diverse syndrome with the potential to affect virtually any organ system (Table 8). Some of the clinical manifestations of ARC are due directly to the effects of HIV infection (Table 1), while others are due to the interplay of the immunosuppressed host and its indigenous flora. The immune disturbances seen in ARC are qualitatively identical to those described in AIDS, although quantitatively not as severe.

Constitutional symptoms may occur soon after infection by HIV (as documented by seroconversion) and may either remit or persist (133). This illness may be clinically indistinguishable from acute mononucleosis or CMV infection. Patients report low-grade fevers, myalgias, arthralgias, vague pharyngeal discomfort, lassitude, and profound fatigue. Modest weight loss may occur in the absence of diarrhea, but severe unexplained weight loss has been termed the "wasting syndrome" and is accepted as criteria for AIDS (46).

The reticuloendothelial system is affected in the course of HIV infection. "Progressive generalized lymphadenopathy" (PGL), formerly known as the lymphadenopathy syndrome (LAS), involves multiple noninguinal lymph node chains. The adenopathy persists, although it may wax and wane. The nodes are greater than 1 cm in size, nonmatted, mobile, and sometimes mildly tender. The most common sites of involvement are the posterior cervical, posterior auricular, and axillary regions (134). Early in the course of this condition the lymph node architecture is preserved with benign-appearing hyperplasia (135). Electron microscopy of the nodal lymphocytes may reveal unusual tubular-reticular cytoplasmic forms that may be HIV-associated structures (136). As the disease progresses, the lymphadenopathy may become less prominent clinically, and histology will reveal lymphoid depletion with absent germinal centers and sinus histiocytosis (135). Significant intrathoracic or intraabdominal lymphadenopathy is unusual in the absence of AIDS-associated opportunistic infection. Splenomegaly may be seen in as many as 25% of persons with ARC. Recently, intraparotid lymphoepithelial lesions have been reported (137).

There are many mucocutaneous manifestations of ARC. Most of these are caused by infectious agents that normally reside within the ecologic niches of the integumentary structures or mucosa.

Oral candidiasis (thrush) is the most common oral manifestation of ARC. It presents as small white plaques that may be scraped easily from the buccal and lingual surfaces. There are no symptoms associated with mild or moderate thrush and this condition is effectively managed with nonabsorbable antifungal agents, such as nystatin or clotrimazole. More recalcitrant cases require ketoconazole. It has been observed that the appearance of thrush connotes a serious prognosis, with progression from ARC to AIDS of 40 to 60% of cases within several years (138). Severe monilial involvement of the skin, especially the intertriginous regions, also is a common finding in ARC.

Hairy leukoplakia is a newly described entity. On examination, white, painless fibriated strands that resist

**TABLE 7.** *Current infectious diseases accepted by the CDC as criteria for AIDS surveillance purposes*

| Laboratory evidence of HIV infection *not* required | Laboratory evidence of HIV infection required* |
|---|---|
| Candidiasis of esophagus, trachea, bronchi, or lungs | Coccidiomycosis, disseminated |
| Cryptococcosis, extrapulmonary | HIV encephalopathy (subacute encephalopathy) |
| Cryptosporidiosis, lasting > 1 month | Histoplasmosis, disseminated |
| Cytomegalovirus of an organ other than liver, spleen, or lymph node | Isosporiasis (with diarrhea lasting >1 month) |
| Herpes simplex virus infection causing persistent (>1 month) mucocutaneous ulcer, bronchitis, pneumonitis, or esophagitis | Mycobacterium tuberculosis, extrapulmonary |
| Mycobacterium avium-intercellulare or M. kansasii disease, disseminated | Other mycobacterial disease (not M. avium-intercellulare or M. kansasii), disseminated |
| Pneumocystis carinii pneumonia | Salmonella (nontyphoid) septicemia, recurrent |
| Progressive multifocal leukoencephalopathy | HIV wasting syndrome (emaciation, "slim's disease") |
| Toxoplasmosis of brain | |

Adapted from ref. 46.

* Laboratory evidence for HIV infection include: HIV Ab + Elisa, Western blot, or immunofluorescence assay; positive test for HIV serum antigen; positive HIV culture.

**TABLE 8.** *Some manifestations of AIDS-related complex*

Constitutional
  Fevers, myalgias, fatigue
Reticuloendothelial
  Progressive generalized lymphadenopathy
  Splenomegaly
  Other lymphoepitheloid lesions
Mucocutaneous—Infectious
  Oral candidiasis (thrush)
  Monilial intertrigo—severe
  Lingual hairy leukoplakia
  Localized varicella-zoster
  Seborrheic dermatitis
  Molluscum contagiosum
  Folliculitis, impetigo, acne vulgaris,
    furunculosis, paronychiae
  Cheilitis, apthous stomatitis
  Herpes simplex stomatitis
  Severe Tinea cruris, T. pedis, onycholysis
  Condyloma accuminata, common warts
Mucocutaneous—Noninfectious
  Psoriasis
  Urticaria
  Papulosquamous pruritis
  Alopecia
  Xeroderma
  Eczema
Ophthalmologic
  "Cotton-wool" exudates
  Anterior uveitis
Hematologic
  Immune thrombocytopenia
    purpura
  Anemia of chronic disease
Endocrine
  Adrenal insufficiency
Renal
  Focal sclerosing
    glomerulonephritis
Neurologic
  Aseptic meningitis
  Peripheral sensory neuropathy
  Polyradiculopathy/myopathy
  Vacuolar myopathy
Gastrointestinal
  GI ulceration
  Unexplained diarrhea
Cardiac
  Cardiomyopathy
  Myocardial fibrosis

removal by scraping are seen on the lateral lingual surfaces. Electron microscope studies of biopsy material have implicated both the Epstein-Barr virus and the human papilloma virus in the pathogenesis of these lesions (139). Of interest is that resolution of hairy leukoplakia has been observed in patients on high-dose acyclovir, and a recent study of successful treatment with topical acyclovir has been reported (140). The relatively poor prognosis associated with thrush also is seen with hairy leukoplakia.

Other oral manifestations of ARC include angular stomatitis (cheilitis), aphthous stomatitis, and recurrent and severe herpes simplex stomatitis. Angular stomatitis usually responds to antifungal and topical corticosteroid therapy. Herpes simplex stomatitis may be disabling enough to warrant therapy with oral acyclovir, which is highly effective.

Cutaneous infections associated with ARC can dominate the clinical picture. Localized varicella-zoster has been seen with increasing frequency in persons at risk for AIDS (141). Despite the rarity of disseminated or visceral involvement, zoster may be locally invasive. High-dose acyclovir usually is effective in hastening the healing of active lesions.

Dermatophytic infection of the integument and nails are common in persons with ARC. Severe Tinea cruris, Tinea versicola, Tinea pedis, and fungal oncyholysis are all frequently encountered (142). Intensive topical therapy is successful in most cases of dermal infection. Systemic therapy (ketoconazole or griseofluvin) for nail infections usually is reserved for symptomatic patients, or those for whom the infection interferes with their professional activities.

Seborrheic dermatitis can be especially severe in persons with ARC. This condition may be caused by a local inflammatory reaction to the spores of pityrosporum (143). There is a predilection for the malar and forehead areas of the face. Topical ketoconazole in combination with a corticosteroid cream is effective in controlling quickly the signs and symptoms of this condition.

Bacterial infections of the skin and integumentary structures also are manifestations of ARC. Impetigo, furunculosis, acne vulgaris, and paronychiae have all been problematic in this patient population. Orally administered antistaphylococcal antibiotics may control these skin diseases but relapse is extremely common. A search for chronic nasal staphylococcal carriage is warranted.

Viral infections of the skin may pose a significant challenge to the clinician. Molluscum contagiosum appears as multiple large, umbilicated vesicles. In especially virulent cases, large areas of the face or lower trunk may be covered with lesions (144). They are treated by curetting, electrodessication, or thermal injury with liquid nitrogen.

Condyloma accuminata may be aggressive in persons with ARC, even years after sexual activity has ceased. Common skin warts and plantars warts also are seen in this group.

There are severe noninfectious diseases of the skin that are common features of ARC. Psoriasis may present *de novo* with the onset of ARC, or a previously known case may exacerbate (145). Xeroderma of a generalized type with eczematouslike eruptions and severe pruritis is common. Similarly, unexplained giant or papular urticaria is frequently encountered. Some relief with antihistamines and topical corticosteroids is expected, but these frustrating skin conditions usually fail to remit entirely.

Ophthalmologic changes may be seen at some point in the course of ARC in over 50% of patients (146). Cotton-wool exudates are "soft" retinal lesions that may wax and wane and rarely cause significant visual loss. They are felt to be due to immune complex-induced vascular leakage with retinal edema. There is no specific treatment for this condition.

The hematologic manifestations of ARC include a moderate normocytic, normochromic anemia, and immune thrombocytopenic purpura. The anemia has all the characteristics of "anemia of chronic disease". The immune thrombocytopenia (ITP) associated with HIV infection is due to peripheral platelet destruction (27,147). Bone marrow aspirates reveal megakaryocytosis. Nonspecific binding of HIV-anti-HIV $f(ab)_2^1$ immune complexes to platelet membranes has been shown to be the cause of platelet destruction (148). The treatment with corticosteroids is less effective than expected based on experience in nonHIV associated ITP. In addition, corticosteroids carry significant risks in this group of immunosuppressed patients. Intravenous gammaglobulin, danazol, and vincristine have shown limited usefulness in the treatment of this disorder. Splenectomy has been performed in individuals who have had bleeding episodes because of profound thrombocytopenia (10,000 to 20,000 cells/mm$^3$). Of interest are two patients with HIV-associated immune thrombocytopenia treated by the authors with Zidovudine (Retrovir, AZT), who showed normalization of the platelet counts.

Adrenal insufficiency may occur in the course of HIV infection. Most clinically significant episodes of adrenal failure have occurred in patients with advanced AIDS (149). However, it is probable that relative adrenal insufficiency may appear in patients with ARC, and the constitutional symptoms of lassitude, mild diarrhea, low-grade fever, and weight loss should prompt an ACTH stimulation test to exclude this treatable diagnostic possibility.

There are numerous neurologic manifestations of ARC. Early in the course of infection, recurrent aseptic meningitis may be seen, possibly due to direct central nervous system invasion by HIV (150). Another common illness is distal sensory polyneuropathy. Patients will present with pain or hyperaesthesia of the feet (or less commonly hands). There may be no demonstrable neurologic deficit by exam or on electromyographic studies. In patients with severe symptoms, relief with low-dose amitriptylline has been observed (150). In contrast, a predominantly motor polyneuropathy resembling Guillain-Barre syndrome has been reported. Nerve biopsies reveal demyelination with little inflammation, and muscle biopsies show denervation myopathy. Most rare is a transverse myelitis that is associated with vacuolar myelopathy. In the majority of these cases HIV is the probable cause of the syndrome (151).

Other organ systems have been diseased in the course of ARC. A rapid progression to renal failure has been observed due to a focal sclerosing glomerulonephritis (152). Gastrointestinal ulcerations recently have been shown to harbor HIV without other recognizable pathogens. It is also likely that the mild diarrhea associated with ARC may be directly attributable to HIV.

Idiopathic cardiomyopathy and myocardial fibrosis have been reported in association with HIV infection, raising the possibility of direct viral effects on myocardial function (153).

## THERAPEUTIC APPROACH TO HIV INFECTION

There is no definite therapy for persons infected by the HIV. The rapid expansion of knowledge about the basic biology of HIV, however, has opened the road toward meaningful therapies. Some major approaches include immunostimulation/immune restoration, antiretroviral therapy, combination antiretroviral and immunostimulant therapy, and preventative vaccine development.

The earliest attempts at treatment of patients with AIDS involved various agents directed at immune restoration (Table 9). While some of these substances could be demonstrated to result in modest improvement in various immune parameters (e.g., skin-test reactivity, $CD_{4+}$ cell population), little evidence for significant, long-term clinical improvement was forthcoming.

Once the discovery of the HIV as the pathogenetic agent of AIDS was reported, investigators began looking at drugs with antiretroviral activity (Table 10). Suramin and antimoniotungstate (HPA-23) were some of the earliest drugs studied (154,155). Both exhibited significant inhibition of the HIV-associated enzyme, reverse tran-

**TABLE 9.** *Immunorestorative Agents*

| | |
|---|---|
| Isoprinosine (Inosiplex) | Increases N-K cells and T-cell subsets |
| Interleukin-2 (IL-2) | A lymphokine causing proliferation of T-cell subsets |
| Gamma-interferon | Antiviral, antiproliferative, and immunomodulator properties |
| Imreg-1 | A natural leukocyte-derived substance that increases MIF, LIF, and IL-2, from $T_4$ cells |
| Naltrexone (Trexan) | Opiate antagonist that up modulates the lymphocyte opiate receptors and increases circulating endorphins and enkephalins. Decreases acid-labile alpha-interferon. |
| TP-5 (Thymopentane) | Synthetic pentapeptide simulating thymopoietin-induced phenotypic differentiation |

scriptase *in vitro,* although their clinical usefulness was limited by significant toxicities.

Phosphonoformate (Foscarnet®) is another inhibitor of reverse transcriptase with a broad *in vitro* antiviral spectrum (156). This drug is difficult to administer because of its extremely short serum half-life, its need for parenteral administration, and its significant toxicities (especially renal).

Ribavirin (Virazole-ICN Pharmaceuticals) is a synthetic nucleotide derivative that acts as an analog of guanosine, interfering with the 5′-capping of viral messenger RNA (157). Transient suppression of HIV replication has been demonstrated and this agent is usually well tolerated, with occasional reversible microcytic anemia. Several clinical trials have been reported with conflicting results.

The interferons (alpha, beta, gamma) possess indirect antiviral activity by stimulating immune nodulators (e.g., interleukin-2), and by interfering with transcription, translation, assembly, and release of viral particles. Early studies of alpha-interferon in patients with Kaposi's sarcoma showed some clinical response of the tumor to this agent (158). However, a major therapeutic role of the various interferons as sole agents in ARC and AIDS have not been realized.

Drugs that interfere with the binding and penetration of HIV into the $CD_{4+}$ lymphocytes have attracted interest in the past year. Peptide-T is an octapeptide that is derived from a small segment of HIV envelope protein (gp120) (159). It is postulated that it potentially can block binding of the intact virus to the $CD_4$ antigen on the helper cell membrane. Early studies of this agent have yielded contrasting results but further experiments are underway. Another agent directed at inhibition of HIV-$CD_4$ antigen binding is AL-721 (160). This active lipid component (glycerides, phosphatidylcholine, and phosphatidyl ethanokimine in a 7:2:1 ratio) can extract cholesterol from cellular membranes and may inhibit HIV infection of $CD_{4+}$ lymphocytes by altering the HIV binding sites. This drug is well tolerated and is now being tested in various clinical studies.

The most important antiretroviral therapy to date is azidothymidine (3′-azido-3′-deoxythymidine, Retrovir, Zidovudine, Burroughs-Wellcome). This thymidine analog inhibits HIV replication after it is phosphorylated by cellular enzymes. The mode of action appears to be early termination of viral DNA-chain elongation (161). A double-blind, placebo-controlled trial in ARC and AIDS patients was initated in February 1986 (162). There are measurable improvements in $CD_4$ cell counts and circulating p24 antigen levels in the drug recipients. Furthermore, drug recipients exhibited significantly fewer opportunistic infections as compared with the placebo group, and a four-to-sixfold reduction in mortality (162). This agent is given orally at 4-hour intervals because of a short serum half-life. It penetrates the blood-brain barrier well, achieving 50% of the serum levels in the CSF (161). There is significant toxicity, most commonly a macrocytic anemia (163). This drug has now been licensed (only two years since the first human trials) for the treatment of severe ARC and

**TABLE 10.** *Antiretroviral agents*

| Agent | Mechanism of action | Toxicity |
|---|---|---|
| AL-721 | Extracts cholesterol from cell membrane altering HIV binding site and preventing infection | Unknown |
| Azidothymidine (AZT, Zidovudine) | Pyrimidine analog that decreases viral replication by inhibiting reverse transcriptase | Macrocytic anemia, neutropenia, and headaches |
| Foscarnet (Phosphonoformate) | Inhibits reverse transcriptase | Renal failure |
| HPA-23 | Inhibits reverse transcriptase | Thrombocytopenia |
| Peptide T | Interferes with binding of HIV to $CD_4$ receptor site | Unknown |
| Ribavirin (Virazole) | Guanosine analog that interferes with 5′ capping of viral mRNA | Microcytic anemia, hemolysis |
| Suramin | Inhibits reverse transcriptase | Fever, thrombocytopenia, adrenal insufficiency, hepatic failure |
| Alpha-interferon | May inhibit viral production, assembly, and budding | Fever, bone marrow suppression |

AIDS. A derivative of AZT, 2'3'dideoxycytidine, is now being tested for toxicity in phase I human trials (164).

Antiviral therapy theoretically must be employed indefinitely because it would be inactive against latent HIV that is nonreplicative. The combining of antiviral agents with immune stimulants would be desirable since stimulation of HIV-infected $CD_{4+}$ lymphocytes promotes viral replication. Other avenues of antiviral research will be exploring the combination of two or more antivirals with different sites of action. A study in identical twins of intense AZT therapy followed by synergeneic bone-marrow transplantation is currently underway at the National Institutes of Health.

An HIV vaccine has been considered for the prevention and treatment of HIV infection (165). Development of an effective vaccine may be rendered difficult by the antigenic heterogeneity of HIV and related viruses, and by the capacity for cell-to-cell spread of HIV through syncytial cell formation. Suggested target antigens might be the HIV envelope glycoprotein (gp120) and the transmembrane glycoprotein (gp41), both of which have neutralizing epitopes (165). Early attempts at vaccine development currently are underway.

The study of HIV treatment modalities has been organized by the National Institutes of Health. Through major granting 17 AIDS Treatment Evaluation Units throughout the United States have been created to gain experience systematically and comprehensively in large numbers of patients with new agents as they become available. The Food and Drug Administration has committed to giving highest priority to approval of drugs used in the treatment of AIDS.

## REFERENCES

1. Centers for Disease Control (1981): Pneumocystis pneumonia—Los Angeles. *M.M.W.R.*, 30:250–252.
2. Hymes, K. B., Cheung, T., Greene, J. B., et al. (1981): Kaposi's sarcoma in homosexual men—A report of eight cases. *Lancet*, II:598.
3. Masur, H., Michaels, M. A., Greene, J. B., et al. (1981): An outbreak of community acquired pneumocystis carinii pneumonia—Initial manifestation of cell-mediated immune dysfunction. *N. Engl. J. Med.*, 143:305.
4. Centers for Disease Control (1987): Update: Acquired immunodeficiency syndrome—United States. *M.M.W.R.*, 36:522b.
5. Centers for Disease Control (1986): Update: Acquired immunodeficiency syndrome—United States. *M.M.W.R.*, 35:757–760.
6. City Health Information (1987): Special AIDS Issue #2. 6:1–4.
7. Pitchenik, A. E., Fisch, M. A., Dickinson, G. M., et al. (1983): Opportunistic infections and Kaposi sarcoma among Haitians: Evidence of a new acquired immunodeficiency state. *Ann. Intern. Med.*, 98:277–284.
8. Piot, P., Quin, T., Taelman, H., et al. (1984): Acquired immunodeficiency syndrome in a heterosexual population in Zaire *Lancet*, 2:65–69.
9. Centers for Disease Control (1986): Update: Acquired immunodeficiency syndrome—Europe. *M.M.W.R.*, 35:358–436.
10. Gallo, R. C. (1987): The AIDS Virus. *Sci. Am.* 256:46–56.
11. Kuritsky, J. N., Rastog, S. C., Faich, G. A., et al. (1986): Results of nationwide screening of blood and plasma for antibodies to human T-cell lymphotropic III virus, type III. *Transfusion*, 265:205–207.
12. Burke, D. S., Brundage, J. F., Herbld, J. R., et al. (1987): Human immunodeficiency virus infections among civilian applicants for United States military service, October 1985 to March 1986: Demographic factors associated with seropositivity. *N. Engl. J. Med.*, 317:31–36.
13. Jaffe, H., Hardy, A., Morgan, W., and Darrow, W. (1985): The acquired immunodeficiency syndrome in gay men. *Ann. Intern. Med.*, 103:662–664.
14. Drucker, E. (1986): AIDS and addiction in New York City. *Am. J. Drug Alcohol Abuse*, 12:165–181.
15. Evatt, B., Gomperts, E., McDougal, J., and Rasey, R. (1985): Coincidental appearance of LAV/HTLV-III antibodies in hemophiliacs and the onset of the AIDS epidemic. *N. Engl. J. Med.*, 312:483–486.
16. Hessol, N. A., Rutherford, G. W., O'Malley, P. M., et al. (1987): The natural history of human immunodeficiency virus infection in cohort of homosexual and bisexual men: A 7-year prospective study. Abstracts of the III International Conference on Acquired Immunodeficiency Syndrome. Washington, D.C.
17. Centers for Disease Control (1986): Apparent transmission of human T-lymphotropic virus III/lymphadenopathy—Associated virus (HTLV-III/LAV) from a child to a mother providing care. *M.M.W.R.*, 35:76–79.
18. Friedland, G. H., Saltzman, B. R., Rogers, M. R., et al. (1986): Lack of household transmission of HTLV-III. *N. Engl. J. Med.*, 314:344–349.
19. Hirsch, M. J., Wormser, G. P., Schooley, R. T., et al. (1985): Risk of nosocomial infections with human T-lymphotrophic virus III (HTLV-III). *N. Engl. J. Med.*, 312:1–4.
20. Centers for Disease Control (1987): Update on human immunodeficiency virus infections in health care workers exposed to blood of infected patients. *M.M.W.R.*, 36:285–289.
21. Gottlieb, M. S. (1986): Immunologic aspects of AIDS and male homosexuals. *Med. Clin. N. Am.*, 70:651–664.
22. Laurence, J. (1985): The immune system in AIDS. *Sci. Am.*, 254:85–93.
23. Bowen, D. L., Lane, H. C., and Fauci, A. S. (1985): Immunopathogeneisis of AIDS. *Ann. Intern. Med.*, 103:704–709.
24. Fauci, A. S. (1984): Immunologic abnormalities in AIDS. *Clin. Res.*, 32:491–499.
25. Destefano, E., Friedman, R. N., Friedman-Kien, A. G., et al. (1982): Acid labile human leukocyte interferon in homosexual men with Kaposi's sarcoma and lymphadenopathy. *J. Infect. Dis.*, 146:451–459.
26. Lane, H. C., and Fauci, A. S. (1985): Immunologic abnormalities in AIDS. *Ann. Rev. Immunol.*, 3:477–500.
27. Morris, L., Distenfeld, A., Amorosi, E., and Karpatkin, S. (1982): Autoimmune thrombocytopenia purpura in homosexual men. *Ann. Intern. Med.*, 96:714–717.
28. McDougal, J. S., Kennedy, M. S., Sligh, J. M., et al. (1986): Binding of HTLV-III/LAV to $T_4$ cells by a complex of the 110K viral protein and the $T_4$ molecule. *Science*, 231:382–385.
29. Hoxie, J. A., Alpers, J. D., Rackovski, J. L., et al. (1986): Alterations in $T_4(CD_4)$ protein and MRNA synthesis in cells infected with HIV. *Science*, 234:1123–1127.
30. Sodroski, J., Chun Goh, W., Rosen, C., et al. (1986): Role of HTLV-III/LAV envelope in syncytium formation and cytopathicity. *Nature*, 322:470–474.
31. Gallo, R. C. (1986): The first human retrovirus. *Sci. Am.*, 255:88–98.
32. Barre-Sinoussi, S., Chermann, J. C., Rey, F., et al. (1983): Isolation of a T-lymphotrophic retrovirus from a patient at risk for acquired immunodeficiency syndrome (AIDS). *Science*, 220:868–871.
33. Popovic, M., Sarngadharan, M. G., Read, E., and Gallo, R. C. (1984): Detection, isolation and continuous production of cytopathic retroviruses (HTLV-III) from patients with AIDS and pre-AIDS. *Science*, 224:497–500.
34. Montagnier, L. (1985): Lymphadenopathy associated virus: From molecular biology to pathogenecity. *Ann. Intern. Med.*, 103:689–693.
35. Ho, D. D., Pomerantz, R. J., and Kaplan, J. C. (1987): Pathogenesis of infection with human immunodeficiency virus. *N. Engl. J. Med.*, 317:278–286.
36. Alizan, M., and Montagnier, L. (1986): Lymphadenopathy/

AIDS virus: Genetic organization and relationship to animal lentiviruses. *Anti-cancer Res.,* 6:403–412.
37. Clavel, S., and Francois, M. D., et al. (1987): Human immunodeficiency virus type 2 infection associated with AIDS in West Africa. *N. Engl. J. Med.,* 316:1180–1185.
38. Gallo, R. C., Salahuddin, S. Z., Popovic, M., et al. (1984): Frequent detection and isolation of cytopathic retroviruses (HTLV-III) from patients with AIDS and at risk for AIDS. *Science,* 224:500–503.
39. Melbye, M., Biggar, R. J., Ebbesen, P., et al. (1986): Long-term seropositivity for human T-lymphotropic virus type III in homosexual men without the acquired immunodeficiency syndrome: Development of immunologic and clinical abnormalities: A longitudinal study. *Ann. Intern. Med.,* 104:496–500.
40. Kannagi, M., Kiyotaki, M., Desrosiers, R. C., et al. (1986): Humoral immune responses to T-cell tropic virus type III in monkeys with experimentally induced acquired immune deficiency-like syndrome. *J. Clin. Invest.,* 78:1229–1236.
41. Seligmann, M., Pinching, A. J., Rosen, F. S., et al. (1987): Immunology of human immunodeficiency virus infection and the acquired immunodeficiency syndrome: An update. *Ann. Intern. Med.,* 107:234–242.
42. Chang, K. S., Wang, L., Alexander, S., et al. (1987): Concomitant HTLV-I and HTLV-III infections—A serological survey in Washington D.C. Area abstracts of the Third International Conference on AIDS. Washington, D.C.
43. Jeffries, D. (1986): Virological aspects of AIDS. *Clin. Immunol. Allergy,* 6:627–644.
44. Centers for Disease Control (1982): Update: Acquired immune deficiency syndrome (AIDS)—United States. *M.M.W.R.,* 31:507–514.
45. Centers for Disease Control (1985): Revision of the case definition of acquired immunodeficiency syndrome for national reporting—United States. *M.M.W.R.,* 34:101–103.
46. Centers for Disease Control (1987): Revision of the CDC Surveillance case definition of acquired immunodeficiency syndrome. *M.M.W.R.,* 36(Suppl):1S–14S.
47. Mills, J. (1986): Pneumocystis carinii and Toxoplasma gondii infections in patients with AIDS. *Rev. Infect. Dis.,* 8:1001–1011.
48. Kramer, E. L., Sanger, J. J., Garay, S. M., et al. (1987): Gallium-67 scans of the chest in patients with acquired immunodeficiency syndrome. *J. Nucl. Med.,* 28:1107–1114.
49. Garay, S. M., and Greene, J. B. (1987): Prognostic implications serum LDH in pneumocystis carinii pneumonia. *Am. Rev. Respir. Dis.,* 135(Suppl 1):172A.
50. Broaddus, C., Dake, M. D., Stulbarg, M. S., et al. (1985): Bronchoalveolar lavage and transbronchial biopsy for the diagnosis of pulmonary infections in acquired immunodeficiency syndrome. *Ann. Intern. Med.,* 102:747–752.
51. Wharton, J. M., Coleman, D. L., Wofsy, C. B., et al. (1986): Trimethoprim—Sulfamethoxazole or pentamidine for pneumocystis carinii pneumonia in the acquired immunodeficiency syndrome. *Ann. Intern. Med.,* 105:37–44.
52. Gordin, F. M., Simon, G. L., Wofsy, C. B., and Mills, J. M. (1984): Adverse reaction to trimethoprim-sulfmethoxazole in patients with the acquired immunodeficiency syndrome. *Ann. Intern. Med.,* 100:495–499.
53. Anderson, R., Boedicker, M., Ma, M., and Goldstein, E. J. (1986): Adverse reactions associated with pentamidine isethionate in AIDS patients: Recommendations from monitoring therapy. *Drug Intell. Clin. Pharm.,* 20:862–868.
54. DeLorenzo, L. J., Maguire, G. P., Wormser, G. P., Davidian, M. M., and Stone, D. J. (1985): Persistence of pneumocystis carinii pneumonia in the acquired immunodeficiency syndrome. Evaluation of therapy by follow-up transbronchial lung biopsy. *Chest,* 88:79–83.
55. Broder, S. (1987): Identification of therapies against the retroviruses. In: Devita, V. T., Jr. (Moderator): Developmental therapeutics and the acquired immunodeficiency syndrome. *Ann. Intern. Med.,* 106:568–571.
56. Hughes, W. T., Kuhn, S., Chaudhary, S., et al. (1977): Successful chemoprophylaxis for pneumocystis carinii pneumonitis. *N. Engl. J. Med.,* 297:1419–1426.
57. Metroka, C. E., Lange, M., Braun, N., et al. (1987): Successful chemoprophylaxis for pneumocystic carinii pneumonia with Dapsone in patients with AIDS and ARC. Abstracts of Third International Conference on AIDS. Washington, D.C.
58. Gottlieb, M. S., Knight, S., Mitsuyusav, R., et al. (1984): Prophylaxis of pneumocystis carinii infection in AIDS with pyrimethamne-sulfadoxine (letter) *Lancet,* 2:398–399.
59. Bernard, E. M., Pagel, L., Schmitt, R. J., Donnelly, H., and Armstrong, D. (1987): Clinical trials with aerosolized pentamidine for prevention of pneumocystis carinii pneumonia. *Clin. Res.,* 35:468a.
60. Conlman, C. V., Greene, I., and Archibald, R. W. R. (1987): Cutaneous pneumocystis. *Ann. Intern. Med.,* 106:396–398.
61. Schinella, R., Breda, S. D., and Hammerschlag, P. E. (1987): Otic infection due to pneumocystis carinii in an apparently healthy man with antibody to the human immunodeficiency virus. *Ann. Intern. Med.,* 106:399–400.
62. Kwok, S., O'Donnell, S. S., and Wood, I. S. (1982): Retinal cotton-wool spots in a patient with pneumocystis carinii infection. *N. Engl. J. Med.,* 307:1845.
63. Feldman, H. A. (1968): Toxoplasmosis. *N. Engl. J. Med.,* 279:1370–1375.
64. Luft, B. J., Brooks, R. G., Conley, F. K., McCabe, R. E., and Remington, J. S. (1984): Toxoplasmic encephalitis in patients with acquired immune deficiency syndrome. *J.A.M.A.,* 252:913–917.
65. Potasman, I., Resnick, L., Luft, B. J., and Remington, J. S. (1987): Intrathecal production of antibodies against T-gondii in patients with toxoplasmic encephalitis and AIDS. Abstracts of the Third International Conference on AIDS. Washington, D.C., p. 159.
66. Ferguson, J. G., Jr. (1981): Clindamycin therapy for toxoplasmosis. *Ann. Ophthalmol.,* 13:95–100.
67. Allegra, C. J., Kovacs, J. A., Drake, J. C., et al. (1987): Potent *in vitro* and *in vivo* antitoxoplasma activity of the new lipid-soluble antifolate trimetrexate. *J. Clin. Invest.,* 79:478–482.
68. Zuger, A., Louie, E., Holzman, R. S., Simberkoff, M. S., and Rahal, J. J. (1986): Cryptococcal disease in patients with the acquired immunodeficiency syndrome: Diagnostic features and outcome of treatment. *Ann. Intern. Med.,* 104:235–240.
69. Bennett, J. E., Dismukes, W. E., Dume, R. J., et al. (1979): Amphoterian-B and 5-fluorocytosine in cryptococcal meningitis. *N. Engl. J. Med.,* 301:126–131.
70. Dupont, B., and Drouhet, E. (1987): Cryptococcal meningitis and fluconazole. *Ann. Intern. Med.,* 106:778.
71. Soave, R., and Ma, P. (1985): Cryptosporidiosis: Travelers' diarrhea in two families. *Arch. Intern. Med.,* 145:70–72.
72. Soave, R., Danner, R. L., Honig, C. L., et al. (1984): Cryptosporidiosis in homosexual men. *Ann. Intern. Med.,* 100:504–511.
73. Margulis, S. J., Honig, C. L., Soave, R., Govoni, A., and Jacobson, I. M. (1986): Biliary tract obstruction in the acquired immunodeficiency syndrome. *Ann. Intern. Med.,* 105:207–210.
74. Ma, P., Villanueva, T. G., Kaufman, D. G., and Illhooley, J. F. (1984): Respiratory cryptosporidiosis in the acquired immune deficiency syndrome. *J.A.M.A.,* 252:1298–1301.
75. Sheatner, A. L. (1953): The detection of intestinal protozoa and mange parasites by rotation technique. *J. Comp. Pathol.,* 36:268–275.
76. Hendricksen, S. A., and Pholenz, J. F. L. (1981): Staining of cryptosporidia by a modified Ziehl-Neelson technique. *Acta Vet. Scand.,* 22:594–596.
77. Portnoy, D., Whiteside, M. E., Buckley, E., III, and MacLeod, C. L. (1984): Treatment of intestinal cryptosporidiosis with spiramycin. *Ann. Intern. Med.,* 101:202–204.
78. Louie, E., Borkowsky, W., Klesius, P. H., et al. (1986): Treatment of cryptosporidiosis with oral bovine transfer factor. Abstracts of the Second International Conference on AIDS. Paris.
79. Drew, W. L., Mintz, L., Miner, R. C., Sands, M., and Ketterer, B. (1981): Cytomegalovirus infection in homosexual men. *J. Infect. Dis.,* 143:188–192.
80. Holland, G. N., Gottlieb, M. S., et al. (1982): Ocular disorders associated with a new severe acquired cellular immunodeficiency syndrome. *Am. J. Ophthalmol.,* 93:393–402.
81. Holland, G. N., Salcamote, M. J., Hardy, D., et al. (1986): Treatment of cytomegalovirus retinopathy in patients with ac-

quired immunodeficiency syndrome. Use of experimental drug 9-[2-hydroxy-1-(hydroxymethyl) ethoxymethyl] guanine. *Arch. Ophthalmol.,* 104:1794–1800.
82. Jacobson, M. A., Brodie, H. R., O'Donnell, et al. (1987): Randomized prospective trial of ganciclovir. Maintenence therapy for cytomegalovirus (CMV) retinitis. Abstracts of the Third International Conference on AIDS. Washington, D.C.
83. Chachoua, A., Dieterich, D., Krasinski, K., et al. (1987): 9-(1,3-dihydroxy-2-propoxymethyl) guanine (Ganciclovir) in the treatment of cytomegalovirus gastrointestinal disease with the acquired immunodeficiency syndrome. *Ann. Intern. Med.,* 107:133–137.
84. Wollinsky, E. (1979): Nontuberculous mycobacteria and associated diseases. *Am. Rev. Respir. Dis.,* 119:107–159.
85. Maayan, S., Wormser, G. P., Hewlett, D., et al. (1985): Acquired immunodeficiency syndrome (AIDS) in an economically disadvantaged population. *Arch. Intern. Med.,* 145:1607–1612.
86. Pierce, P. F., DeYound, D. R., and Roberts, G. D. (1983): Mycobacteremia and the new blood culture systems. *Ann. Intern. Med.,* 99:786–789.
87. Greene, J. B., Sidhu, G. S., Lewin, S., et al. (1982): Mycobacterium avium-intracellulare: A cause of disseminated life-threatening infection in homosexuals and drug abusers. *Ann. Intern. Med.,* 97:539–546.
88. Hawkins, C. C., Gold, J. W. M., Whimbey, E., et al. (1986): Mycobacterium avium complex infections in patients with the acquired immunodeficiency syndrome. *Ann. Intern. Med.,* 105:184–188.
89. Centers for Disease Control (1987): Diagnosis and management of mycobacterial infection and disease in persons with human immunodeficiency virus infection. *Ann. Intern. Med.,* 106:254–256.
90. Navia, B. A., Jordan, B. D., and Price, R. W. (1986): The AIDS dementia complex. I. Clinical Features. *Ann. Neurol.,* 19:517–524.
91. Ho, D. D., Rota, Jr., Schooley, R. J., et al. (1985): Isolation of HTLV-III from cerebrospinal fluid and neural tissue of patients with neurologic syndromes related to AIDS. *N. Engl. J. Med.,* 313:1493–1497.
92. Gyorkey, F., Melnick, J. L., and Gyorkey, P. (1987): Human immunodeficiency virus in brain biopsies of patients with AIDS and progressive encephalopathy. *J. Infect. Dis.,* 155:870–877.
93. Kennedy, C. J., Teschke, R. S., Messelink, J., et al. (1987): Clinical evaluation of the central nervous system in HIV infected patients on AZT. Abstracts of the Third International Conference on AIDS. Washington, D.C., p. 58.
94. Safai, B., and Good, R. A. (1980): Kaposi's sarcoma: A review and recent developments. *Clin. Bull.,* 10:62–69.
95. Taylor, J. F., Templeton, A. C., Vogel, C. I., et al. (1971): Kaposi's sarcoma in Uganda: A clinicopathologic study. *Int. J. Cancer,* 8:125–135.
96. Slavin, G., Cameron, H. M., Forbes, C., et al. (1970): Kaposi's sarcoma in East African children: A report of 51 cases. *J. Pathol.,* 10:187–199.
97. Penn, I. (1979): Kaposi's sarcoma in organ transplant recipients: A report of 20 cases. *Transplantation,* 27:8–11.
98. Gague, R. W., and Wilson-Jones, E. (1978): Kaposi's sarcoma and immunosuppressive therapy: A reappraisal. *Clin. Exp. Dermatol.,* 3:135–146.
99. Rubenstein, O., Walker, N., Moller, N., et al. (1983): Immunogenetic aspects of epidemic Kaposi's sarcoma in homosexual men. In: Friedman-Kien, A., Laubenstein, L., (eds). *AIDS: The Epidemic of Kaposi's Sarcoma and Opportunistic Infections.* Masson, New York, pp. 139–146.
100. Haverkos, H. W., Pinsky, P. F., Drotman, D. P., and Bregman, D. J. (1985): Disease manifestation among homosexual men with acquired immunodeficiency syndrome: A possible role of nitrites in Kaposi's sarcoma. *Sex. Transm. Dis.,* 12:203–208.
101. Drew, W. L., Miner, R. C., Ziegler, J. L., et al. (1982): Cytomegalovirus and Kaposi's sarcoma in young homosexual men. *Lancet,* 1:125–127.
102. Gottlieb, G., and Ackerman, A. B. (1982): Kaposi's sarcoma. An extensively disseminated form in young homosexual men. *Hum. Pathol.,* 13:882–892.
103. Nadjii, M., Morales, A. R., Ziegles-Weisman, J., et al. (1981): Kaposi's sarcoma: Immunohistologic evidence for an endothelial origin. *Arch. Pathol. Lab. Med.,* 105:274–275.
104. Beckstead, J. H., Wood, G., and Fletcher, V. (1985): Evidence for the origin of Kaposi's sarcoma from lymphatic endothelium. *Am. J. Pathol.,* 119:294–300.
105. Freidman, S. L., Wright, T. L., and Altman, D. F. (1985): Gastrointestinal Kaposi's sarcoma in patients with acquired immunodeficiency syndrome—Endoscopic and autopsy findings. *Gastroenterology,* 89:102–108.
106. Niedt, G., and Schinella, R. A. (1985): Acquired immunodeficiency syndrome: Clinicopathologic study of 56 autopsies. *Arch. Pathol. Lab. Med.,* 109:727–734.
107. Murray, J. F., Felton, C. P., Garay, S. M., et al. (1984): Pulmonary complications of the acquired immunodeficiency syndrome: Report of a national heart, lung and blood institute workshop. *N. Engl. J. Med.,* 310:1682–1688.
108. Garay, S. M. (1986): Fiberoptic bronchoscopic findings in patients with the acquired immune deficiency syndrome. *Chest.*
109. McCauley, D. I., Naidich, D. P., Leitman, B. S., et al. (1982): Radiographic patterns of opportunistic lung infections and Kaposi's sarcoma in homosexual men. *Am. J. Roentgenol.,* 139:661–666.
110. Kriegel, R. L., Laubenstein, L. J., and Muggia, F. M. (1983): Kaposi's sarcoma: A new staging classification. *Cancer Treat. Rep.,* 67:531–534.
111. Safai, B., Johnson, K. G., Myskowski, P. L., et al. (1985): The natural history of Kaposi's sarcoma in the acquired immune deficiency syndrome. *Ann. Intern. Med.,* 103:744–750.
112. Taylor, J., Afrasiabi, R., Fahey, J. L., et al. (1986): Prognostically significant classification of immune changes in AIDS with Kaposi's sarcoma. *Blood,* 67:666–671.
113. Lewis, B. J., Abrams, D. I., Zigler, J., et al. (1983): Single agent or combination chemotherapy of Kaposi's sarcoma in AIDS. *Proc. Am. Soc. Clin. Oncol.,* 2:59.
114. Mintzer, D. M., Ral, F. X., Jonno, L., et al. (1985): Treatment of Kaposi's sarcoma and thrombocytopenia with vincristine in patients with the acquired immunodeficiency syndrome. *Ann. Intern. Med.,* 102:200–202.
115. Laubenstein, L. J., Kreigel, R. L., Odajnyk, C. M., et al. (1983): Treatment of epidemic Kaposi's sarcoma with VP-16-213 (etoposide) and a combination of doxoribicin, bleomycin and vinblastine (ABV). *J. Clin. Oncol.,* 2:1115–1120.
116. Volberding, P. A., and Mitsuyasu, R. (1985): Recombinant interferon alpha in the treatment of acquired immune deficiency syndrome-related Kaposi's sarcoma. *Semin. Oncol.,* 12(*Suppl 5*):2–6.
117. Centers for Disease Control (1982): Diffuse undifferentiated lymphomas among homosexual males—United States. *M.M.W.R.,* 31:277–279.
118. Ziegler, J. L., Beckstead, J. A., Volberding, P., et al. (1984): NonHodgkins lymphoma in homosexual men. *N. Engl. J. Med.,* 311:565–570.
119. Binx, D. L., and Redfield, R. (1986): Defective regulation of Epstein-Barr virus infection in patients with acquired immunodeficiency syndrome (AIDS) or AIDS related disorders. *N. Engl. J. Med.,* 314:874–879.
120. Non-Hodgkins lymphoma pathologic classification project (1982): National Cancer Institute Sponsored Study of Classification of Non-Hodgkins Lymphomas: Summary and Description of a Working Formulation for Clinical Usage. *Cancer,* 49:2112–2135.
121. Dugan, M., Subar, M., Odajnyk, C., et al. (1985): Multiagent chemotherapy for AIDS related diffuse large cell lymphomas. *Blood,* 68(*Suppl 1*); 1242.
122. Subar, M., Chamulak, G., Della-Favera, R., et al. (1986): Clinical and pathologic characteristics of AIDS associated Hodgkins disease. *Blood,* 86(*Suppl 1*):135a.
123. Levine, A. M., Gill, P. S., Krails, M., et al. (1986): Natural history of persistent generalized lymphadenopathy in gay men: Risk of lymphoma and factors associated with the development of lymphoma. *Blood,* 86(*Suppl 1*):130a.
124. Bryne, R. K., Chan, W. C., Spire, T. J., et al. (1983): Value of

lymph node biopsy in unexplained lymphadenopathy in homosexual men. *J.A.M.A.*, 250:1313–1316.
125. Bermudez, M. A., Grant, K. U., and Rodlsen, R. (1986): Lymphoma in a population with or at risk for AIDS. A single institution experience. *Blood*, 86(*Suppl 1*):121a.
126. Skarin, A., Canellos, G., Rosenthal, D., et al. (1983): Moderate dose methotrexate combined with bleomycin, adrianmycin, cyclophosphamide and dexaethasone in advanced diffuse histiocytic lymphoma. *Proc. Am. Soc. Clin. Oncol.*, 2:220.
127. Fisher, R. I., DeVita, V. T., Hubbard, S. M., et al. (1983): Diffuse aggressive lymphomas: Increased survival after alternating sequences of pro-MACE and MOPP chemotherapy. *Ann. Intern. Med.*, 98:304–309.
128. Laurence, J., Coleman, M., Allen, S., et al. (1985): Combination chemotherapy of advanced diffuse histiocytic lymphoma with Mx-drug COP-BLAM regimen. *Ann. Intern. Med.*, 102:596–609.
129. Odaynyk, C., Subar, M., Dugan, M., et al. (1986): Clinical features and correlation with immunopathology and molecular biology in a large group of patients with AIDS associated small non-cleaved cell lymphoma, Burkitt's and nonBurkitts type. *Blood*, 86(*Suppl 1*):131a.
130. Peters, R. K., and Mack, T. M. (1986): Patterns of anal carcinoma by gender and marital status in Los Angeles. *Dis. Colon Rectum*, 28:402–404.
131. Longo, W. E., Ballantyne, G. E., Gerald, W. I., et al. (1986): Squamous cell carcinoma *in situ* in condyloma accuminatum. *Dis. Colon Rectum*, 29:503–506.
132. Gol, A. A., Meyer, P. R., and Taylor, C. R. (1987): Papilloma virus in anorectal condyloma and carcinoma in homosexual men. *J.A.M.A.*, 257:337–340.
133. Cooper, D. A., Gold, J., and MacLean, P. (1985): Acute AIDS retrovirus infection. Definition of a clinical illness associated with sarconversion. *Lancet*, 1:537–540.
134. Gottlieb, M. S., Wolfe, P. R., Fahey, J. L., et al. (1985): The syndrome of persistent generalized lymphadenopathy: Experience with 101 patients. *Adv. Exp. Med. Biol.*, 187:85–91.
135. Burns, B. F., Wood, G. S., and Dorfman, R. F. (1985): The varied histopathology of lymphadenopathy in the homosexual male. *Am. J. Surg. Pathol.*, 9:287–297.
136. Sidhr, G. S., Stahl, R. E., el-Sadr, W., et al. (1985): The acquired immunodeficiency syndrome: An ultrastructural study. *Hum. Pathol.*, 16:377–386.
137. Ryan, J. R., Ioachin, H. L., Marmer, J., and Loubeav, J. M. (1985): Acquired immune deficiency syndrome—Related lymphadenopathies presenting in the salivary gland lymph nodes. *Arch. Otolaryngol.*, 111:554–556.
138. Klein, R. S., Harris, C. A., Butkassmall, C., et al. (1984): Oral candidiasis in high-risk patients as the initial manifestation of AIDS. *N. Engl. J. Med.*, 311:354–358.
139. Greenspan, J. S., Greenspan, D., Lennette, E. T., et al. (1985): Replication of Epstein-Barr virus within the epithelial cells of oral "hairy" leukoplakia, an AIDS-associated lesion. *N. Engl. J. Med.*, 313:1564–1571.
140. Conant, M. A., Newlin, B., and Illeman, M. (1987): Topical acyclovir for treatment of hairy leukoplakia. Abstracts of the Third International Conference on AIDS. Washington, D.C., p. 146.
141. Melbye, M., Grossman, R. J., Goedert, J. J., Eyster, M. E., and Biggar, R. J. (1987): Risk of AIDS after Herpes Zoster. *Lancet*, I:728–730.
142. Farthing, C. (1986): Non-malignant cutaneous disease in AIDS and related conditions. *Clin. Immunol. Allergy*, 6:559–567.
143. Skinner, R. B., Jr., Noah, P. W., Zanolli, M. D., and Rosenberg, E. W. (1986): The pathogenic role of microbes in seborrheic dermatitis. *Arch. Dermatol.*, 122:16–17.
144. Redfield, R. R., James, W. D., Wright, C. D., et al. (1985): Severe molluscum contagiosum infection in a patient with human T-cell lymphotropic (HTLV-III) disease. *J. Am. Acad. Dermatol.*, 13:821–823.
145. Johnson, T. M., Duvic, M., Rapini, R. P., and Rios, A. (1985): AIDS exacerbates psorlasis. *N. Engl. J. Med.*, 313:1415.
146. Pepose, J. S., Holland, G. N., Nestor, M. S., Cochran, A. J., and Foos, R. Y. (1985): Acquired immune deficiency syndrome. Paogenic mechanisms of ocular disease. *Ophthalmology*, 92:472–484.
147. Walsch, C., Krigel, R., Lennette, E., and Karpatkin, S. (1985): Thrombocytopenia in homosexual patients. Prognosis, response to therapy, and prevalence of antibody to the retrovirus associated with the acquired immunodeficiency syndrome. *Ann. Intern. Med.*, 103:542–545.
148. Yu, J. R., Lennette, E. T., and Karpatkin, S. (1986): Anti-F-(ab')$_2$ antibodies in thrombocytopenic patients at risk for acquired immunodeficiency syndrome. *J. Clin. Invest.*, 77:1756–1761.
149. Greene, I. W., Cole, W., Greene, J. B., et al. (1984): Adrenal insufficiency as a complication of the acquired immunodeficiency syndrome. *Ann. Intern. Med.*, 101:497.
150. Navia, B. A., and Price, R. W. (1986): Central and peripheral nervous system complications of AIDS. *Clin. Immunol. Allergy*, 6:543–558.
151. Petito, C. K., Navia, B. A., Cho, E. S., et al. (1985): Vacuolar myelopathy pathologically resembling subacute combined degeneration in patients with the acquired immunodeficiency syndrome. *N. Engl. J. Med.*, 312:874–879.
152. Rao, T. K. S., Filippone, E. J., Nicastri, A. D., et al. (1984): Associated focal and segmental glomerulosclerosis in the acquired immunodeficiency syndrome. *N. Engl. J. Med.*, 310:669–673.
153. Anderson, D. W., Virmani, R., Macher, A. M., et al. (1987): Cardiac pathology and cardiovascular cause of death in patients dying with the acquired immunodeficiency syndrome (AIDS). Abstracts of the Third International Conference on AIDS. Washington, D.C., p. 9.
154. Kaplan, L. D., Wolfe, P. R., Volberging, P. A., et al. (1987): Lack of response to suramin in patients with AIDS and AIDS related complex. *Am. J. Med.*, 82:615–620.
155. Rozenbaum, W., Dormont, D., Spire, B., et al. (1985): Antimoniotungstate (HPA-23) treatment of three patients with AIDS and one with prodrome. *Lancet*, I:450–451.
156. Sandstrom, E. G., Kaplan, J. C., Byington, R. E., and Hirsch, M. S. (1985): Inhibition of human T-cell lymphotropic virus type III *in vitro* by phosphonoformate. *Lancet*, 1:1480–1482.
157. Vogt, M., and Hirsch, M. S. (1986): Prospects for prevention and therapy of infections with the human immunodeficiency virus. *Rev. Infect. Dis.*, 8:991–1000.
158. Krown, S. E., Real, F. X., Cunningham-Rundles, S., et al. (1983): Preliminary observations on the effect of recominant leukocyte. Interferon in homosexual men with Kaposi's sarcoma. *N. Engl. J. Med.*, 308:1071–1076.
159. Wetterberg, Z., Alexius, B., Saaf, J., et al. (1987): Peptide in treatment of AIDS. *Lancet*, I:159.
160. Sarrin, P. S., Gallo, R. C., Scheer, D. I., Crews, F., and Lippa, A. B. (1985): Effect of a novel compound (AL-721) on HTLV-III infectivity *in vitro*. *N. Engl. J. Med.*, 313:1289–1290.
161. Yarchoan, R. Y., and Broder, S. (1987): Development of antiretroviral therapy for the acquired immunodeficiency syndrome and related disorders: A progress report. *N. Engl. J. Med.*, 316:557–564.
162. Fischl, M. A., Richman, D. D., Grieco, M. H., et al. (1987): The efficacy of azidothymidine (AZT) in the treatment of patients with AIDS and AIDS-related complex: A double-blind placebo-controlled trial. *N. Engl. J. Med.*, 317:185–191.
163. Richman, D. D., Fischl, M. A., Grieco, M. H., et al. (1987): The toxicity of azidotrymidine (AZT) in the treatment of patients with AIDS and AIDs-related complex: A double-blind placebo-controlled study. *N. Engl. J. Med.*, 317:192–197.
164. Mitsuya, H., and Broder, S. (1987): Stratgies for anti-viral therapy in AIDS. *Nature*, 325:773–778.
165. Franeis, D. F., and Petricciani, J. C. (1985): The prospects for and pathways toward a vaccine for AIDS. *N. Engl. J. Med.*, 315:1586–1590.

CHAPTER 2

# Neuroradiology of AIDS

Walter L. Olsen and Wendy Cohen

Neurological signs and symptoms in patients with human immunodeficiency virus (HIV) infection have become common features of the disease. Neuroimaging studies therefore are frequently requested in these patients. Because AIDS is ultimately a fatal disease, the principal goal is to identify treatable components of the HIV infection in order to prolong the time that a patient spends outside of the hospital.

## INCIDENCE OF NEUROLOGICAL MANIFESTATIONS

The reported frequency of neurological complications in patients infected with HIV reflects the type of clinical manifestation, the sensitivity of the observer to the types of possible diseases, and the increasing specificity in documenting HIV infection in the brain and spinal cord. An early report identified 50 patients with acquired immune deficiency syndrome (AIDS) in a group of 160 persons who had identifiable neurological disease (41). In a more recent study, Levy et al. (21) found that 39% of 352 AIDS patients had neurological complaints. Of this group, 10% presented with neurological symptoms prior to other manifestations of HIV infection.

Reported figures of neurological manifestations during life may underestimate the involvement of the neuroaxis. Autopsy series have found histologically significant neuropathologic lesions in 73 to 80% of cases (2,23,26). Recent studies document the presence of HIV in the central nervous system (CNS). Ho et al. (13) examined 56 specimens of brain, spinal cord, or cerebrospinal fluid (CSF) in 45 patients who were seropositive for HIV. Thirty-three of these patients had neurological symptoms and HIV was cultured from 24 of these specimens. Levy et al. (19) isolated and cultured HIV from the CSF and brain of AIDS and AIDS-related complex (ARC) patients with neurological symptoms. These results suggest that the AIDS virus is neurotropic and attacks CNS tissue as well as T lymphocytes. Similar observations of the neurotropism of HIV have been made by others (5,39). It is unclear which cells within the CNS are attacked by the AIDS virus, but a current hypothesis places the viral particles within cells of monocyte-macrophage derivation, but this remains controversial (11,12). Direct infection of glial cells is still considered to be a possibility, as is the potential disruption of neural cell function either from secretion of toxic substances by the infected cells, competition for binding sites by the virus, or direct interference with neuronal function (3). The overlying impression engendered by these studies is that there is a significant involvement of the CNS by the AIDS virus that may produce neurological symptoms irrespective of opportunistic infections or tumors.

## SPECTRUM OF DISEASE

As mentioned, neurological syndromes are prominent features of HIV infection. As described elsewhere in this volume, patients with AIDS have a profound defect in T-cell lymphocyte function. There is an absolute lymphopenia selective for the T4 subset of the helper-inducer lymphocytes. There is a depletion of these lymphocytes as well as qualitative defects in T-cell function that prevent a normal response to antigenic material. There is also decreased antibody production. Thus, in addition to the potential direct effects of the HIV agent, the patient is susceptible to opportunistic infections and neoplasms. A variety of neurological manifestations of AIDS have been described, including viral syndromes, nonviral infections, neoplasms, cerebral vascular accidents, myelopathy, and peripheral neuropathies (21). Viral syndromes include subacute encephalitis caused by the HIV virus (the AIDS dementia complex; ADC), cytomegalovirus (CMV) encephalitis, herpes virus encephalitis, progressive multifocal leukoencephalopathy, and aseptic meningitis. Nonviral infections include toxoplasmosis, tuberculosis, and fungal infections. Meningovascular syphilis also has been reported. Primary CNS lymphoma is the most common neoplasm encountered in AIDS patients, although gliomas and metastases occasionally may be encountered. All of these disease processes will be discussed in subsequent sections on radiological manifestations. Rather than being grouped according to etiology, we have chosen to group the intracranial diseases according to the radiological manifestation, that is, according to whether the disease produces atrophy, mass lesion(s), white matter disease, or leptomeningeal disease.

## RADIOLOGICAL MANIFESTATIONS

### Indications

Approximately 39% of all AIDS victims have neurological symptoms, and a significant percentage of them are referred for neuroimaging studies. Since various diseases may affect the brains of AIDS victims, these patients may present with a variety of clinical symptoms that prompt a neuroimaging study. Unfortunately, the symptoms may be focal or diffuse and often are nonspecific. Probably the most common symptom is progressive dementia, a part of ADC (28). Although ADC is a diffuse pathological process, focal neurological symptoms also may be seen with this condition, including focal motor deficits, headache, and seizures (21,28). Focal neurological symptoms and signs are common with the mass lesions that may affect the brains of AIDS patients. For instance, focal neurological deficits and seizures are frequent in patients with toxoplasmosis. However, nonfocal symptoms, such as an altered level of consciousness and confusion, are seen commonly in patients with toxoplasmosis, especially early in the course of the disease (27). Hence, the clinical features may not always point to the etiology of the neurological abnormality in AIDS patients. Neuroimaging studies are required to help make the diagnosis and guide therapy.

The most common indications for neuroimaging in patients with AIDS include decreased mental status, altered level of consciousness, headache, seizures, focal motor or sensory deficits, and cranial nerve palsies. The neuroradiological findings that may account for these symptoms generally fall into four patterns. The most common finding is cerebral atrophy, which is often striking in these generally young patients. The second pattern is single or multiple mass lesions that may be caused by either infectious or neoplastic diseases. The third pattern is focal or diffuse white matter disease. The fourth and least commonly observed pattern is leptomeningeal or ependymal disease. (These four patterns are discussed in detail below. Myelopathy and head and neck manifestations are discussed separately.)

### Technique

Both computed tomography (CT) and magnetic resonance imaging (MR) have been shown to screen effectively for neurological manifestations of AIDS. No large study comparing CT and MR in AIDS patients has been performed. However, several smaller studies have suggested that MR may be more sensitive than CT in detecting intracranial lesions in AIDS. (22,35,44; Fig 1). Our preliminary experience also suggests that MR is more sensitive than CT but it does not provide more specificity. MR is more sensitive than CT in detecting white matter abnormalities. Conversely, leptomeningeal abnormalities currently are better detected with contrast-enhanced CT than with MR, although even with CT, patients with leptomeningeal disease usually have a normal study. Therefore, MR and CT probably complement each other in the study of AIDS patients (35). Although specific recommendations cannot be made at this time, if MR and CT are equally available, it is reasonable to screen patients with MR unless the clinical symptoms clearly suggest meningitis. If MR is not readily available, CT is a reasonable alternative.

The optimal screening technique with MR for most indications is a T2-weighted technique. With a standard spin echo sequence, a T2-weighted image is achieved by using a long repetition time (TR) (2,000 msec or greater) and a long echo time (TE) (60 msec or greater). Other pulsing sequences, such as gradient echo techniques, also may provide T2 weighting but this is beyond the scope of this chapter. In general, all T2-weighted techniques are sensitive to changes in brain water content. Virtually all of the focal brain lesions described below increase the brain water content; therefore, T2-weighted MR images reveal the lesion(s) as areas of high-signal intensity that contrast significantly with normal brain. This is especially true for white matter lesions, since normal white matter has relatively low signal intensity on T2-weighted images. T1-weighted images using a short TR (600 msec or less) and short TE (30 msec or less) spin echo technique may be used to supplement the T2-weighted screening technique. T1-weighted images are less sensitive to changes in brain water content. However, anatomic resolution is generally better with T1-weighted images and subacute hemorrhage is well detected with this technique. We obtain T1-weighted images only when the T2-weighted study shows an abnormality because the T1-weighted imaging is a much less sensitive technique.

The optimal technique for imaging AIDS patients with CT requires intravenous (i.v.) contrast material. Noncontrast CT is optional in the nonacute setting, but should be employed with the patient who has an acute neurological event. There are three contrast studies that may be performed: the standard contrast-enhanced CT scan involves administering approximately 40 gm of iodine prior to the scan. Double-dose techniques using 80

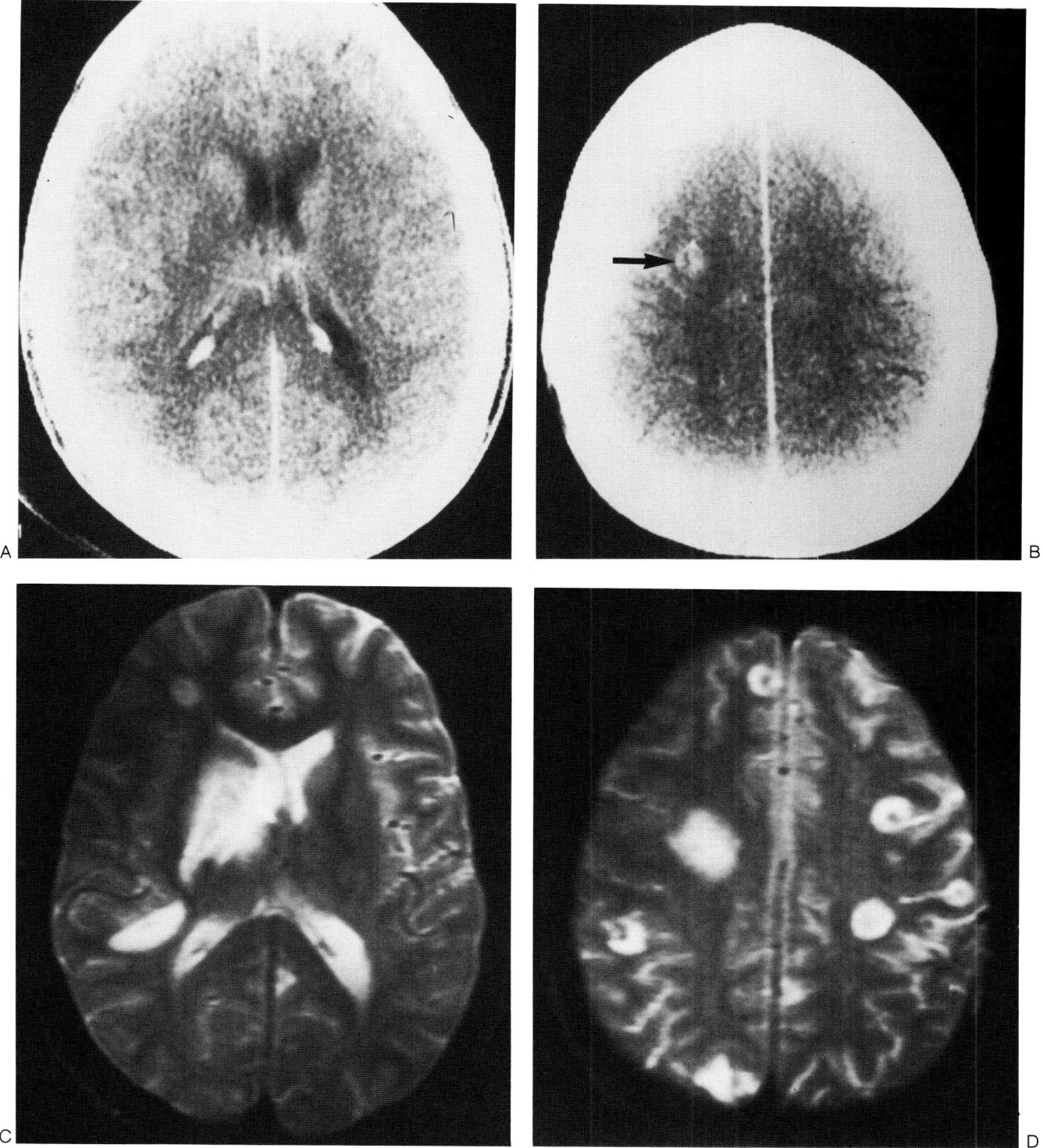

**FIG. 1.** Superiority of MR compared with CT: Toxoplasmosis. The lower contrast enhanced CT image (**A**) shows slight mass effect on the frontal horn of the right lateral ventricle but no enhancing lesion is seen. The upper section (**B**) shows an enhancing lesion in the right corona radiata (*arrow*). This is the only lesion seen. **C, D:** These T2-weighted MR images (SE 2000/80) were obtained 2 days after the CT scan. Multiple mass lesions are identified. There is a large right basal ganglia lesion that compresses the right frontal horn. In addition, lesions in the right frontal white matter and right temporal lobe also are seen. Near the convexity, multiple lesions are seen at the gray-white junction and cortex. The significantly increased sensitivity of T2-weighted MR compared with CT is evident.

gm of iodine are described as being more sensitive than the standard technique (34,35; Fig 2). The immediate double-dose technique involves scanning the patient immediately following administering i.v. contrast. The delayed double-dose technique involves waiting 1 hour after administering the contrast before scanning the patient. The delayed double-dose technique has been reported to be more sensitive than either the standard or the immediate double-dose technique for detecting intracranial lesions in AIDS patients (34,35). If MR is not readily available, the delayed double-dose CT technique appears to be the next most sensitive screening study.

## ATROPHY

The most common abnormal intracranial finding in AIDS is diffuse cerebral atrophy (Fig. 3): this was found in 75 of 200 consecutive AIDS patients with neurological symptoms studied by Levy et al. (22). Only 81 of these 200 patients had normal scans. Of interest, 12 of the 75 patients demonstrating diffuse cerebral atrophy developed focal CNS disease. However, only four of the 81 patients with initially normal CT scans progressed to focal CNS disease. This suggests that patients with atrophy are at greater risk for subsequently developing other CNS manifestations.

The etiology of the diffuse cerebral atrophy in these patients is unclear. There is accumulating evidence that HIV is neurotropic and infects the brains of AIDS victims, resulting in a subacute encephalitis syndrome (13,19,28,29). Clinically, there is impaired memory and concentration with psychomotor slowing. This progresses to dementia, and the syndrome is now more properly termed ADC (28,29). In an autopsy review of 70 demented AIDS patients, Navia et al. (29) found only five brains that were histologically normal. Seventy-six percent of the brains examined had evidence of gross cerebral atrophy. This finding correlated with dementia prior to death. Unfortunately, dementia is a common clinical finding in AIDS patients, occurring in over half of all AIDS victims (28). ADC probably results from infection of the brain by the HIV, which may account for the common finding of diffuse atrophy on imaging studies.

Other diffuse disease states also may afflict these patients. CMV is seen pathologically in the brains of 25% of AIDS victims (33). CMV causes a diffuse encephalitis that may also lead to loss of brain substance. AIDS patients frequently are cachectic and may be dehydrated from bowel disease, which also might result in an appearance of diffuse cerebral atrophy. The enlarged ventricles and sulci of atrophy are equally well detected by CT and MR.

## MASS LESIONS

Intracranial mass lesions are common in patients with AIDS. In one study, mass lesions were found in 44 of 200 (22%) AIDS patients with neurological symptoms (22). In another study, 35 of 153 (23%) AIDS patients who underwent autopsy had focal, macroscopic CNS disease (33). Of these 35 patients, 16 had toxoplasmosis and 9 had CNS lymphoma. Other reports have similarly shown that toxoplasmosis and primary CNS lymphoma account for the large majority of mass lesions found in AIDS patients (2,21,30). Other less common mass lesions include Candida abscesses, tuberculomas, cryptococcomas, and herpes simplex encephalitis. In our experience, these diseases are very uncommon. Even rarer are metastatic Kaposi's sarcoma and bacterial infections. Occasionally, a peripheral nonHodgkin's lymphoma will metastasize to the brain or spine.

As indicated above, the most common intracranial mass lesion in patients with AIDS is toxoplasmosis, occurring in approximately 10% of all AIDS patients (21,33). Moreover, toxoplasmosis represents the most common treatable form of CNS involvement in AIDS. The organism, toxoplasma gondii, is an obligate intracellular protozoan. It is ubiquitous throughout the world and causes subclinical or mild infection in a large percentage of the population. In the United States, 20 to 70% of adults are seropositive for toxoplasmosis (21). The seropositivity rate varies in different parts of the country, as does the rate of clinical infection in AIDS (21). In immunodeficient patients, especially those with impaired cellular immunity, as is seen in AIDS, life-threatening infection may occur. This usually results from reactivation of previously acquired infection (27). In the brain, a necrotizing encephalitis that may be focal or diffuse ensues. Usually, several well-defined toxoplasma abscesses are present that have thin capsules and necrotic centers (27,33).

Clinically, these patients usually present with a subacute onset of headache, fever, and focal neurological findings. As the lesions may involve the cortex, central gray matter, and sometimes brainstem and cerebellum, a large variety of neurological findings may be encountered. Nonfocal findings also are common, including confusion, decreased level of consciousness, lethargy, and sometimes coma (27). The diffuse findings often precede the focal findings, simulating the subacute encephalitis syndrome of primary HIV infection.

The typical appearance on neuroimaging studies of cerebral toxoplasmosis is that of multiple mass lesions with surrounding edema. Solitary lesions are less common. With CT, the lesions usually enhance with i.v. contrast in either a ring or nodular pattern (34,43; Fig. 4). No enhancement was seen in only two of 31 cases of toxoplasma encephalitis reported by Post et al. (34).

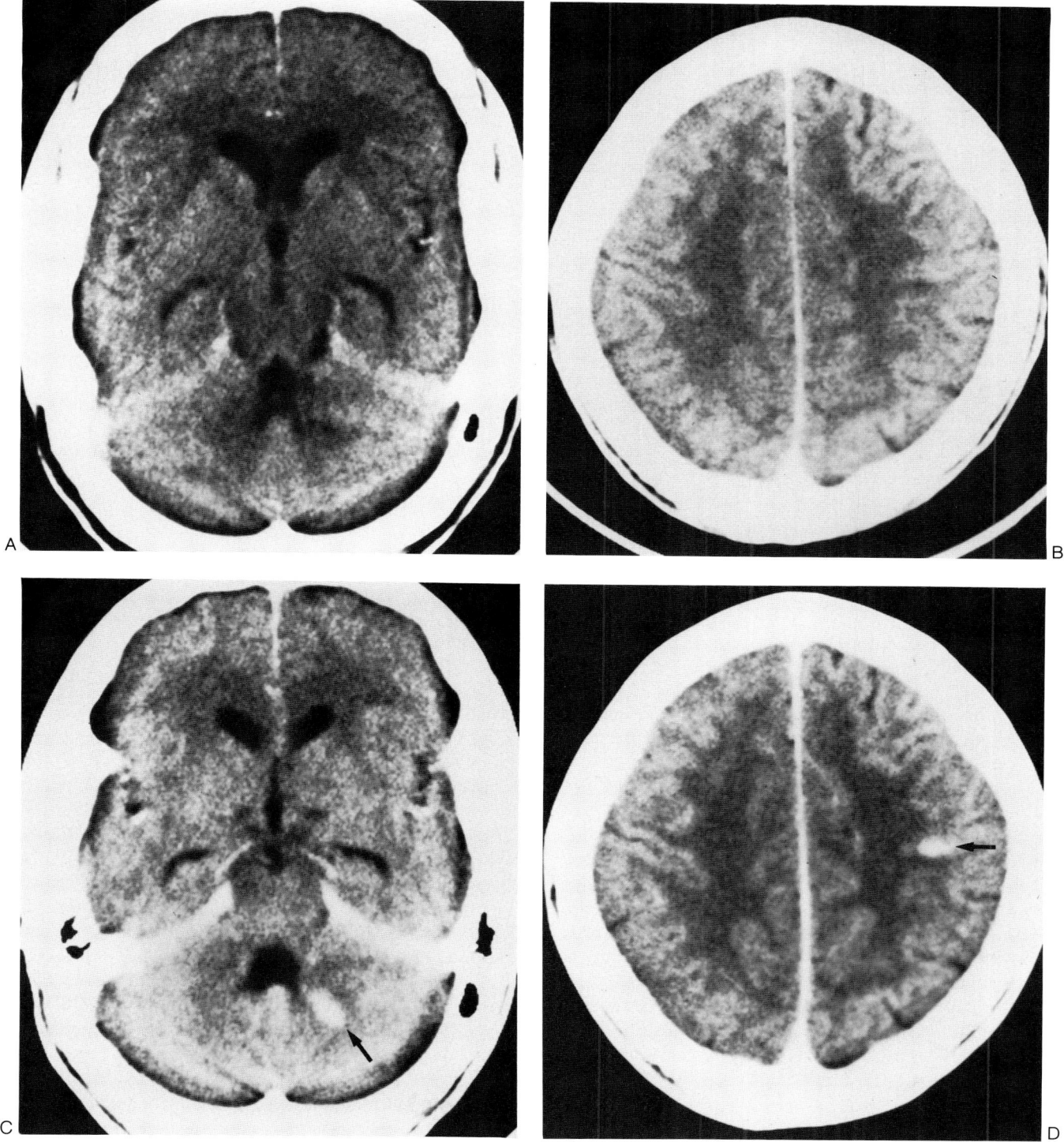

**FIG. 2.** Superiority of double dose compared with single dose contrast CT: Toxoplasmosis. **A, B:** The single-dose CT images performed with 40 gm of iodine show no areas of abnormal enhancement. **C, D:** The double-dose CT study performed with 80 gm of iodine was performed 2 days later. Enhancing lesions in the left cerebellum and at the gray-white junction in the left posterior frontal lobe are evident (*arrows*).

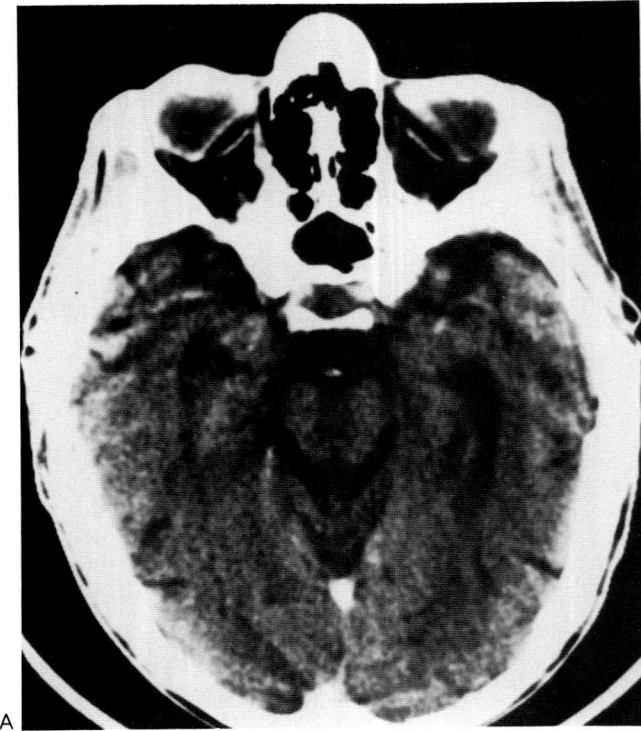
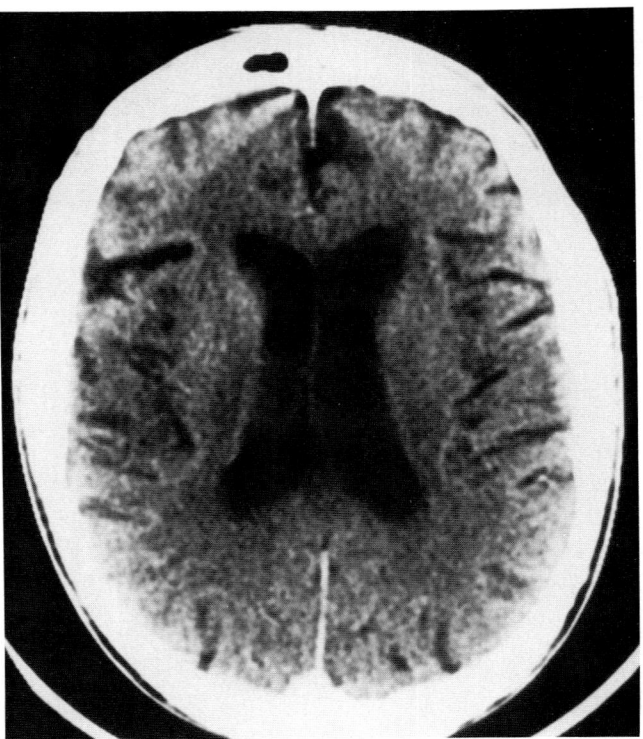

FIG. 3. Atrophy. A, B: These noncontrast head CT images show diffuse cerebral atrophy in a 35-year-old homosexual man with AIDS. The sulci and ventricles, including the temporal tips, are enlarged. No focal lesions are identified. Atrophy is the most common finding on neuroimaging studies of patients with AIDS.

Surrounding edema is common and usually is moderate to marked. Occasionally, periventricular or leptomeningeal enhancement is seen from involvement of the meninges or ependyma (6). With MR, toxoplasmosis lesions usually are of low-signal intensity on T1-weighted images and medium high-signal intensity on T2-weighted images (Fig. 5). The capsule may be low in signal. The lesions often are round in shape and are surrounded by a significant high signal from vasogenic edema that may obscure the margins of the abscess. Following treatment, the central portion of the abscess may be high in signal on the T1-weighted images, possibly from subclinical hemorrhage (Fig. 5). It is not uncommon for MR to demonstrate more lesions than CT (22,44). As with CT, the lesions usually are seen with MR in the cortex and in the subcortical deep gray matter.

Because toxoplasmosis is the most common treatable intracranial disease in AIDS, it is currently not recommended to biopsy all patients with mass lesions (7,27). Effective treatment with a variety of antibiotics (usually sulfadiazine and pyrimethamine) is available. Clinical and radiologic improvement usually are seen within two weeks (27; Figs. 5 and 6). Biopsy is reserved for patients who fail therapy or who are clinically atypical for toxoplasmosis. Patients who have atypical findings on CT or MR, such as solitary or nonenhancing lesions, are still usually treated empirically with antitoxoplasma antibiotics (Fig. 6). An occasional patient will have both toxoplasmosis and lymphoma, and it has been recommended to biopsy all patients with suspected toxoplasmosis in order to detect these patients (21). However, since this is an unusual occurrence and since lymphoma has a grave prognosis, most centers reserve biopsy for patients who have failed antibiotic therapy.

After toxoplasmosis, the next most common mass lesion found in patients with AIDS is primary CNS lymphoma. This is found in approximately 6% of all AIDS patients (33). Before the AIDS epidemic, primary CNS lymphoma occurred with increased frequency in immunosuppressed patients, but was still a rare disease. However, in the past several years this disease is being seen with increased frequency in AIDS patients. The clinical findings of primary CNS lymphoma in AIDS patients are variable and include encephalopathy, seizures, cranial nerve palsies, and focal neurological symptoms (42). The prognosis is extremely poor, with most patients surviving less than 2 months. Radiation therapy sometimes produces regression (42).

The CT findings of primary CNS lymphoma in AIDS and nonAIDS patients have been reviewed in two recent series (15,18). The classic CT appearance of primary CNS lymphoma is that of a solitary, iso- or hyperdense mass precontrast that enhances homogeneously follow-

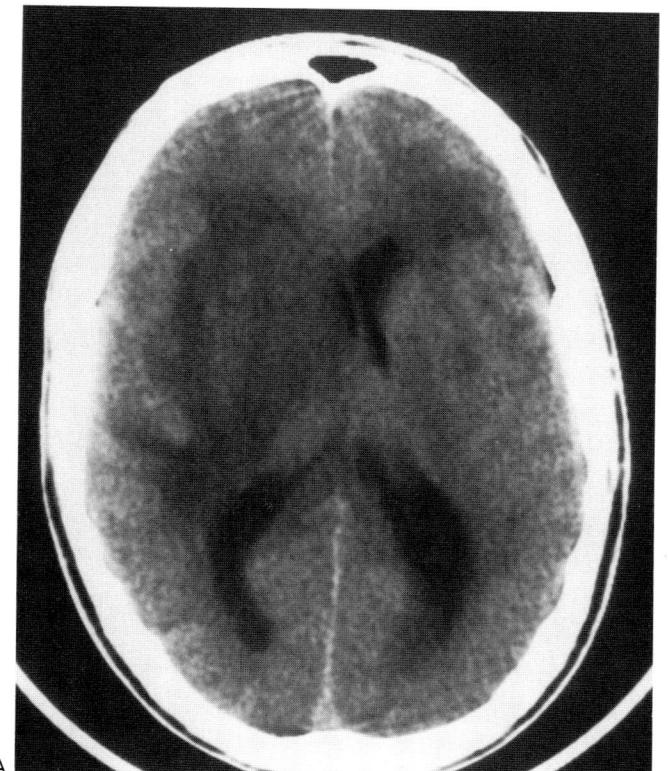 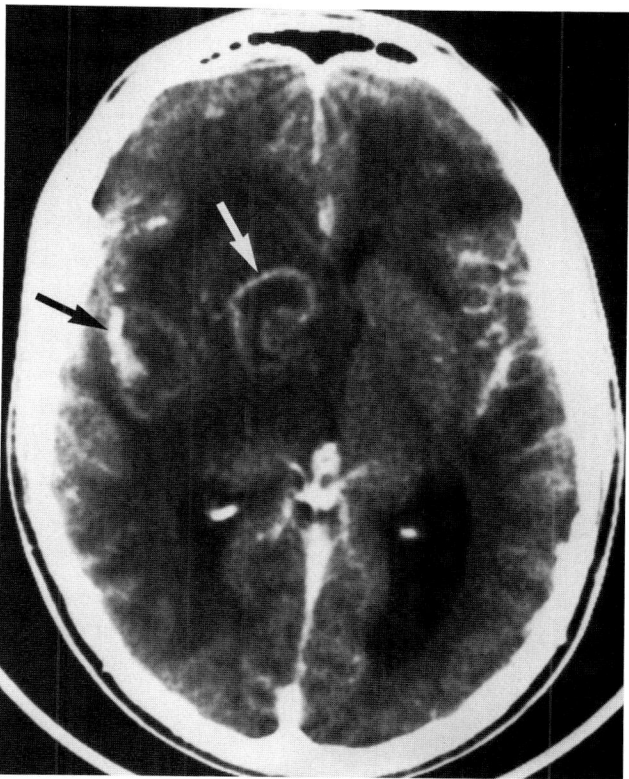

**FIG. 4.** Toxoplasmosis. **A, B:** Pre- (**A**) and postcontrast (**B**) CT scans show two large masses in the right basal ganglia (arrows). The lesions are of low attenuation precontrast and there is ring enhancement following contrast administration. There is marked mass effect and surrounding vasogenic edema. The location, enhancement pattern, multiplicity, and amount of edema of these lesions are typical of toxoplasmosis. However, lymphoma sometimes can have a similar appearance.

ing contrast administration (Fig. 7). This appearance is seen in the majority of nonAIDS patients, and in about half of AIDS patients. Ring enhancement is unusual in nonAIDS patients with primary CNS lymphoma. However, almost half of primary CNS lymphoma lesions in patients with AIDS show ring enhancement with central hypodensity (18; Fig. 8). The central area of hypodensity correlates with central necrosis at pathology, a rare feature of primary CNS lymphoma in nonAIDS patients. In nonAIDS patients, primary CNS lymphoma tends to be solitary, whereas about half of AIDS patients will have multiple lesions (42). Most lesions tend to be peripheral rather than deep, with the majority located in the supratentorial gray or white matter (15). The posterior fossa is involved in approximately 13% of cases (15). In a minority of patients these lesions may spread diffusely along subependymal or white matter routes. With MR imaging, primary CNS lymphoma usually is low in signal on T1-weighted images and medium to high in signal on T2-weighted images. We have seen some cases where there was relatively low signal on T2-weighted images, possibly reflecting the densely packed cellular structure of the tumor (Fig. 9).

Mass lesions other than toxoplasmosis or primary CNS lymphoma are unusual in patients with AIDS. The lesions that have been reported include fungal abscesses, tuberculomas, and metastatic tumors (21). Infections with herpes simplex or zoster virus also may give the appearance of mass lesions.

Fungal infections are common in patients with AIDS, occurring in up to 15% of all AIDS patients (2,21,33). Cryptococcal meningitis is the most common fungal infection. Rarely, a fungal abscess may present as a mass lesion in the brain. Levy et al. (21) reported two cases of Candidal abscess and one case of a cryptococcoma out of 128 AIDS patients with neurological symptoms. Unfortunately, the CT findings were not reported. Other autopsy series also report rare focal fungal lesions (2,26,33). Again, the imaging characteristics of these lesions are not reported. In a review of 51 AIDS patients with CNS pathology, Post et al. (34) reported one case of a fungal abscess proven by autopsy that was missed by a contrast-enhanced CT scan. Despite the paucity of radiology literature on the imaging characteristics of fungal abscesses in AIDS, it is known that these lesions are well evaluated by CT. Fungal abscesses may have a variable appearance, including solid, nodular, or ring enhancement with a variable amount of surrounding edema.

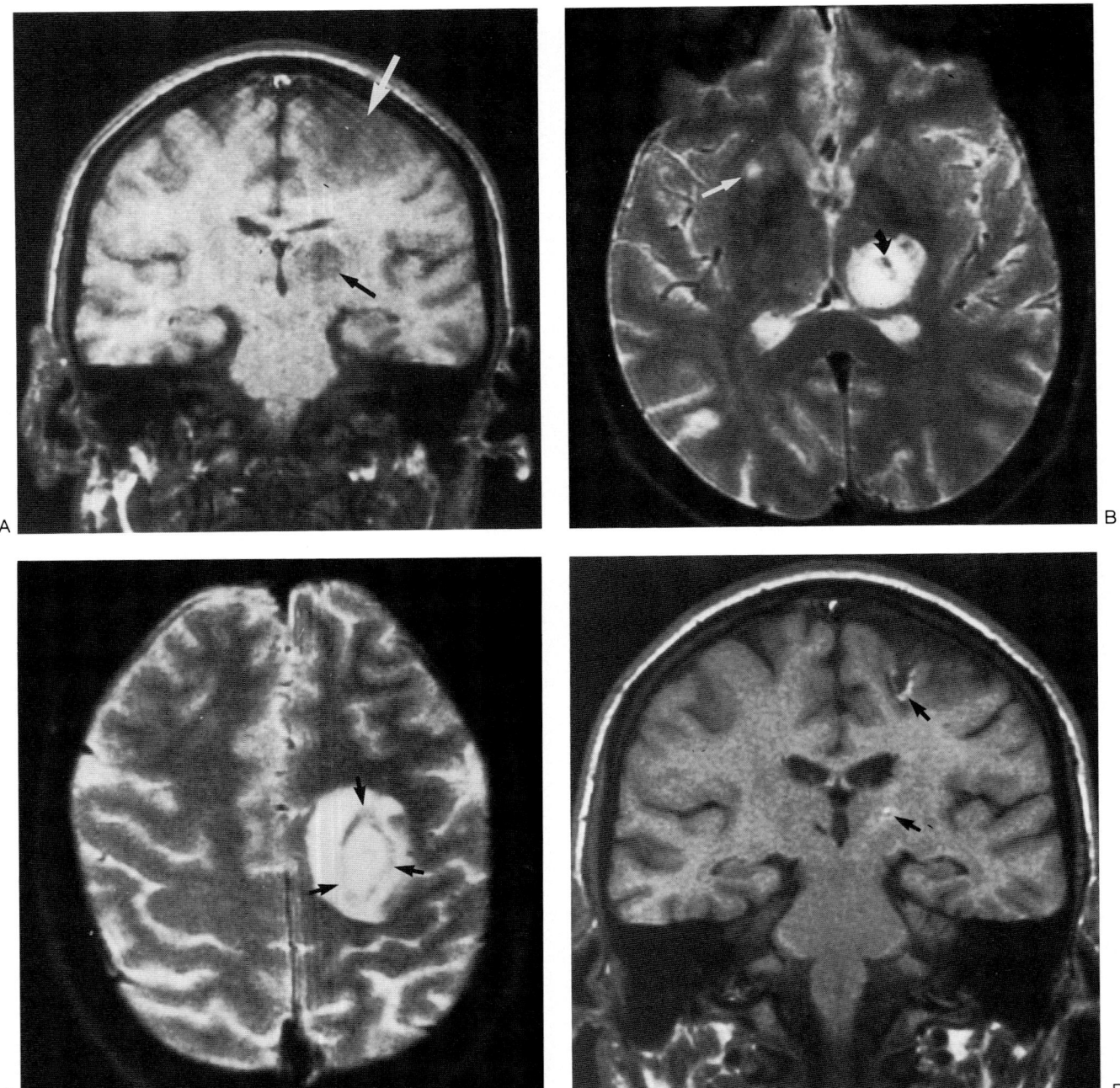

**FIG. 5.** Toxoplasmosis before and after therapy. **A:** The T1-weighted (PS 600/20) coronal MR image reveals two areas of abnormal low-signal intensity. There is a low-signal mass in the left thalamus (*black arrow*) and a second mass in the left parietal lobe (*white arrow*). The left thalamic lesion causes mild compression of the third and lateral ventricles. **B:** A T2-weighted (SE 2000/70) image shows the left thalamic lesion to be of high-signal intensity. Centrally there is an area of relatively low-signal intensity (*curved arrow*), that probably is the capsule of the abscess. A lesion within the right putamen (*straight arrow*) also is identified. **C:** The upper T2-weighted (SE 2000/70) section shows a mass of high-signal intensity with a relatively low-signal rim (*arrows*). This is surrounded by a higher signal zone that probably represents edema. The low-signal rim most likely represents the capsule of the toxoplasmosis abscess. **D:** Following 3 weeks of treatment with sulfadiazine and pyrimethamine, the thalamic and parietal lesions have decreased in size. However, both lesions contain small areas of high-signal intensity (*arrows*) on this T1-weighted coronal image (PS 600/20). These high-signal areas represent subclinical hemorrhage. However, this is rarely seen with noncontrast CT scanning. **E, F:** The T2-weighted (SE 2000/70) axial MR images following treatment show that the high-signal masses largely have disappeared. The low-signal area within the thalamus persists and may represent an area of fibrous scar. The right putamen lesion appears smaller in size. There is also significant reduction in size of the left parietal convexity lesion. The reduction in the size of these lesions following antibiotic therapy correlated with improvement in clinical status, which is typical of the response to therapy for toxoplasmosis.

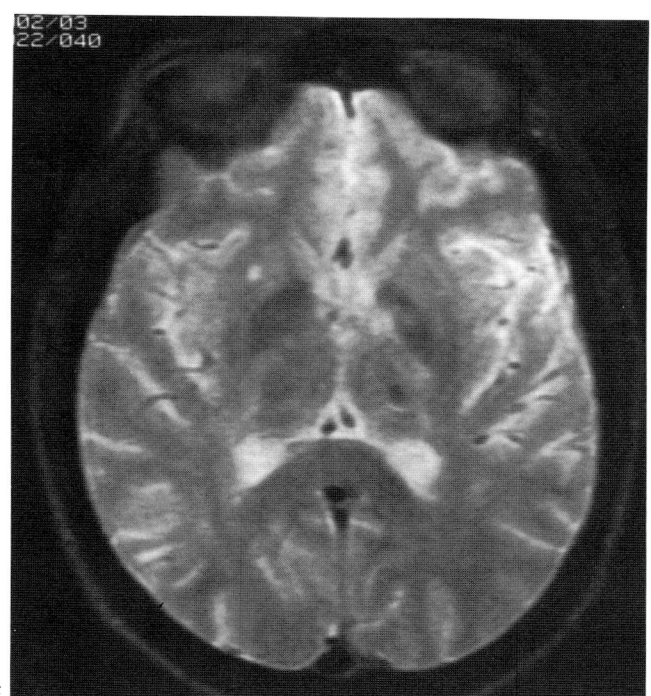
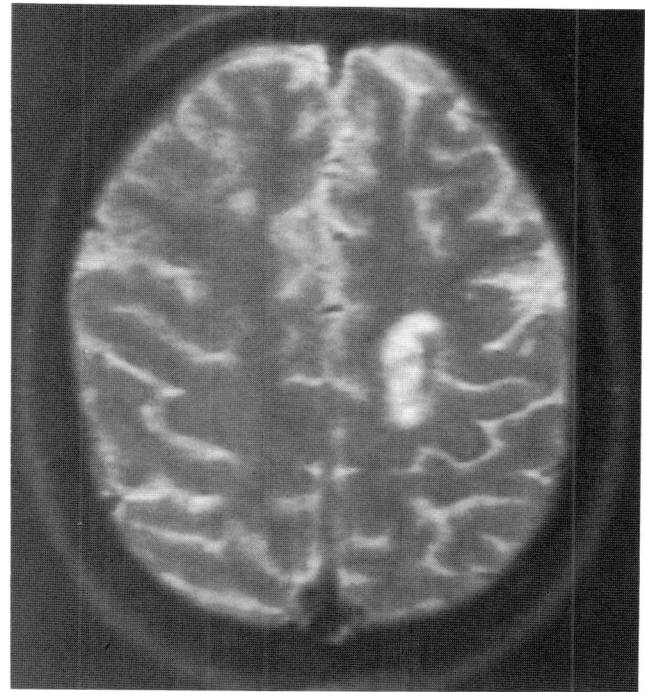

**FIG. 5.** *(Continued)*

They may occur anywhere in the brain parenchyma and may be associated with abnormal leptomeningeal enhancement from associated meningitis. Infarcts also may be seen from involvement of vessels. Hydrocephalus is common, especially with cryptococcal meningitis. Fungal infections will be discussed further under the section of leptomeningeal disease, since the usual manifestation of fungal infection in AIDS is that of meningitis.

Intracranial tuberculosis is a rare manifestation of AIDS. In several large autopsy series, no cases of intracranial tuberculosis in AIDS patients were found (2,21,33). Only one of 51 patients with documented CNS pathology had tuberculosis as reported by Post et al. (34). However, a series of 10 cases of intracranial tuberculosis in patients with AIDS was recently reported (4). Nine of these patients were i.v. drug abusers and one was a Haitian. Three of the patients had AIDS and seven had ARC. Seven of the patients had normal chest roentgenograms. CT scans of the head revealed ring-enhancing lesions in five patients. One of these five patients had multiple ring-enhancing lesions that proved to be acute tuberculous abscesses by brain biopsy. The other four solitary lesions were tuberculomas containing caseous material. Three other patients showed hypodense non-enhancing cortical areas that are not characterized further. These may have represented infarcts secondary to tuberculous meningitis. CNS tuberculosis may manifest as meningitis, indolent tuberculoma, or as acute tuberculous abscesses. Abnormal leptomeningeal enhancement may be seen with tuberculous meningitis, and infarcts from narrowing of arteries at the base of the brain sometimes are seen. Tuberculomas typically show solid enhancement when small, and ring enhancement when large (Fig. 10). Surrounding edema is common. The one case reported by Post et al. (34) showed a multiloculated ring-enhancing mass with surrounding edema. Acute tuberculous abscesses are seen in immunocompromised patients as is seen in AIDS patients. These lesions frequently are multiple and usually show ring enhancement with marked surrounding edema. Although rare, tuberculoma or tuberculous abscess should be considered in the differential diagnosis of an intracranial mass lesion, especially in an i.v. drug abuser or a Haitian with AIDS. A history of previous tuberculosis usually can be elicited (4).

Intracranial mass lesions caused by neoplasms other than lymphoma in patients with AIDS are very uncommon. Most large autopsy series show no nonlymphomatous involvement of the brain (2,26,33). Metastatic Kaposi's sarcoma has been reported by Levy et al. (20) in two patients with AIDS. One of these patients had a CT scan that showed a mass lesion. The paucity of other literature on metastatic Kaposi's sarcoma to the brain indicates the rarity of this occurrence. The only neoplasm that appears to metastasize to the brain with some frequency is peripheral non-Hodgkin's lymphoma. At autopsy, metastases from non-Hodgkin's lymphoma to the brain is present in approximately 2% of cases (33). However, metastatic spread to the brain from systemic

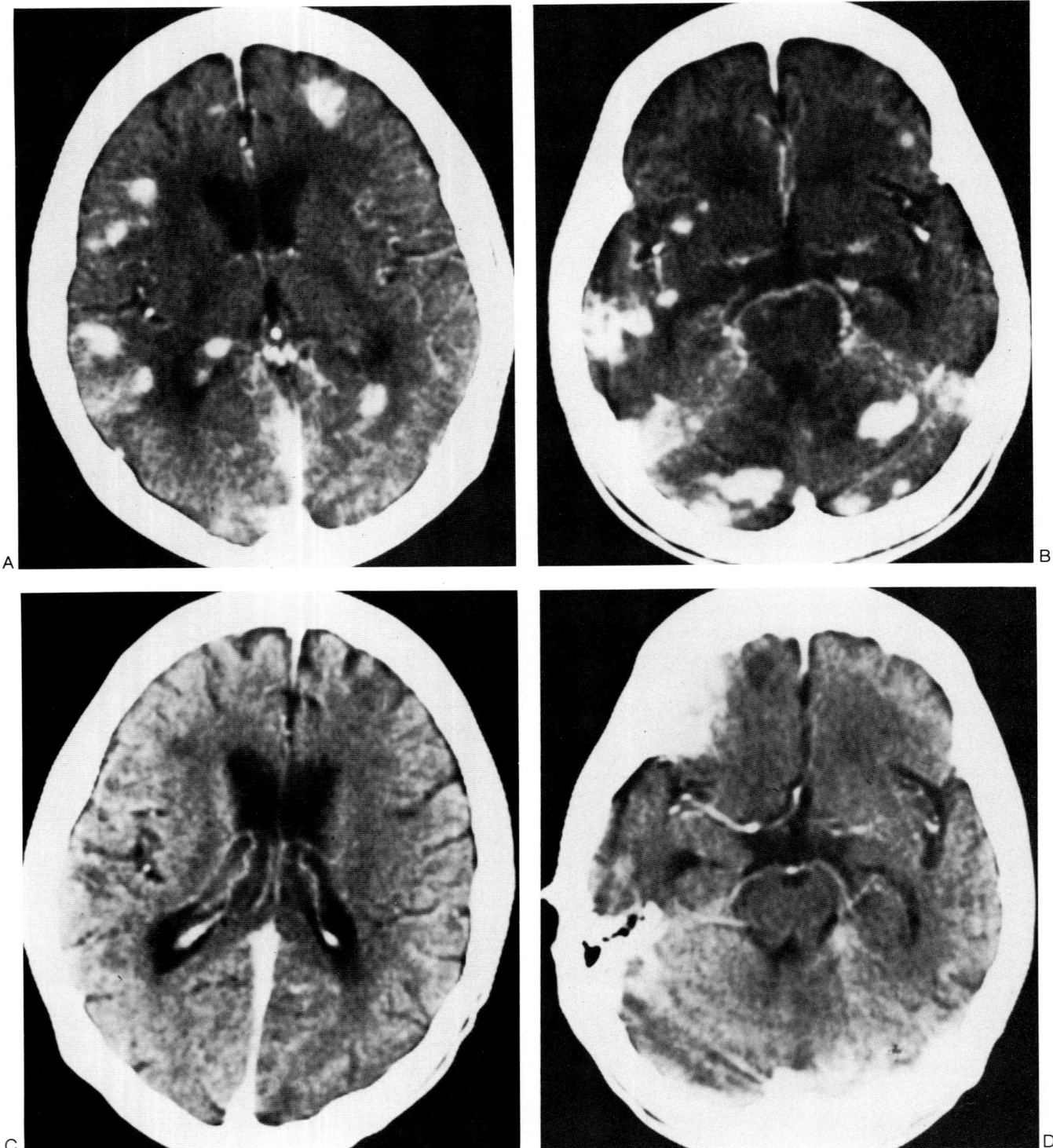

**FIG. 6.** Toxoplasmosis before and after treatment. **A, B:** Contrast-enhanced CT images show multiple enhancing mass lesions scattered throughout the supra- and infratentorial parenchyma. The lesions are not surrounded by significant edema and demonstrate diffuse enhancement. This is an atypical appearance for toxoplasmosis, which usually shows ring enhancement with significant vasogenic edema. However, the patient was treated empirically for toxoplasmosis with sulfadiazine and pyrimethamine. **C, D:** Contrast-enhanced CT scans obtained one month following treatment demonstrate complete resolution of the lesions. The patient's clinical course matched the CT resolution. This case illustrates that it is usually worthwhile giving a trial of antitoxoplasmosis antibiotics even if the CT appearance is atypical.

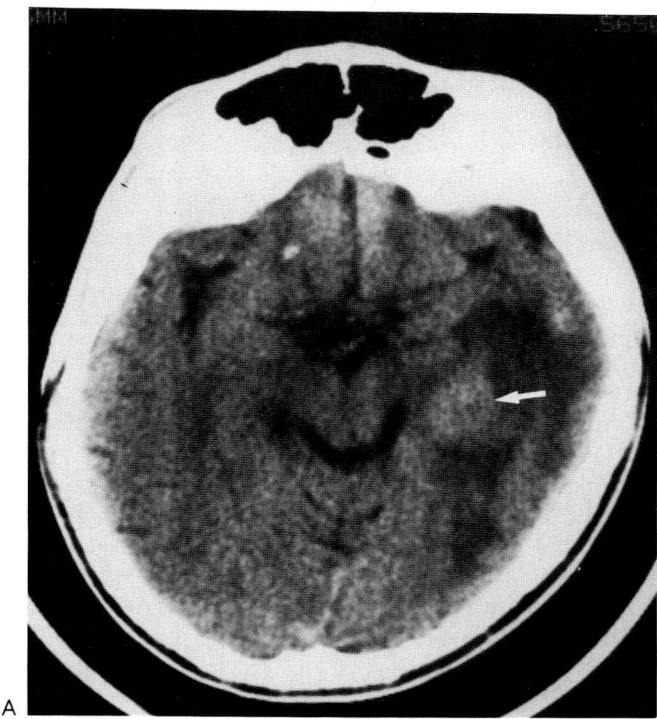 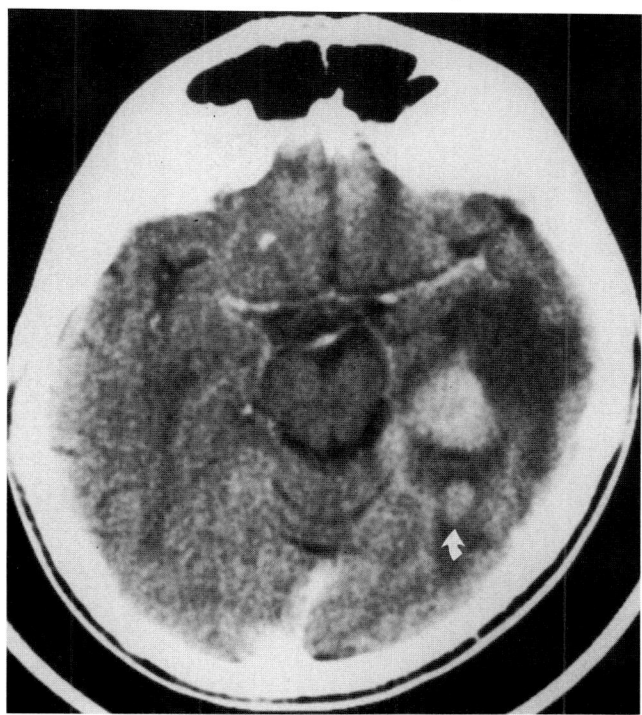

FIG. 7. Primary CNS lymphoma. **A:** A noncontrast CT scan shows a left temporal mass (*arrow*) with surrounding edema. The mass is slightly hyperdense compared to the brain. **B:** Following contrast administration, the mass enhances homogeneously. A second lesion (*curved arrow*) posterior to the larger mass also enhances homogenously. Similar lesions were noted in the right frontal cortex and near the splenium of the corpus callosum on the right. The homogeneous enhancement of these lesions is more typical of lymphoma than toxoplasmosis.

lymphoma usually manifests as leptomeningeal or ependymal disease rather than as mass lesions. The rare case of metastatic carcinoma to the brain may be encountered. We have seen one such case of rectal carcinoma metastatic to the skull base in a patient with AIDS. We also have encountered a patient with AIDS in whom a glioblastoma multiforme developed. Again, these occurrences are rare, and it is worth reiterating that intracranial mass lesions in AIDS are likely to represent either toxoplasmosis or primary CNS lymphoma.

Vascular events may be included in the differential diagnosis of mass lesions in patients with AIDS. Infarcts and hemorrhages are not infrequent at autopsy but usually are not apparent clinically (2). Infarcts may be secondary to vascular occlusion from disseminated intravascular coagulopathy and from emboli from endocarditis. Meningovascular syphilis is another cause of infarcts in AIDS patients. This form of neurosyphilis appears with increased frequency in HIV-infected patients (16). It also occurs sooner after initial infection in AIDS patients (months) than the general population (5 to 12 years). CT or MR will show multiple small or large vessel infarcts (14), whereas angiography will demonstrate narrowing or occlusion of major intracerebral vessels. Herpes zoster encephalitis and meningitis from cryptococcus or tuberculosis also may rarely cause cerebral infarction. Hemorrhage occurs and may be related to the thrombocytopenia that is frequently seen in patients with AIDS (21). The clinical presentation and imaging characteristics of infarcts and hemorrhages usually are distinguishable from mass lesions.

## WHITE MATTER DISEASE

White matter disease in patients with AIDS is common, although it is often seen only at autopsy. Most often, white matter lesions are caused by viral infections. The most common virus to cause white matter disease is probably the AIDS virus (HIV) itself (29,33). Other agents that attack the white matter include CMV, papova virus (the agent that causes progressive multifocal leukoencephalopathy), varicella zoster, and herpes simplex. Nonspecific white matter changes of uncertain etiology also are frequently seen at autopsy (2,33). Patchy or diffuse white matter changes of ischemic encephalopathy are sometimes found at autopsy in patients with severe hypoxia from opportunistic pneumonia (2). White matter lesions frequently are seen with neuroimaging studies of AIDS patients. MR is much more sensitive to abnormalities of white matter than CT. We have observed white matter changes in approximately 30% of

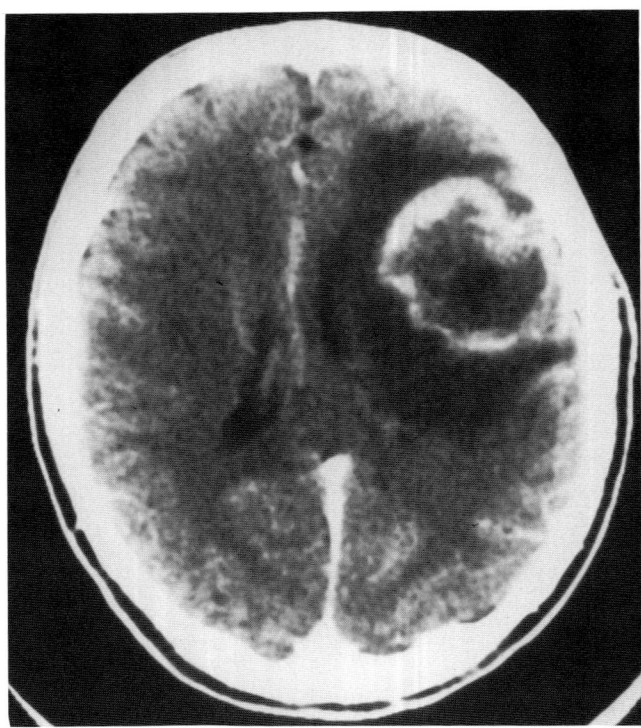

**FIG. 8.** Primary CNS lymphoma. This contrast-enhanced CT scan shows a ring-enhancing mass in the left frontal area with marked surrounding vasogenic edema. There is central low density within the mass. This was the only mass lesion identified. The patient was biopsied and primary CNS lymphoma was found. This appearance, which is similar to toxoplasmosis, is seen in approximately 30% of primary CNS lymphoma lesions in AIDS patients.

AIDS patients imaged with MR. In most cases, the cause of the white matter disease is probably the result of HIV encephalitis or nonspecific encephalitis of unknown cause.

As described previously, HIV is a neurotropic virus. Pathologically, HIV encephalitis is diagnosed by the presence of multinucleated giant cells that are usually found in the white matter of the cerebral and cerebellar hemispheres (29). HIV particles have been demonstrated within these multinucleated cells on electron microscopy (33). Associated histologic abnormalities in the white matter include diffuse or focal areas of demyelination, focal inflammation containing macrophage infiltrates, and vacuolation (29,33). Myelin pallor was found in 64 of 70 autopsied patients with ADC studied by Navia et al. (29). There is variability in the degree of white matter involvement but frequently there is diffuse involvement of large irregular areas of the white matter. The centrum semiovale is most severely affected, but internal capsules, brain stem, and cerebellum also may be involved. The subcortical gray matter may show infiltration by macrophages, multinucleated giant cells, and lymphocytes, but there usually is relative sparing of the cerebral cortex (29). At autopsy, these findings occur in approximately 28% of all AIDS patients (33).

There are few reports of the imaging characteristics of HIV encephalitis. The most common finding is that of cortical atrophy as described previously. Two of the 70 patients described by Navia et al. (28) underwent T2-weighted MR examination which showed focal areas of high-signal intensity images in the white matter that were not shown with CT. Because of the prominent white matter involvement on neuropathological examination, it is reasonable to assume that much of the white matter disease seen with MR in patients with AIDS is due to HIV encephalitis. We have imaged several patients shown to have subacute encephalitis with multinucleated cells and no other white matter disease. MR revealed diffuse or patchy areas of increased signal intensity on T2-weighted images in the periventricular white matter (Fig. 11). Abnormalities are sometimes seen in the brain stem, cerebellum, and in the internal capsules. T1-weighted images are much less sensitive to white matter abnormalities and show either a slight decrease in signal intensity or normal signal in the white matter. White matter abnormalities also may be seen by CT, although much less sensitively (Fig. 12). Diffuse low density in the periventricular white matter is a common observation in patients with AIDS and although unproven in most cases, probably is secondary to HIV encephalitis in many patients.

Progressive multifocal leukoencephalopathy (PML) is another viral infection producing white matter disease in patients with AIDS. PML may afflict other immunosuppressed patients, such as patients with cancer or on immunosuppressive medications. The incidence of PML in patients with AIDS ranges from 2 to 7% (2,17,21,33). The disease is caused by a papova virus (the J-C virus). Pathologically, there is demyelination and necrosis of the white matter. Microscopically, oligodendrocytes with eosinophilic viral inclusions are seen (2). The white matter lesions are most prominent in the subcortical areas of the cerebral hemispheres and centrum semiovale. Clinical features correlate with the site of involvement and include mental status changes, visual loss, aphasia, hemiparesis, ataxia, and other focal findings (17). The disease relentlessly progresses to death. The mean time to death following diagnosis is approximately 18 weeks (17). Cytosine arabinoside has antiviral activity against the J-C virus, but there is usually no clinical response to therapy. Radiologically, abnormalities are seen in the white matter without significant mass effect. With CT, focal zones of decreased density in the cerebral white matter that may be single or multiple are seen (Fig. 13). These lesions progress with time to involve enlarging areas of white matter. Any portion of the cerebral hemisphere may be involved, but there is a slight parietoccipital predominance. There is

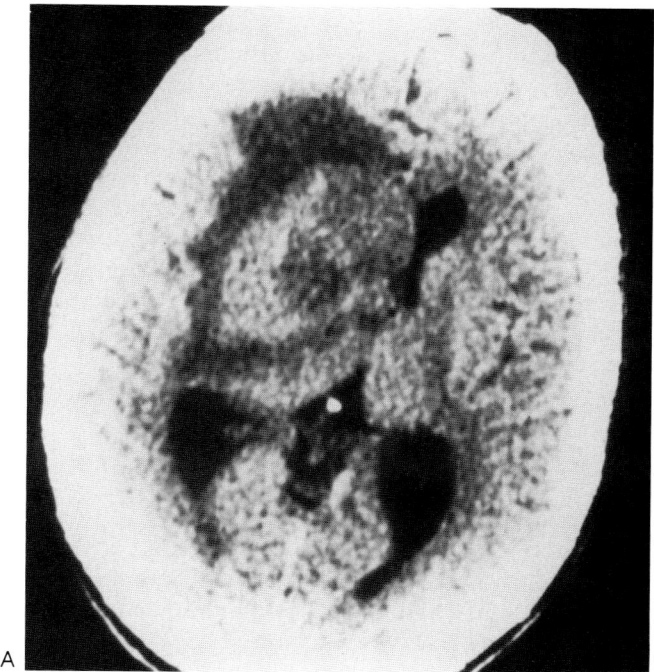 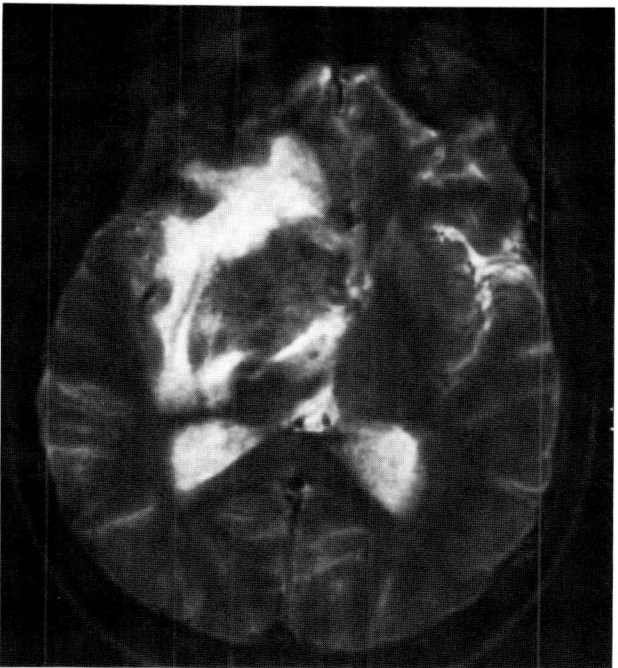

**FIG. 9.** Primary CNS lymphoma. **A:** A noncontrast CT scan shows a large mass in the right basal ganglia with surrounding edema. There is mixed density within the lesion with areas that are iso- and hypodense relative to brain. There is significant compression of the right frontal horn. Intravenous contrast could not be given to this severely ill patient. **B:** T2-weighted MR (SE 2000/70) shows that the mass is isointense with brain parenchyma. The vasogenic edema is of high-signal intensity, similar to CSF in the ventricles. The compact cellular structure of this lymphoma probably accounts for its relatively low-signal intensity. However, lymphoma also may appear hyperintense on T2-weighted images.

usually no mass effect or contrast enhancement (Fig. 14). The CT findings usually underestimate the degree of neurological impairment (17). MR reveals focal areas of increased signal intensity on T2-weighted images in the subcortical white matter and centrum semiovale (Figs. 13, 14). There may be multiple areas of abnormality that are usually asymmetric. MR usually shows more lesions than CT. In our experience, focal white matter lesions on either MR or CT strongly suggest PML, while a diffuse or patchy white matter process is more consistent with HIV encephalitis.

Another cause of white matter disease in patients with AIDS is infection with CMV. Disseminated CMV infection involving the brain and other parts of the body is common in AIDS patients. Pathological evidence of CMV infection of the brain is found in approximately 25% of all AIDS patients (2,33). Multiple glial nodules in the gray and white matter that sometimes contain CMV intranuclear inclusions are the pathological hallmark of CMV encephalitis. However, frank tissue necrosis is rare (33). For this reason, symptomatic CMV infection is probably uncommon and is overshadowed by the subacute encephalitis caused by HIV (30). However, an occasional patient will present with symptoms that are clearly attributable to CMV encephalitis. Gross demyelinative changes have been reported (25). Other changes that may be seen with severe CMV infection include ventriculitis, subependymal necrosis, and myelitis in the spinal cord.

Patients infected with CMV usually have a normal head CT or MR study, or there may be evidence of cortical atrophy (36). This is not surprising since most often the CMV infection is microscopic without gross histological abnormalities. In severe cases, evidence of demyelination may be seen on CT or MR (36). Low-density white matter lesions on CT and high-signal white matter lesions on T2-weighted MR are present that are indistinguishable from other white matter diseases. Abnormal periventricular enhancement also may be seen rarely with CMV infection, as will be discussed below. Unfortunately, there is no treatment proven to be effective for severe CMV encephalitis (21). Vidarabine and several experimental drugs related to acyclovir show some promise (21,30).

Although rare, herpes simplex virus (HSV; I and II) and varicella zoster virus (VZV) infections can cause CNS disease in patients with AIDS. Herpes simplex encephalitis can occur in normal and immunosuppressed

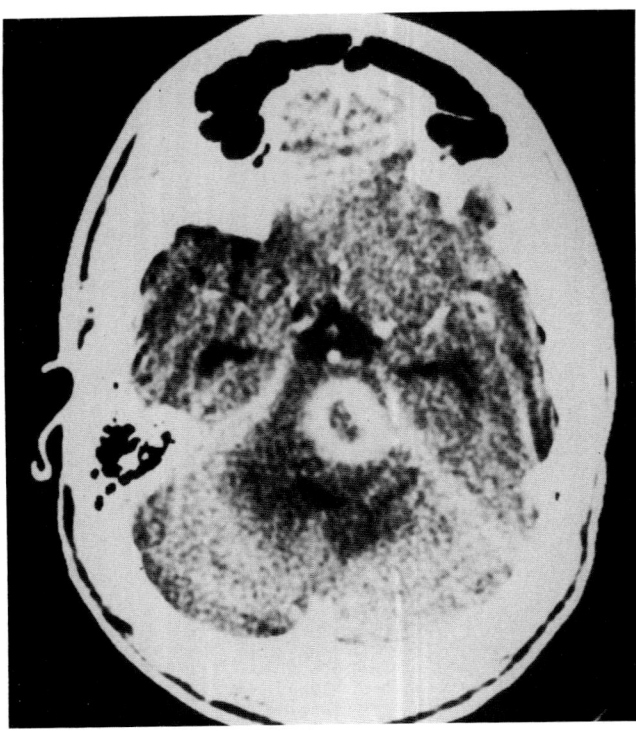

**FIG. 10.** Tuberculoma. A contrast-enhanced CT scan shows a ring-enhancing lesion with surrounding edema in the upper pons. This was the only lesion present. At surgery this proved to represent a tuberculoma with caseous material centrally. Although unusual, CNS tuberculosis sometimes may be seen in AIDS patients who are i.v. drug abusers.

patients. The incidence in patients with AIDS is quite low in most autopsy series (2,26,33). Levy et al. (21) reported eight cases of herpes encephalitis in patients with AIDS or ARC. The two patients with ARC had an acute illness typical of herpes simplex virus encephalitis as is seen in normal patients, except that HSV-II was cultured from the temporal lobes rather than the usual HSV-I. The more immunosuppressed patients with AIDS had an atypical encephalitis with symptoms much milder than usually seen with herpes encephalitis in normal patients. An MR scan in one of these patients showed white matter abnormalities in both frontal lobes, despite a normal CT scan. It is evident that in AIDS and other immunosuppressed patients herpes simplex encephalitis may be a more diffuse process with less severe symptoms and white matter changes on MR imaging.

VZV infection may cause CNS disease in three forms (37): it may cause a multifocal encephalitis affecting primarily white matter; it may cause a vasculitis in the setting of ophthalmic zoster that can lead to infarcts; and it may infect the spinal cord leading to myelopathy. These are very rare occurrences, with most large autopsy series showing the VZV infection in 2% or less of cases (2,33). In the three cases discussed by Petito et al. (33), a multifocal demyelinating encephalitis involving the brain and the spinal cord was found pathologically. The imaging characteristics of VZV encephalitis have not been described. White matter lesions, more effectively demonstrated with T2-weighted MR than with CT, might be expected. With the vasculitis associated with zoster ophthalmicus, infarcts may be seen. Herpes simplex encephalitis and varicella zoster encephalitis can respond to treatment with acyclovir.

## LEPTOMENINGEAL AND EPENDYMAL DISEASE

Although pathologic evidence of disease of the leptomeningeal and ependymal linings is common in patients with AIDS, this usually is not evident on neuroimaging studies. Therefore, leptomeningeal or ependymal disease is the least common neuroimaging pattern in AIDS patients. In general, contrast-enhanced CT is superior to MR in demonstrating leptomeningeal or ependymal disease, as is the case with nonAIDS patients (8). Contrast-enhanced CT may show abnormal enhancement of the leptomeninges, usually at the base of the brain, or of the ependymal lining of the ventricles (Fig. 15).

Meningeal disease can result in communicating hydrocephalus from obstruction of the arachnoid granulations and infarcts from occlusion of arteries at the base of the brain. Hydrocephalus and infarcts can be diagnosed with either CT or MR. Disease of the ependyma can result in increased protein content of the CSF within the ventricles. This will result in increased density of the CSF on CT and increased signal intensity on both T1- and T2-weighted MR images (Fig. 16).

The infectious agents that cause leptomeningeal or ependymal disease in AIDS patients include HIV, CMV, toxoplasmosis, fungi (especially cryptococcus) mycobacteria, and syphilis. HIV is probably responsible for the syndrome of aseptic meningitis that occurs in up to 13% of AIDS patients (21). Pathologically, the majority of AIDS patients show thickening of the meninges felt to be secondary to HIV (33). Clinically, aseptic meningitis presents as headache, fever, and meningeal signs. Cranial nerve findings are common (21). CSF pleocytosis is present and HIV is frequently cultured from the CSF (13,19). The CT and MR scans of patients with aseptic meningitis, however, almost never show abnormalities of the leptomeninges, but there may be atrophy or white matter changes secondary to HIV infection as described above. CMV also can cause inflammation of

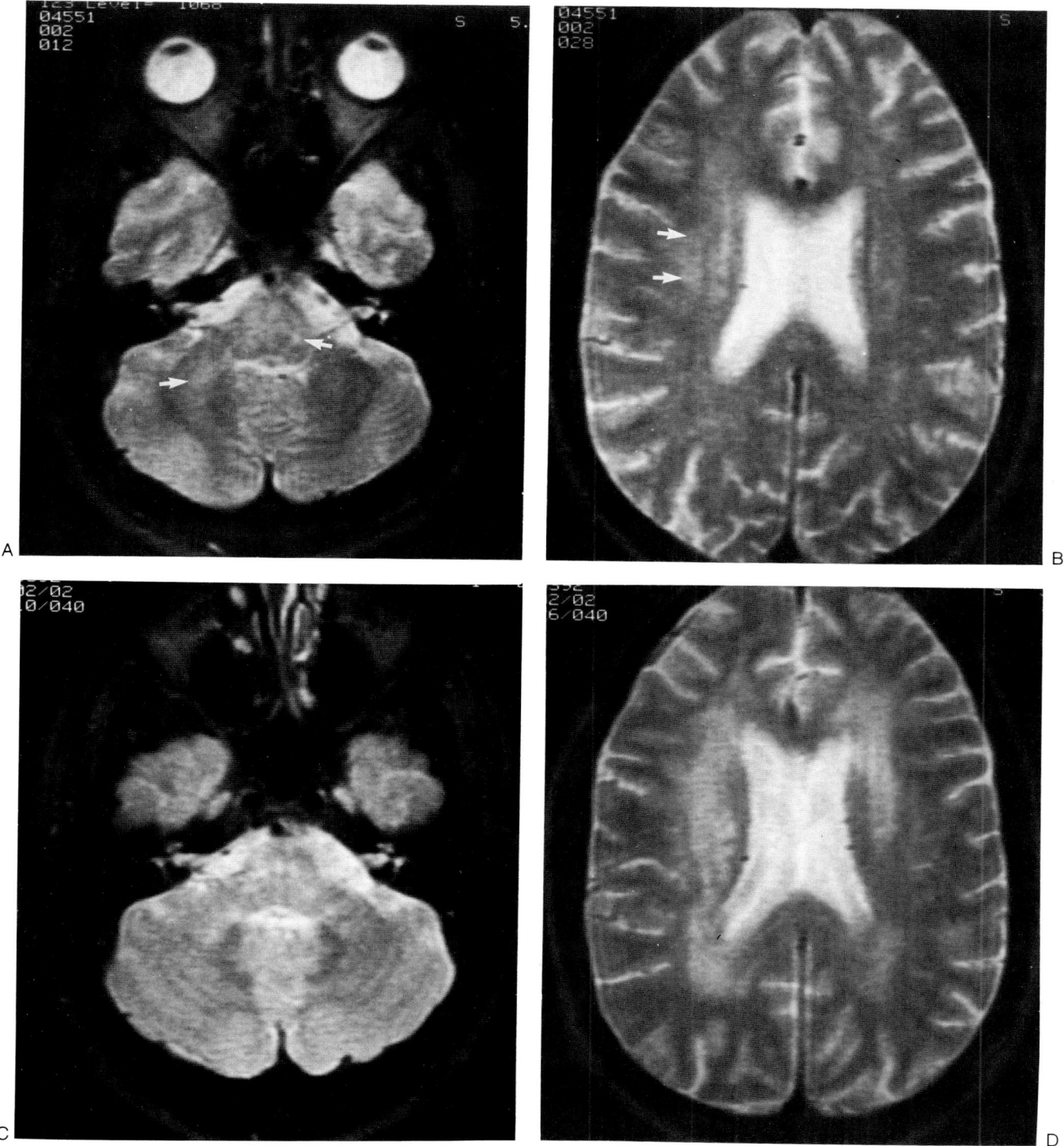

**FIG. 11.** HIV encephalitis. **A, B:** T2-weighted (SE 2000/70) axial MR images at the level of the pons and midlateral ventricles show subtle white matter abnormalities, with areas of high-signal intensity in the pons, right brachium pontis, and the right centrum semiovale (*arrows*). **C, D:** T2-weighted (SE 2000/70) MR images at the same levels corresponding to **A** and **B** were obtained 4 months later. In the interim, the patient underwent progressive deterioration of intellectual function. The lesions in the pons have increased in size and signal intensity. Diffuse bilateral centrum semiovale lesions are now present. This diffuse process is more typical of HIV encephalitis than PML, which is usually focal.

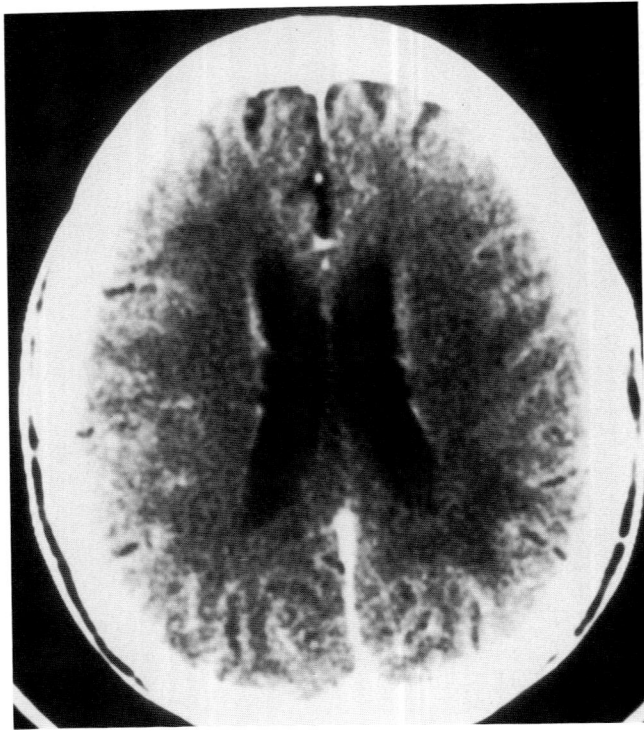

**FIG. 12.** HIV encephalitis. A contrast-enhanced CT scan shows subtle diffuse low density in the periventricular white matter tracts bilaterally. There is slight asymmetry of involvement, with the left occipital area more involved than the right. However, most of the periventricular white matter is abnormal. Mild diffuse atrophy also is present. At autopsy, multinucleated giant cells indicative of HIV infection were found scattered diffusely throughout the brain parenchyma.

the leptomeninges and ependyma. As described above, CMV can cause a ventriculitis and subependymal necrosis. Post et al. (36) described a case of CMV infection that showed marked enhancement of the ependyma that correlated with CMV inclusion bodies in the ependymal cells at autopsy. Toxoplasmosis also may cause ependymitis and ventriculitis which has a similar appearance of abnormal enhancement of the ependymal lining of the ventricle. However, this is an unusual manifestation of toxoplasmosis.

Fungal and mycobacterial infections commonly produce meningitis. Five to 15% of all AIDS patients have pathologic evidence of fungal meningitis (2,21,33). The usual agent is cryptococcus, although histoplasmosis, candida, aspergillus, and coccidioidomycosis also may be encountered. Patients with cryptococcal meningitis present with symptoms similar to immunocompetent patients: headaches, confusion, and meningeal signs. Cryptococcal antigen titers are elevated in the serum and CSF (10). Rarely, focal neurological signs from increased intracranial pressure or infarcts will occur (21). Treatment is with amphothericin B. Neuroimaging studies usually are either normal or show cortical atrophy (43). Abnormal leptomeningeal enhancement, hydrocephalus, or infarcts rarely may be seen.

Mycobacterial infections, including tuberculosis and atypical mycobacteria, can produce meningitis in AIDS patients. As described above, this is relatively rare in most series. Intravenous drug abusers appear to be more at risk for mycobacterial meningitis, and clinical symptoms are similar to those of the other meningitides. Abnormal enhancement of the leptomeninges at the base of the brain may be seen with contrast-enhanced CT (Fig. 15).

The only neoplasm to cause significant leptomeningeal or ependymal disease in AIDS is lymphoma. Peripheral nonHodgkins lymphoma occasionally may metastasize to the CNS, usually to the meninges. This occurs in 1 to 2% of all AIDS patients (2,33). Primary CNS lymphoma also may spread along leptomeningeal or ependymal pathways. Contrast-enhanced CT scans show increased enhancement of the leptomeninges or ependyma that is often nodular or irregular in pattern (Fig. 17). Leukemia and carcinomatous meningitis also may manifest as abnormal leptomeningeal enhancement but these diseases are rare in AIDS patients.

## PEDIATRIC AIDS

AIDS in children is one of the more unfortunate aspects of the AIDS epidemic. Most of these children are born to mothers who are i.v. drug abusers or women who have had bisexual sex partners or were exposed to contaminated blood products (1). Children also may contract AIDS if they themselves receive blood products contaminated with HIV. Neurological symptoms, most prominently a progressive encephalopathy, may be present in these children (38). Longitudinal studies in children with AIDS suggest that there is a childhood equivalent of ADC in adult AIDS patients. Clinically, there is failure to thrive, developmental delay, acquired microcephalus, and long track signs (1). Pathologically, the brains of children with AIDS show varying degrees of low brain weights, inflammatory infiltrates, multinucleated giant cells, and white matter changes similar to the subacute encephalitis pattern caused by HIV in adults. Calcifications in vessel walls and adjacent to vessels also may be seen, especially in the basal ganglia region (38). Intracranial mass lesions have not been reported, but this is not unexpected because there is remarkably little opportunistic infection within the CNS in children with AIDS (39). Older children have a greater chance of acquiring an opportunistic infection

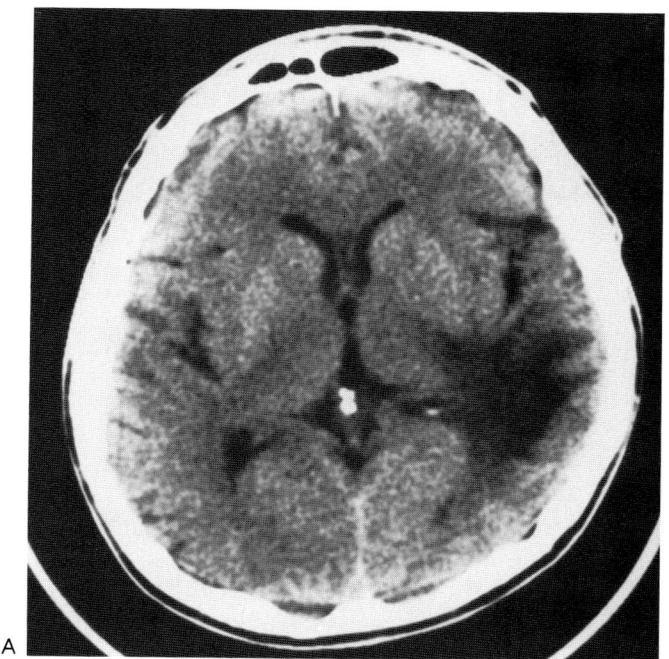
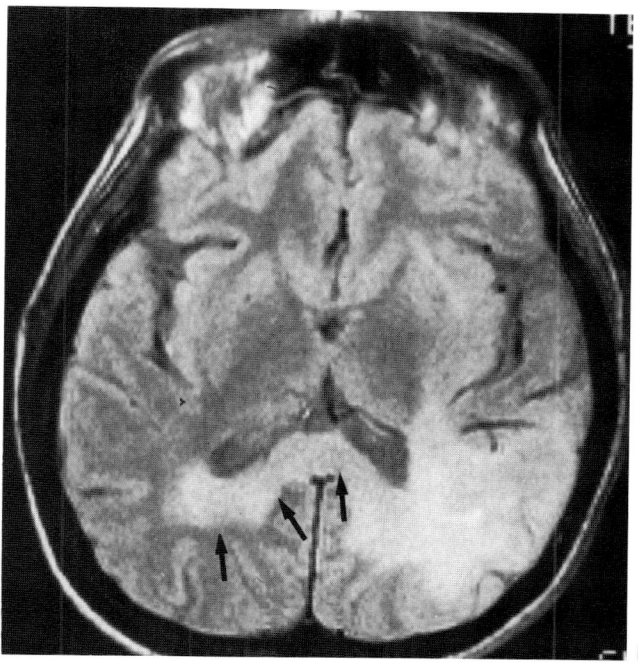

**FIG. 13.** PML. **A:** A noncontrast CT scan shows low density in the left temporal white matter extending to the posterior limb of the left internal capsule. There is no significant mass effect. **B:** T2-weighted (SE 3000/32) MR demonstrates high-signal intensity in the temporo-occipital white matter. There is also high signal in the corpus callosum and right occipital white matter (*arrows*) that was not seen on the CT scan. The asymmetric white matter abnormality without significant mass effect is typical of progressive multifocal leukoencephalopathy, which was proven surgically in this case.

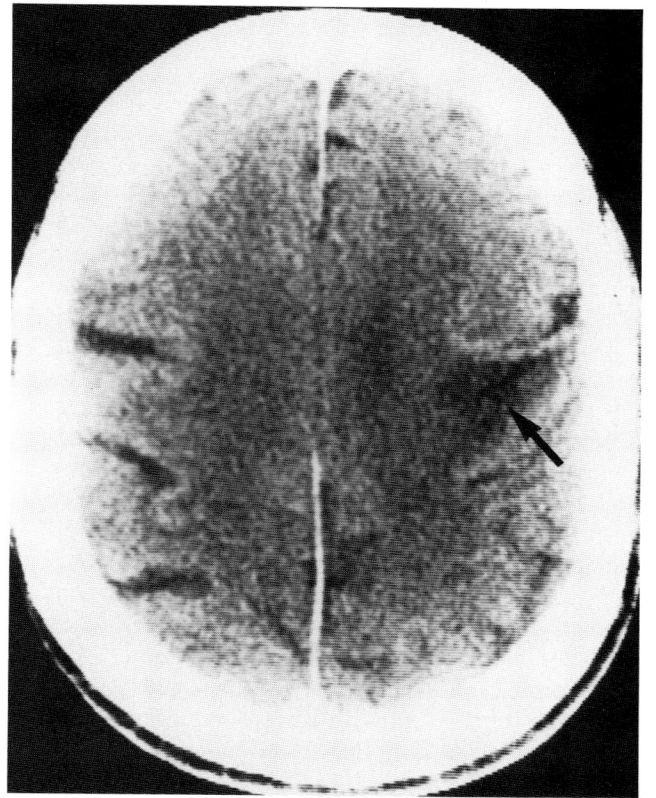
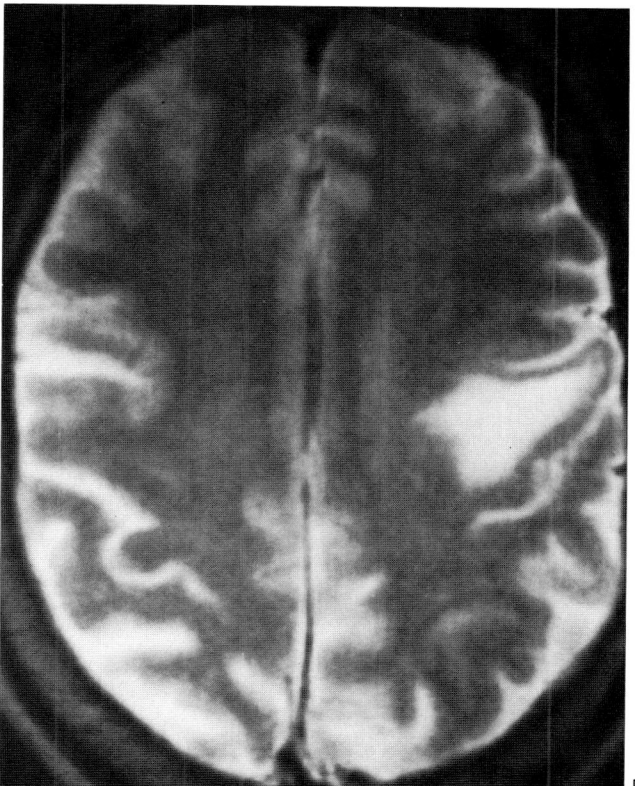

**FIG. 14.** PML. **A:** The contrast-enhanced CT scan shows a focal area of decreased attenuation in the left centrum semiovale (*arrow*) without mass effect or contrast enhancement. The low density extends toward the gray-white junction. **B:** The T2-weighted (SE 2000/70) MR scan shows the white matter abnormality to better advantage. There is high-signal intensity in the involved white matter extending from the centrum semiovale to the gray-white junction. There is no mass effect. At surgery, this proved to be PML.

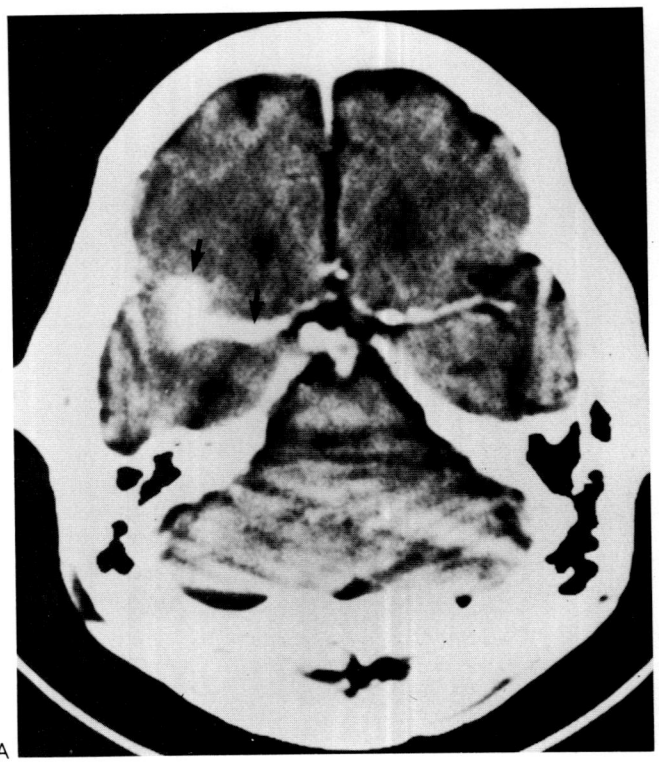 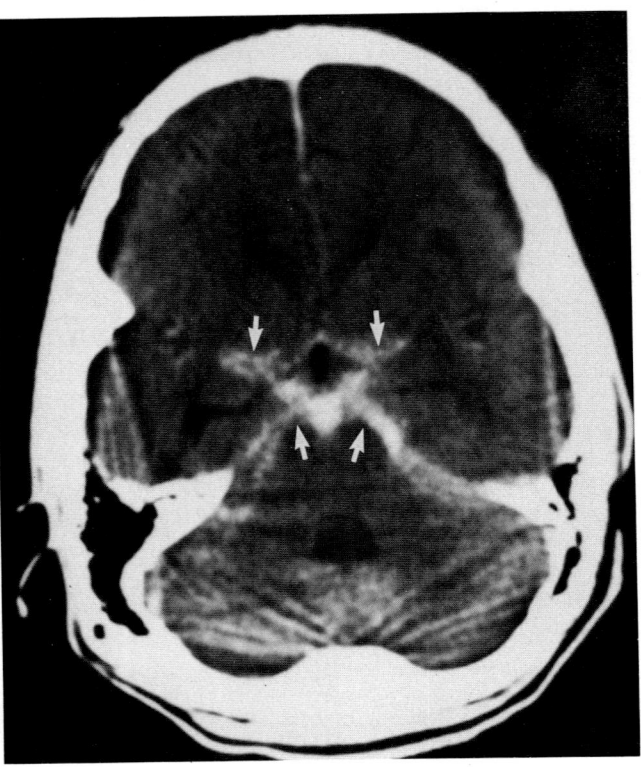

**FIG. 15.** Mycobacterial meningitis. **A, B:** Contrast-enhanced CT scans in two patients show abnormal enhancement in the right sylvian fissure and throughout the basal cisterns (*arrows*). This abnormal meningeal enhancement was secondary to infection with MAI. Tuberculous and other meningitides can have a similar appearance.

(39). CT scans in these patients may be either normal or show cortical atrophy (Fig. 18). Basal ganglia calcifications sometimes may be seen. MR imaging will show the cortical atrophy and possibly white matter changes. MR is much less sensitive to calcification than CT and therefore may not detect basal ganglia calcification.

## MYELOPATHY

The occurrence of myelopathic symptoms in AIDS patients has become, as in other aspects of this disease, another of the initially overlooked but now more obvious components of the total disease. Myelopathy may be caused by cord compression, (usually by metastatic tumors), or by intrinsic cord pathology. The latter is more common. In a study of 89 consecutive patients with AIDS in whom autopsies were performed, Petito et al. (32) found 20 patients with pathologic lesions in the spinal cord. The lesions were characterized by swelling of the myelin sheaths leading to vacuolation similar to that found in subacute combined degeneration. However, serum vitamin $B_{12}$ and folic acid levels were normal in these patients. The clinical findings in these patients correlated with the severity of the vacuolar myelopathy. All five patients with severe myelopathic changes had a progressive spastic-ataxic paraparesis and urinary incontinence that evolved over several weeks to months. The lateral and posterior columns of the thoracic spinal cord were most severely involved. In these 20 patients there was no evidence of infection with HSV, VZV, CMV, or toxoplasma gondii. The etiology of the myelopathy is unclear, but may be the result of direct infection by HIV, which has been cultured from the spinal cord in some patients (13). In other patients, CMV, VZV, and other viruses have been cultured (25,37). Although myelography in these patients usually is normal, CT scans performed after a 12- to 24-hr delay may demonstrate mild to moderate uptake of nonionic contrast agents within the cord (Fig. 19). Presumably, this represents transudation and collection of contrast into areas of vacuolation within the spinal cord, similar to that seen in posttraumatic myelomalacia. T2-weighted MR has promise in demonstrating the cord lesions, since areas of vacuolation should have prolonged T2 compared with normal cord. However, this has not yet been reported.

absent. With axial CT or MR images, abnormal posterior mediastinal tissue that extends into the neuroforamina with relatively little bone destruction strongly suggests the diagnosis of metastatic non-Hodgkin's lymphoma (Fig. 20). Squamous cell carcinomas of the rectum and oronasopharynx also occur with increased frequency in AIDS patients and may metastasize to the spine. Typical findings include destruction of the vertebral body and/or pedicle with an extradural mass compressing the sac and cord. Pyogenic or tuberculous spondylitis appear to be uncommon in patients with AIDS. Myelography, CT, and MR will be expected to show similar findings as in nonAIDS patients.

Peripheral neuropathy accompanying a syndrome of fever, night sweats, and lymphadenopathy has been reported in patients with AIDS (23). Symptoms are primarily a mononeuropathy multiplex, although a distal polyneuropathy also may be seen. Nerve biopsy shows axonal degeneration with segmental demyelination. There are no reported radiological abnormalities in this disorder.

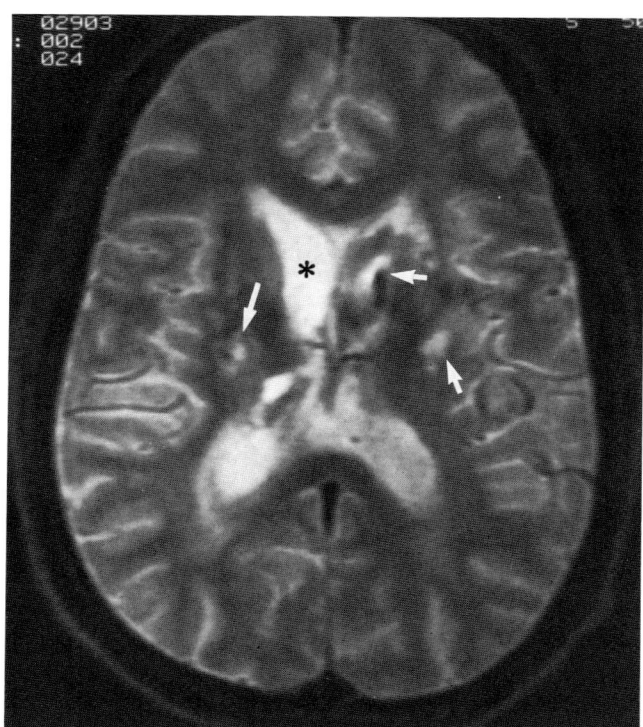

**FIG. 16.** Toxoplasmosis with ventriculitis. The T2-weighted (SE 2000/70) MR study shows multiple lesions of high-signal intensity in the right and left basal ganglia (arrows). There is also significantly increased signal intensity of the CSF in the right lateral ventricle (∗) compared with the left, as well as increased signal intensity surrounding the right lateral ventricle. This patient was status postbiopsy and antibiotic therapy for toxoplasmosis. The basal ganglia lesions are resolving toxoplasma abscesses. The high signal within the right lateral ventricle represents increased protein within the CSF from ventriculitis. Involvement of the ependymal lining of the ventricules is an unusual finding in toxoplasmosis. CMV also may produce this appearance.

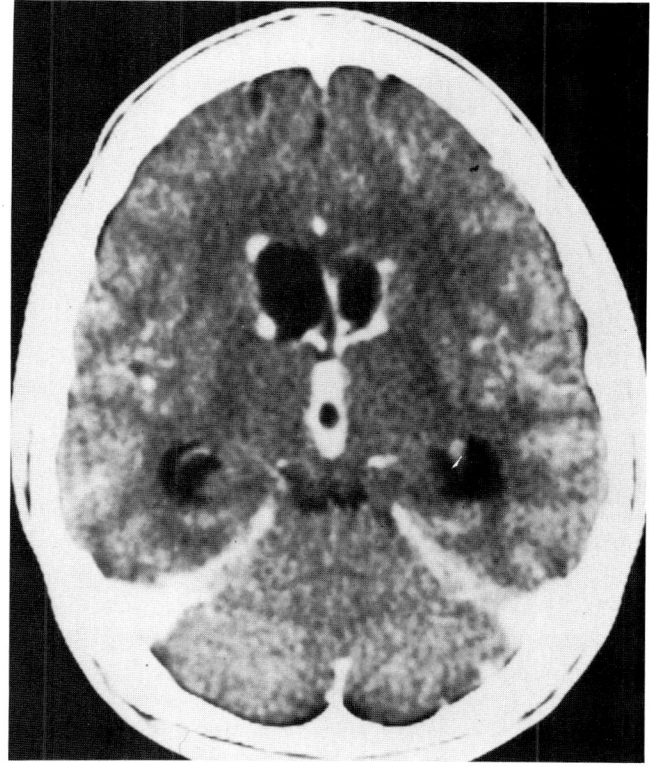

**FIG. 17.** Metastatic non-Hodgkin's lymphoma. The contrast-enhanced CT scan in this patient with non-Hodgkin's lymphoma shows abnormal nodular enhancement around both frontal horns and third ventricle. This represents subependymal spread of lymphoma.

Although less common than intrinsic cord pathology, myelopathy also may be caused by extrinsic compression from epidural tumors or abscesses. In our experience, non-Hodgkin's lymphoma is the most common cause for extrinsic compression of the cord. Lymphoma may metastasize to the vertebra or may extend into the spinal canal via the neuroforamina. Compression of the dural sac and cord may be demonstrated by myelography, intrathecal contrast CT studies, or by MRI. Myelography and intrathecal contrast-enhanced CT studies will show that there is an extradural mass that may cause a complete block to the flow of contrast (Fig. 20). MR may not show that there is a complete block, but the relationship of the tumor to the cord is best shown with this technique. Also, complete block may be inferred if the phase-encoding artifacts on T2-weighted images, that are normally present due to CSF pulsations, are

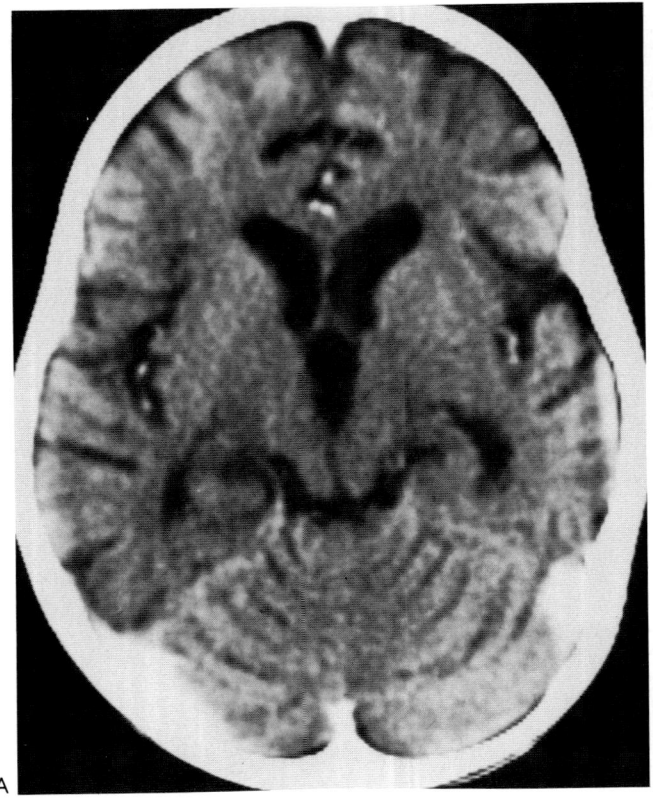 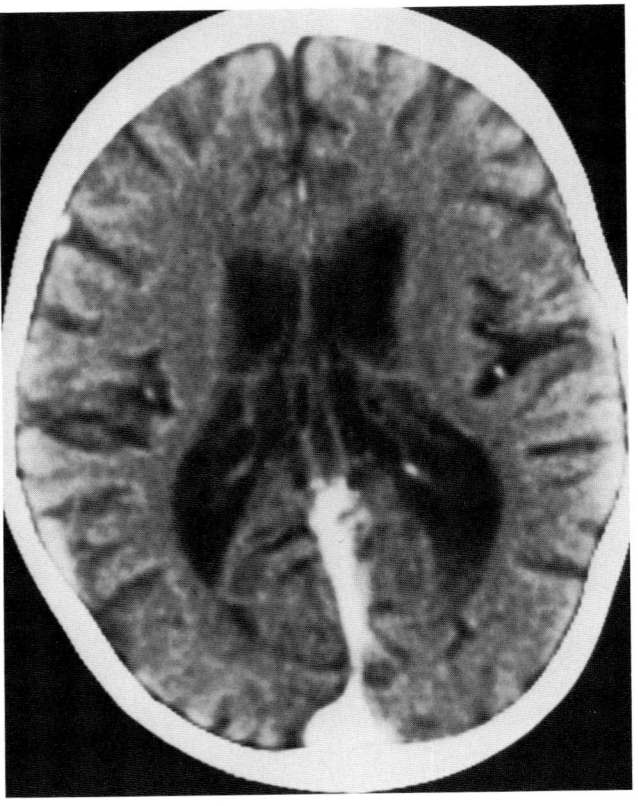

**FIG. 18.** Four-year-old child with AIDS and atrophy. **A, B:** Contrast-enhanced CT images in this 4-year-old AIDS victim with developmental delay show marked enlargement of the ventricles and sulci. No focal lesions are seen. The atrophy is most likely the result of brain infection with HIV.

## HEAD AND NECK DISEASE

Head and neck disease in patients with HIV infection is common: approximately 40% of patients with AIDS have such manifestations on initial evaluation (24). The most common lesions encountered clinically are Kaposi's sarcoma, fungal and viral infections, sinusitis, chronic cough, and rapidly enlarging neck masses. Most of these patients can be adequately evaluated by clinical or laryngoscopic examination. However, a significant number of patients are referred for CT or MR evaluation. Most of these patients have mass lesions that are difficult to evaluate completely by conventional means. In our experience with over 40 patients, three categories of disease are imaged in patients with AIDS or ARC: infections, tumors, and benign lymphoid hyperplasia (31).

A variety of head and neck infections may be encountered in patients with AIDS or ARC. The most common are deep neck infections, caused by bacteria or mycobacteria. We have also seen unusual infections such as pneumocystis of the external auditory canals and rhinosporidium of the nasal cavity. Uncommon bacterial pathogens including Nocardia, Pasteurella, Bacteroides, and Pseudomonas have been cultured. Mycobacterial neck infections may be caused by either tuberculosis or atypical organisms such as mycobacteria avium intracellulare (MAI). Clinically, HIV-infected patients with neck infections respond poorly to antibiotic therapy and frequently require one or more operations to drain the infection adequately. For this reason, early imaging with CT or MR is helpful to the surgeon for preoperative planning. Although there is considerable overlap with the imaging characteristics of tumors, several distinguishing features of infections generally are present. The most important feature of a bacterial neck infection is the presence of overlying cellulitis. This manifests as thickening and infiltration of the overlying subcutaneous fat. With CT, there is thickening and increased density of the subcutaneous fat (Fig. 21). With T2-weighted MR, there is thickening and increased signal intensity within the fat. While there may be a small amount of infiltration of the subcutaneous fat with tumors, there usually is no significant thickening unless there has been radiation treatment. Beneath the cellulitis, the bacterial infection usually is a well-defined mass with a low-density center. However, early in the course

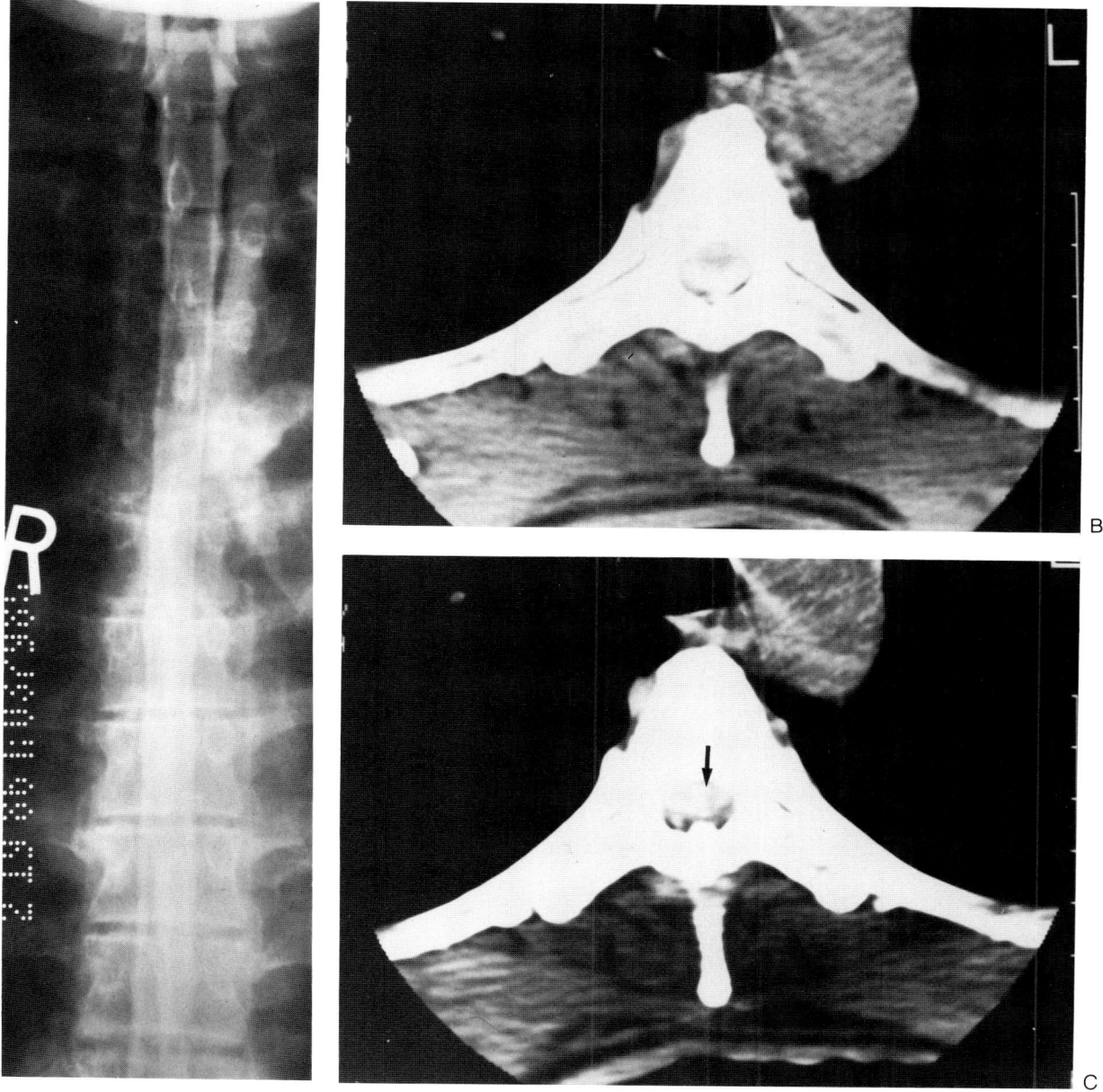

FIG. 19. AIDS myelopathy. A: This patient presented with progressive spastic paraparesis. The AP thoracic myelogram is normal. B: The axial CT scan of T4 was obtained within 2 hours of the myelogram. Although the cord margins are ill-defined, the center of the cord is free of contrast. C: The CT scan obtained 24 hours after the myelogram shows a collection of contrast within the central portion of the cord (arrow). This most likely represents accumulation of contrast within an area of vacuolar myelopathy caused by infection of the cord with the AIDS virus.

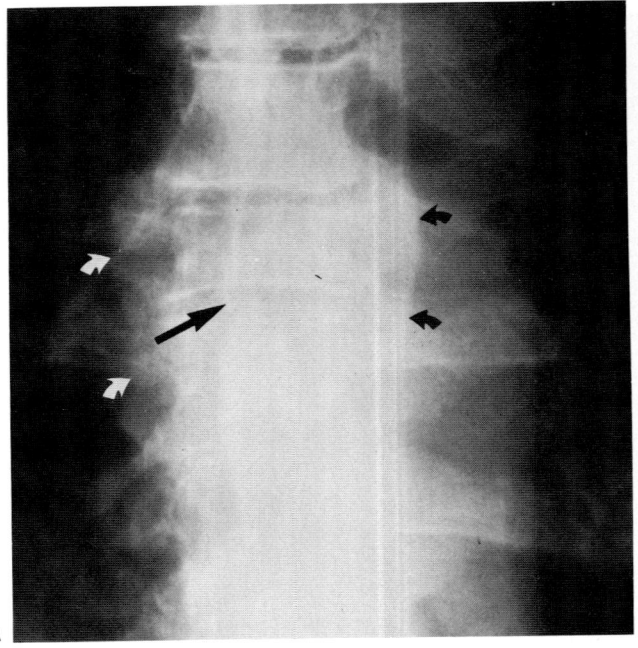
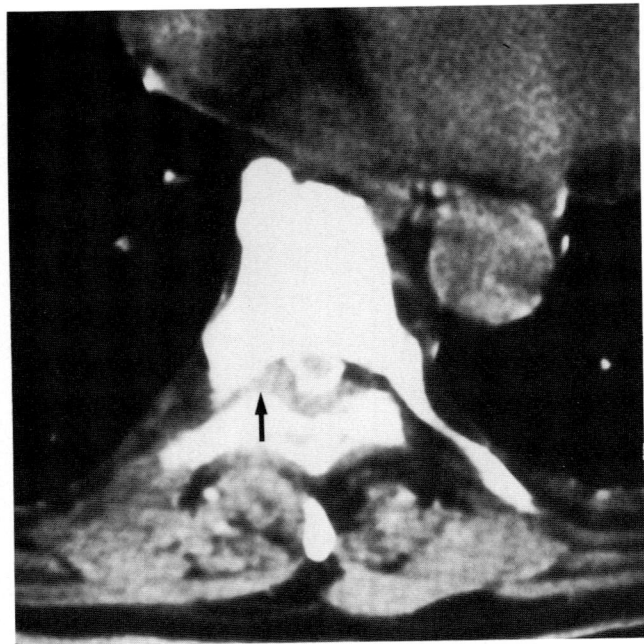
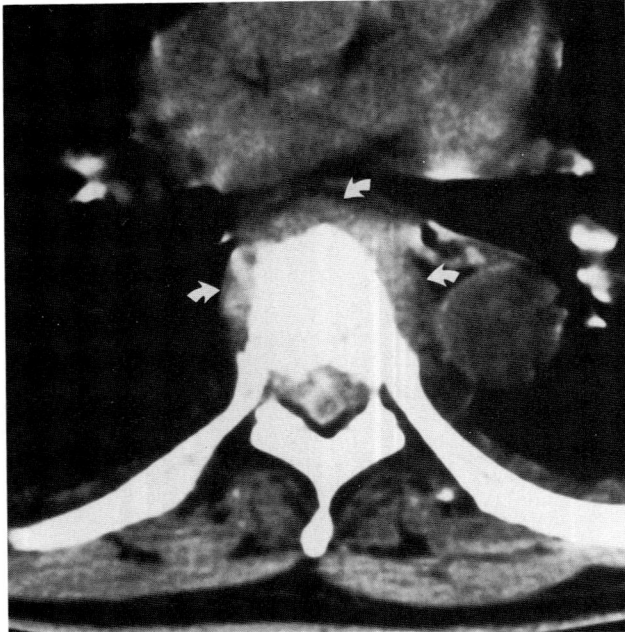

FIG. 20. Non-Hodgkin's lymphoma metastatic to spine. **A:** A PA view of the spine during a lumbar myelogram shows partial collapse of the T7 body. There is complete block to the flow of intrathecal contrast at this level (*straight arrow*). Also note widening of the posterior paraspinal line on the left and posterior mediastinal soft tissue density on the right (*curved arrows*). **B, C:** The CT scan following the myelogram shows abnormal soft tissue material within the spinal canal that surrounds and compresses the sac. The soft tissue material fills the neural foramen on the right (**B;** *arrow*). Also note the soft tissue material anterior to the vertebral body (**C;** *curved arrows*). Diffuse tumor spread that extends through the neural foramina is seen with round cell tumors such as lymphoma, which was proved in this case.

of the infection a phlegmonous ill-defined mass without a low-density center may be present. When lymphadenopathy is present, the nodes usually will not demonstrate low density centrally.

Mycobacterial infections, including infections with MAI, usually differ from bacterial infections in the degree of overlying cellulitis. Mycobacterial neck infections usually are more indolent and therefore elicit less of an inflammatory response, leading to little or no cellulitis on imaging studies. Lymph nodes often are involved with mycobacterial infections. Nodes typically have very low-density centers on CT studies (Fig. 22). Generally, the density is lower than that of nodes involved with tumor.

The most common tumors encountered in the head and neck region of patients with AIDS or ARC are Kaposi's sarcoma and non-Hodgkin's lymphoma (24). There is also a slightly increased incidence of squamous cell carcinomas of the oral and nasopharyngeal areas (40). Kaposi's sarcoma of the head and neck is ex-

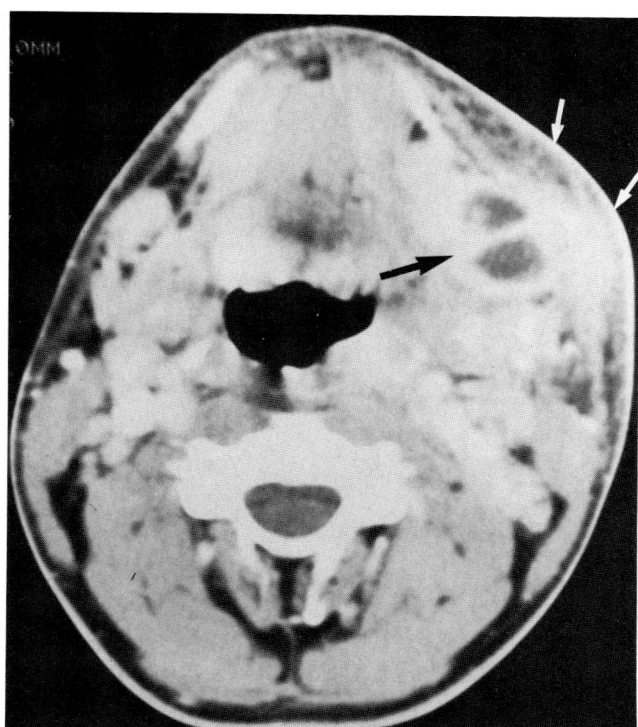

**FIG. 21.** Submandibular space abscess. The contrast-enhanced CT scan shows a mass in the left submandibular space with peripheral enhancement and central low density (*large arrow*). Note the marked thickening and increased density in the adjacent subcutaneous fat (*small arrows*). These findings are typical of a bacterial abscess. Tumors and mycobacterial infections usually do not have this degree of cellulitis. This lesion was surgically drained and Pasteurella (a gram-negative rod) was cultured.

tremely common in AIDS, occurring in 15% of all patients (24). However, usually the lesions involve the cutaneous, oral, or upper pharyngeal areas that can be adequately evaluated by direct inspection or laryngoscopic examination. Occasionally, deep involvement or suspected nodal metastases may lead to radiologic evaluation. Barium pharyngography is usually adequate for demonstrating pharyngeal lesions, showing nodular lesions without ulcerations (9). If metastases to regional lymph nodes are suspected, then CT or MR should be performed. CT will show nodular or polypoid mass lesions of the oral cavity or pharyngeal mucosa. There may be distortion of the vallecula and pyriform sinuses (9). When present, lymph nodes frequently will contain low-density centers (31). There is usually no cellulitis.

Non-Hodgkin's lymphoma of the head and neck region is less common than Kaposi's sarcoma. We have imaged five patients with lymphoma, including two of the nasopharynx, two of the neck, and one of the parotid gland (21). As described elsewhere, non-Hodgkin's lymphoma is increased in incidence in patients infected with HIV. Lymphoma usually presents as large, bulky nodal masses or bulky disease of the nasopharynx. The tumor usually has a homogeneous cellular structure without significant necrosis centrally. With CT, lymphoma is usually of homogeneous density without low-density centers. There may be thin peripheral enhancement. With MR, there is homogeneous signal intensity on both T1- and T2-weighted images (Fig. 23). The tumor usually is of medium-signal intensity on T1-weighted images and of high-signal intensity on T2-weighted images. Lymph node involvement usually does not show necrotic central zones with either CT or MR. There usually is no overlying cellulitis.

Squamous carcinoma in AIDS patients present similarly to patients that are not infected with HIV. Mass lesions with lymph nodes that often have necrotic centers are typical of squamous cell carcinoma. Of interest, we have seen several cases of nasopharyngeal and parotid lymphoepitheliomas in AIDS patients. Lymphoepitheliomas are squamous cell carcinomas that are frequently associated with the Epstein-Barr virus infection.

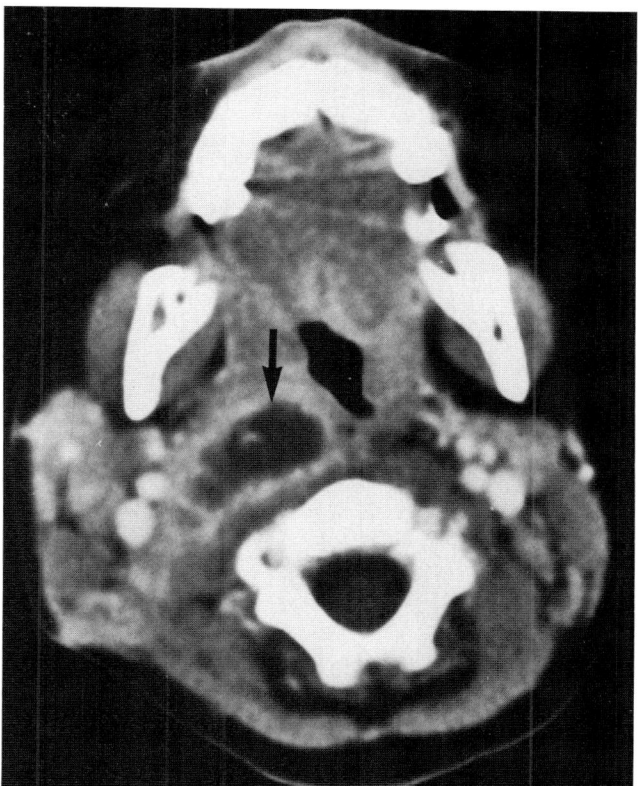

**FIG. 22.** MAI. The contrast-enhanced CT scan shows a large oropharyngeal mass with an enhancing rim and low-density center (*arrow*). The striking low density within the mass is characteristic of mycobacterial infections. Although pyogenic infections and squamous cell nodal metastasis can have low-density centers from necrosis, these are not usually of such low density as in this case.

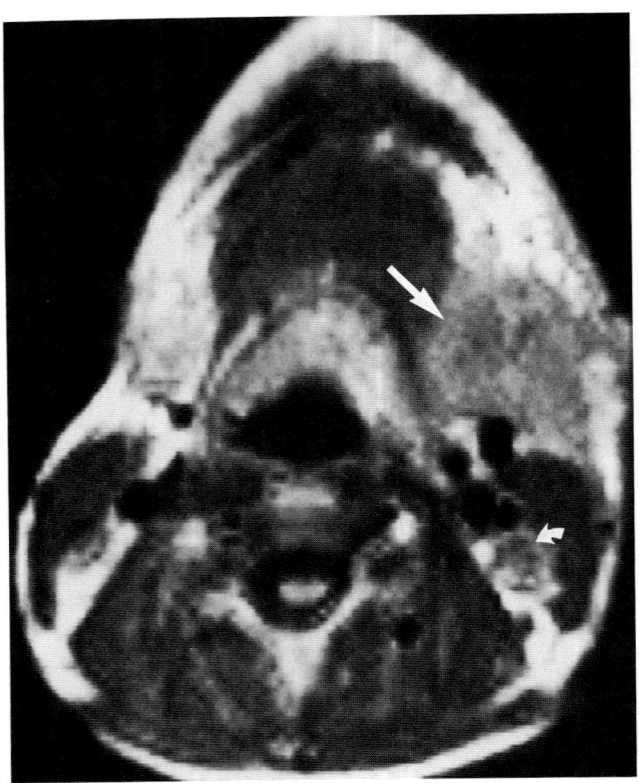 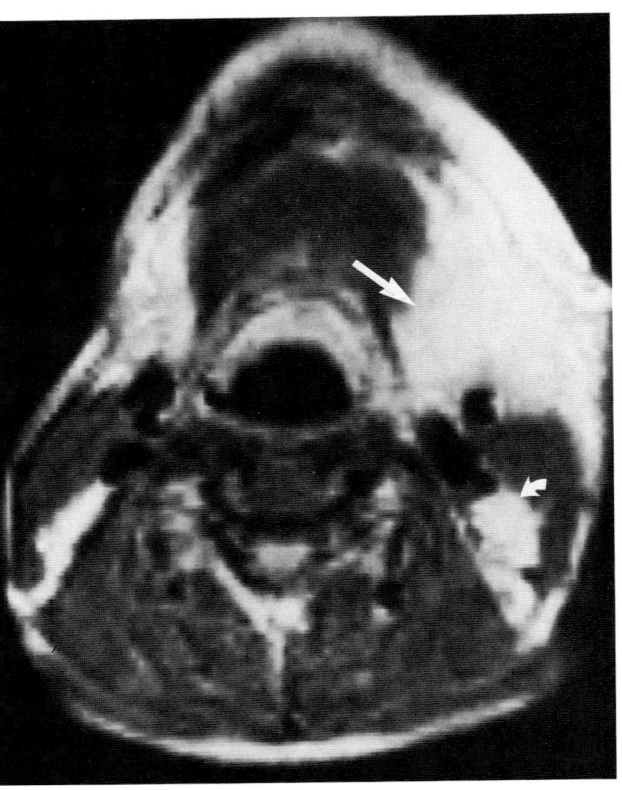

**FIG. 23.** Non-Hodgkin's lymphoma of the neck. **A, B:** T1-weighted (SE 500/30) and T2-weighted (SE 2000/60) MR images reveal a left submandibular mass (*straight arrow*) and a posterior triangular lymph node (*curved arrows*) on the left. On the T1-weighted image (**A**) the mass and node are intermediate in signal between muscle and fat. On the T2-weighted image (**B**) the lesions are of high-signal intensity. The homogeneous signal intensity on both **A** and **B** are typical of lymphomas.

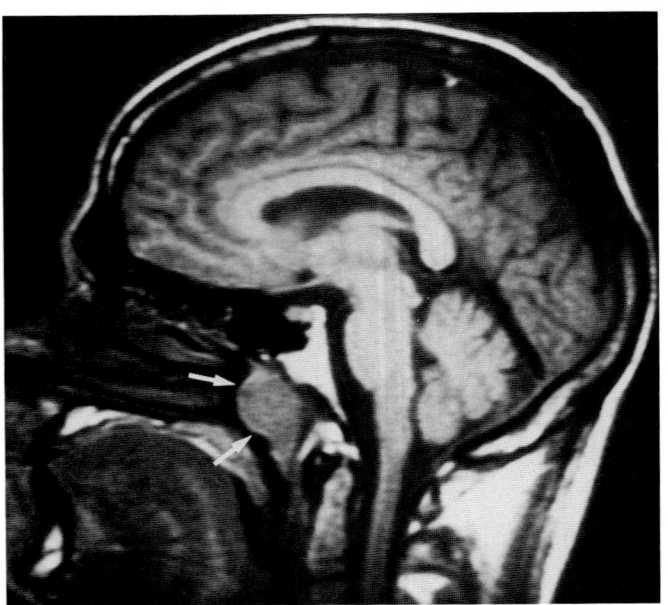 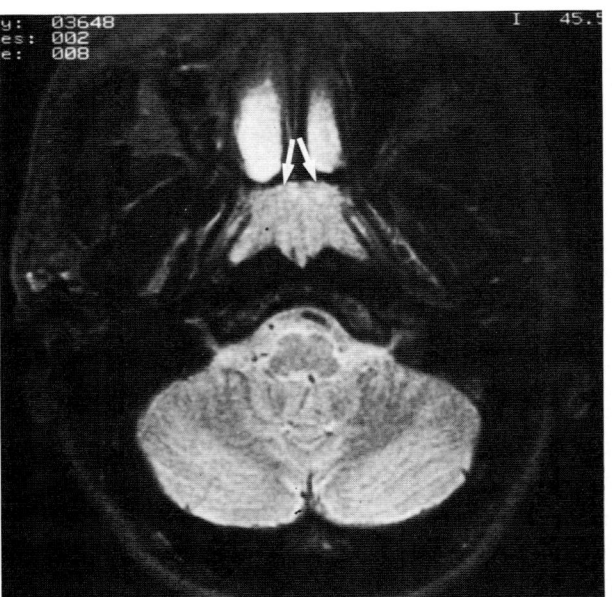

**FIG. 24.** Benign adenoidal enlargement. **A, B:** T1-weighted (PS 600/20) MR (**A**) shows smooth enlargement of the adenoids (*arrows*). The nasopharyngeal airway appears narrowed by the mass. The T2-weighted (SE 2000/60) axial MR (**B**) shows increased signal intensity within the adenoidal tissue. The anterior margin of the adenoidal mass is smooth and flat (*arrows*). These findings are typical of benign adenoidal enlargement. This patient was operated on because of nasal obstruction. Pathology revealed benign lymphoid hyperplasia with no evidence of tumor.

Lymph node enlargement in patients with HIV infection is common, and is a prominent feature of the ARC syndrome. Benign lymph node enlargement is therefore commonly encountered in the head and neck region in patients with AIDS. Also commonly seen is enlargement of the adenoids and tonsillar tissue. The main clinical significance of benign lymphoid tissue enlargement is in distinguishing this from neoplasms. Usually this can be done on physical examination. However, in a patient with a known malignancy, enlarged lymph nodes may be problematic. Also, adenoidal enlargement may become so severe that nasopharyngeal obstruction may result, simulating a tumor. For these reasons, imaging studies may be ordered to evaluate patients with lymph node or adenoidal enlargement.

Benign adenoidal enlargement usually has a very smooth anterior border, best seen with T1-weighted sagittal MR (Fig. 24). On T2-weighted images, there usually is moderately increased signal intensity, greater than muscle but less than CSF. Although the anterior margin is usually flat on both CT and MR images in the axial plane, bulky asymmetric lesions indistinguishable from tumor are occasionally seen (Figs. 25 and 26). Tonsillar

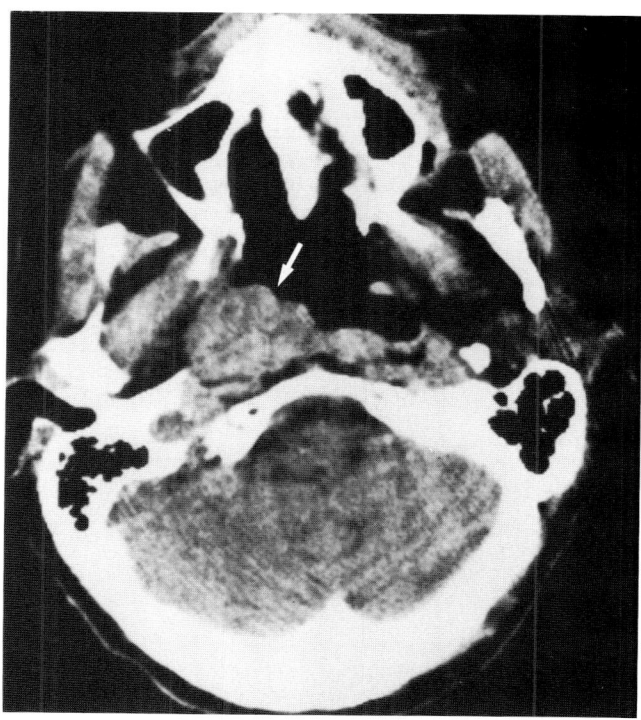

**FIG. 26.** Nasopharyngeal lymphoma. This scan is similar to that of Fig. 25 because there is asymmetric enlargement of the right side of the nasopharynx (*arrow*). However, unlike the prior case, at surgery this lesion proved to be non-Hodgkin's lymphoma.

enlargement usually is symmetrical, with increased signal intensity on T2-weighted MR images. CT images may show fullness in the tonsillar areas but the findings are less striking than with MR. Benign lymph node enlargement is also better detected with MR. Nodes are of high-signal intensity on T2-weighted imaging, and usually are homogeneous. With CT, the lymph nodes usually are homogeneous in density and do not have a central zone of low density. The nodes in benign lymphoid hyperplasia are generally less than 2 cm.

Finally, sinus disease is extremely common in patients with AIDS. This is usually an incidental finding on head imaging studies. Although the true incidence of sinusitis in patients with AIDS is unknown, at least 30% of the head CT scans at our institutions show evidence of sinus mucosal abnormalities. In addition to the usual organisms encountered in nonAIDS patients, AIDS victims may have sinus infections with unusual organisms. We have seen mycobacterial and fungal sinus infections. These were indistinguishable from more routine sinus infections with CT.

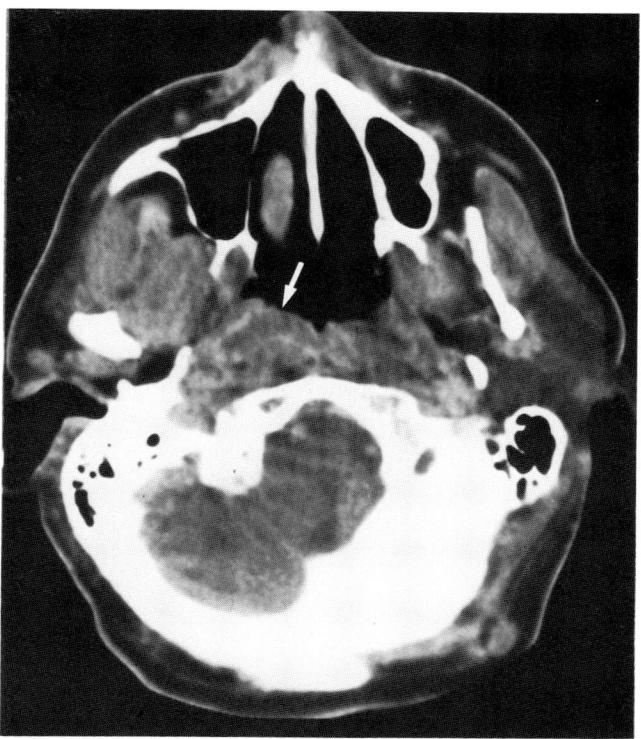

**FIG. 25.** Benign adenoid enlargement. This contrast-enhanced CT scan at the level of the nasopharynx shows asymmetric enlargement of the right side of the nasopharynx (*arrow*) that does not have a smooth flat anterior border. A tumor was suspected and the mass was biopsied. However, the biopsy revealed benign lymphoid hyperplasia with no evidence of neoplasm. Although unusual, benign adenoidal hypertrophy can simulate neoplastic disease.

## REFERENCES

1. Amman, A. (1985): The acquired immunodeficiency syndrome in infants and children. *Ann. Intern. Med.,* 103:734–735.

2. Anders, K. H., Guerra W. F., Tomiyasu, U., Verity, M. A., and Vinters, H. V. (1986): The neuropathology of AIDS. UCLA experience and review. *Am. J. Pathol.*, 124:537–558.
3. Barnes, D. M. (1987): Brain damage by AIDS under active study. *Science*, 235:1574–1577.
4. Bishburg, E., Sunderam, G., Reichman, L. B., and Kapila, R. (1986): Central nervous system tuberculosis with the acquired immunodeficiency syndrome and its related complex. *Ann. Intern. Med.*, 105:210–213.
5. Black, P. H. (1985): HTLV-III, AIDS, and the brain. *N. Engl. J. Med.*, 313:1538–1540.
6. Cohen, W., and Koslow, M. (1985): An unusual CT presentation of cerebral toxoplasmosis. *J. Comput. Assist. Tomogr.*, 9:384–386.
7. Cohn, J., McMeeking, A., Cohen, W., Jacobs, J., and Holzman, R. (1987): Response and survival in patients treated for presumed versus proven CNS toxoplasmosis. Presented at the Third International Conference on Acquired Immunodeficiency Syndrome (AIDS). Washington, D.C.
8. Davis, P. C., Friedman, N. C., Fry, S. M., Malko, J. A., Hoffman, J. C., Braun, I. F. (1987): Leptomeningeal metastases: MR imaging. *Radiology*, 163:449–454.
9. Emery, C. D., Wall S. D., Federle, M. P., and Sooy, C. D. (1986): Pharyngeal Kaposi's sarcoma in patients with AIDS. *A.J.R.*, 147:919–922.
10. Eng, R. H., Bishburg, E., Smith, S. M., and Kapila, R. (1986): Cryptococcal infections in patients with acquired immune deficiency syndrome. *Am. J. Med.*, 81:19–23.
11. Gabuzda, D. H., Ho, D. D., de la Monte, S. M., Hirsch, M. S. et al. (1986): Immunohistochemical identification of HTLV-III antigen in brains of patients with AIDS. *Ann. Neurol.*, 20:289–294.
12. Gartner, S., Markovits, P., Markovitz, D. M., Betts, R. F., et al. (1986): Virus isolation from and identification of HTLV/LAV producing cells in brain tissue in a patient with AIDS. *J.A.M.A.*, 256:2365–2371.
13. Ho, D. D., Rota, T. R., Schooley, R. T., et al. (1985): Isolation of HTLV-III from cerebrospinal fluid and neural tissues of patients with neurologic syndromes related to the acquired immunodeficiency syndrome. *N. Engl. J. Med.*, 313:1493–1497.
14. Holland, B. A., Perrett, L. V., and Mills, C. M. (1986): Meningovascular syphilis: CT and MR findings. *Radiology*, 158:439–442.
15. Jack, C. R., Jr., Reese, D. F., and Scheithauer, B. W. (1986): Radiographic findings in 32 cases of primary CNS lymphoma. *A.J.R.*, 146:271–276.
16. Johns, O. R., Tierney, M., Felsenstein, D. (1987): Alteration in the natural history of neurosyphilis by concurrent infection with the human immunodeficiency virus. *N. Engl. J. Med.*, 316:1569–1572.
17. Krupp, L. B., Lipton, R. B., Swerdlow, M. L., Leeds, N. E., and Llena, J. (1985): Progressive multifocal leukoencephalopathy: Clinical and radiographic features. *Ann. Neurol.*, 87:344–349.
18. Lee, Y. Y., Bruner, J. M., Van Tassel, P., and Libshitz, H. I. (1986): Primary central nervous system lymphoma: CT and pathologic correlation. *A.J.R.*, 147:747–752.
19. Levy, J. A., Shimabukuro, J., Hollander, H., Mills, J., and Kaminsky, L. (1985): Isolation of AIDS-associated retrovirus from cerebrospinal fluid and brain of patients with neurological symptoms. *Lancet*, 2:586–588.
20. Levy, R. M., Pons, V. G., and Rosenblum, M. L. (1984): Central nervous system mass lesions in the acquired immunodeficiency syndrome (AIDS). *J. Neurosurg.*, 61:9–16.
21. Levy, R. M., Bredesen, D. E., and Rosenblum, M. L. (1985): Neurological manifestations of the acquired immunodeficiency syndrome (AIDS): Experience at UCSF and review of the literature. *J. Neurosurg.*, 62:475–495.
22. Levy, R. M., Rosenbloom, S., and Perrett, L. V. (1986): Neuroradiologic findings in AIDS: A review of 200 cases. *A.J.R.*, 147:977–983.
23. Lipkin, W. I., Parry, G., Kiprov, D., Abrams, D. (1985): Inflammatory neuropathy in homosexual men with lymphadenopathy. *Neurology*, 35:1479–1483.
24. Marcusen, D. C., Sooy, C. D. (1985): Otolaryngologic and head and neck manifestations of acquired immunodeficiency syndrome (AIDS). *Laryngoscope*, 95:401–405.
25. Moskowitz, L. B., Gregorios, J. B., Hensley, G. T., and Berger, J. R. (1984): Cytomegalovirus. Induced demyelination associated with acquired immune deficiency syndrome. *Arch. Pathol. Lab. Med.*, 108:873–877.
26. Moskowitz, L. B., Hensley, G. T., Chan, J. C., Gregorios, J., and Conley, F. K. (1984): The neuropathology of acquired immune deficiency syndrome. *Arch. Pathol. Lab. Med.*, 108:867–872.
27. Navia, B. A., Petito, C. K., Gold, J. W. M., Cho, E.-S., Jordan, B. D., and Price, R. W. (1986): Cerebral toxoplasmosis complicating the acquired immune deficiency syndrome: Clinical and neuropathological findings in 27 patients. *Ann. Neurol.*, 19:224–238.
28. Navia, B. A., Jordan, B. D., and Price R. W. (1986): The AIDS dementia complex: I. Clinical features. *Ann. Neurol.*, 19:517–524.
29. Navia, B. A., Cho, E.-S., Petito, C. K., and Price, R. W. (1986): The AIDS dementia complex: II. Neuropathology. *Ann. Neurol.*, 19:525–535.
30. Navia, B. A., and Price R. W. (1986): Central and peripheral nervous system complications of AIDS. *Clin. Immunol. Allergy*, 6:543–557.
31. Olsen, W. L., Dillon, W. P., Lynch, M. A., and Sooy, C. D. (1987): CT and MR of head and neck pathology in patients with AIDS or ARC. Presented at the 25th American Society of Neuroradiology Meeting, New York.
32. Petito, C. L., Navia, B. A., Cho, E.-S., Jordan, B. D., George, D. C., and Price, R. W. (1985): Vacuolar myelopathy pathologically resembling subacute combined degeneration in patients with the acquired immunodeficiency syndrome. *N. Engl. J. Med.*, 312:874–879.
33. Petito, C. L., Cho, E.-S., Lemann, W., Navia, B. A., and Price, R. W. (1986): Neuropathology of acquired immunodeficiency syndrome (AIDS): An autopsy review. *J. Neuropathol. Exp. Neurol.*, 45:635–646.
34. Post, M. J. D., Kursunoglu, S. J., Hensley, G. T., Chan, J. C., Moskowitz, L. B. and Hoffman, T. A. (1985): Cranial CT in acquired immunodeficiency syndrome: Spectrum of diseases and optimal contrast enhancement technique. *A. J. R.*, 145:929–940.
35. Post, M. J. D., Sheldon, J. J., Hensley, G. T., et al. (1986): Central nervous system disease in acquired immunodeficiency syndrome: Prospective correlation using CT, MR imaging and pathologic studies. *Radiology*, 158:141–148.
36. Post, M. J. D., Hensley, G. T., Moskowitz, L. B., Fischl, M. (1986): Cytomegalic inclusion virus encephalitis in patients with AIDS: CT, clinical, and pathological correlation. *A. J. R.*, 146:1229–1234.
37. Ryder, J. W., Croen, K., Kleinschmidt-DeMasters, B. K., Ostrove, J. M., Strauss, S. E., and Cohn, D. L. (1986): Progressive dementia encephalitis three months after resolution of cutaneous zoster in a patient with AIDS. *Ann. Neurol.*, 19:182–188.
38. Sharer, L. R., Epstein, L. G., Cho, E.-S., et al. (1986): Pathologic features of AIDS encephalopathy in children: Evidence for LAV/HTLV-III infection of brain. *Hum. Pathol.*, 17:271–284.
39. Shaw, G. M., Harper, M. E., Hahn, B. H., Epstein, L. G., and Gajdusek, D. C. (1985): HTLV-II infection in brains of children and adults with AIDS encephalopathy. *Science*, 227:177–182.
40. Silverman, S., Migliorati, C. A., Lozada-Nur, F., Greenspan, D., and Conant, M. A. (1986): Oral findings in people with or at high risk for AIDS: A study of 375 homosexual males. *J. Am. Acad. Dermatol.*, 112:187–192.
41. Snider, W. D., Simpson, D. M., Nielsen, S., Gold, J. W. M., et al. (1983): Neurological complications of acquired immune deficiency syndrome: Analysis of 50 patients. *Ann. Neurol.*, 14:403–408.
42. So, Y. T., Beckstead, J. H., and Davis, R. L. (1986): Primary central nervous system lymphoma in acquired immune deficiency syndrome: A clinical and pathological study. *Ann. Neurol.*, 20:566–572.
43. Whelan, M. A., Krichoff, I. I., Handler, M., et al. (1983): Acquired immunodeficiency syndrome: Cerebral computed tomographic manifestations. *Radiology*, 149:477–484.
44. Zee, C.-S., Segall, H. D., Rogers, C., Ahmadi, J., Apuzzo, M., and Rhodes, R. (1985): MR imaging of cerebral toxoplasmosis: Correlation of computed tomography and pathology. *J. Comput. Assist. Tomogr.*, 9:797–799.

# CHAPTER 3

# Pulmonary Manifestations of AIDS

David P. Naidich, Stuart M. Garay, Philip C. Goodman,
Benito J. Rybak, and Elissa L. Kramer

More than 50% of acquired immune deficiency syndrome (AIDS) patients develop pulmonary manifestations at some time in the course of their disease (1–4). For the purpose of surveillance, the Centers for Disease Control (CDC) originally defined the diagnosis of AIDS based on the identification of a reliably diagnosed disease at least moderately predictive of cellular immune dysfunction in the absence of an underlying cause for such immunodeficiency (see Chapter 1). In light of the discovery that AIDS is caused by human immunodeficiency virus (HIV), formerly known as human T-cell lymphotropic virus-type III/lymphadenopathy associated virus (HTLV-III/LAV), a more systematic categorization of the wide range of clinical findings associated with HIV infection has been established (5,6; see also Chapter 1).

Radiographic evaluation plays an important role in the diagnosis and management of these patients (7,8), despite considerable overlap in the clinical and radiographic manifestations of these varied pulmonary disorders.

## OPPORTUNISTIC INFECTIONS

### Pneumocystis carinii

Pneumonia due to Pneumocystis carinii (PCP) is the most common life-threatening infection in patients with AIDS (9,10). PCP occurs at least once in the course of disease in approximately 60% of AIDS patients, and nearly one-quarter of these initial episodes prove fatal.

Significant clinical differences have been documented to occur with PCP in patients with AIDS as compared with patients with other immunodeficiencies (11). In AIDS patients, diagnosis requires a higher than usual degree of clinical suspicion because PCP frequently presents subacutely with fever, cough, and dyspnea, which may persist for 2 weeks or longer. While laboratory studies often reveal lymphopenia and abnormalities in gas exchange, (including a decrease in mean arterial $pO_2$, and an increased $PAO_2\text{-}PaO_2$ gradient), these findings are nonspecific. In addition, as compared with infection in the preAIDS era, traditional drug therapy is complicated by an unusually high frequency of adverse reactions. Adverse reactions to trimethoprim-sulfamethoxazole, including leukopenia, diffuse erythematous skin rashes (including Stevens-Johnson syndrome), hepatotoxicity, thrombocytopenia, azotemia, and drug fever occur in up to 65% of patients (see Chapter 1). Similar reactions, as well as hypoglycemia, orthostatic hypotension, and azotemia also have been documented to occur with greater than expected frequency following administration of pentamidine. These differences in clinical presentation and course have significant implications for the interpretation of radiographic findings in patients suspected of having AIDS.

The radiographic manifestations of PCP both in the pre- and postAIDS era have been reviewed widely (7,8,10–21). Typically, PCP presents as bilateral, perihilar, and/or basilar reticular or reticulonodular infiltrates, which rapidly progress in 3 to 5 days to diffuse air-space consolidation involving the entire lung (Color Plate 1, Fig. 1). Despite its pathologic designation as an interstitial pneumonitis, infection with PCP is typified by the presence of organisms within intraalveolar exudates, if evaluated using appropriate stains such as silver methenamine (Color Plate 2, Fig. 2). The presence of air-space disease is easily confirmed with computed tomography (CT), which can be used to document further the precise distribution of disease as either central or peripheral in patients scanned within 24 to 48 hr of the diagnosis being established (Fig. 3). In our experience, optimal evaluation of parenchymal disease requires the use of thin section (1.5—2 mm) CT scans, whenever

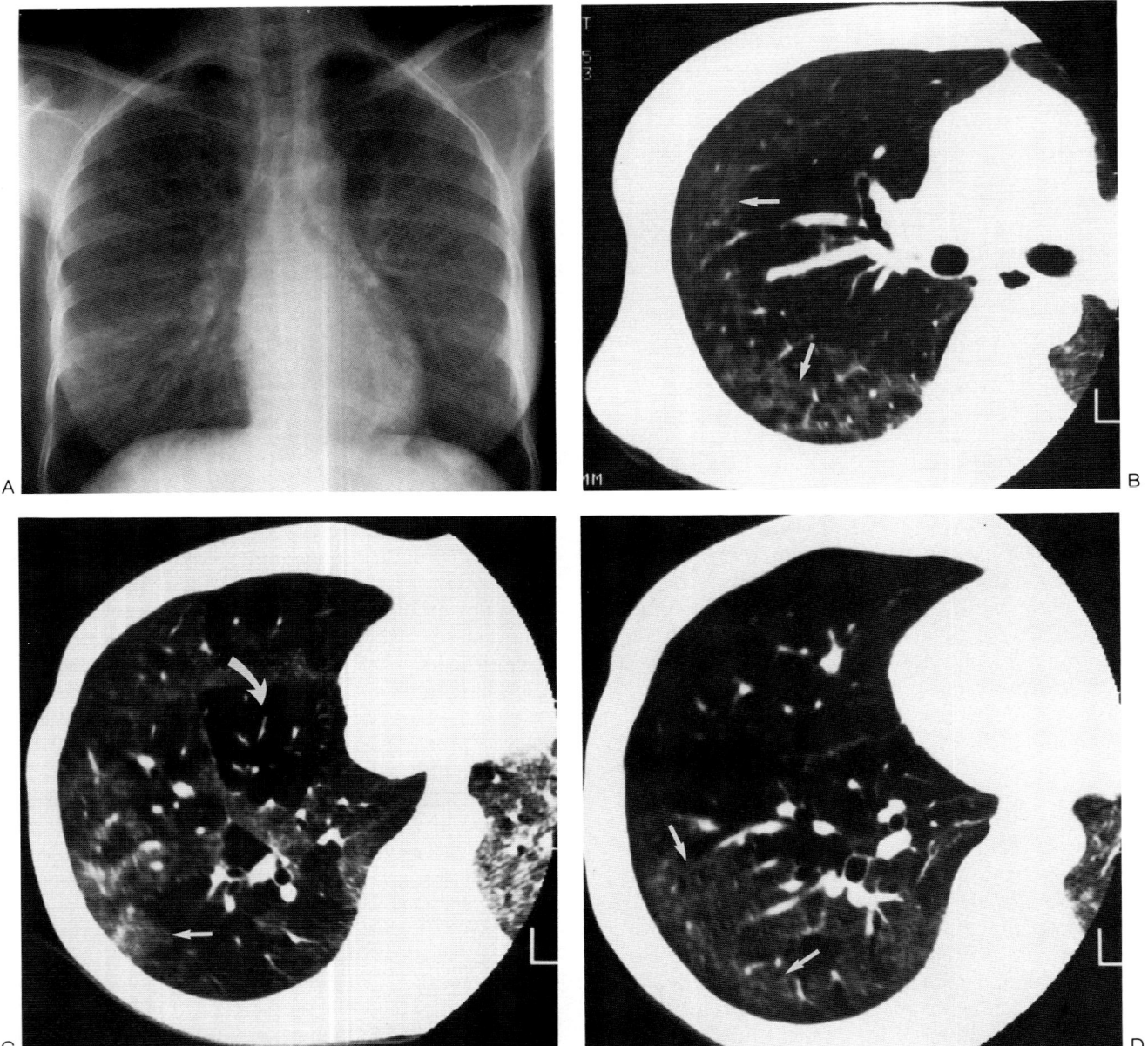

**FIG. 3.** PCP: CT correlation. **A:** PA chest radiograph demonstrates apparently symmetrical, bilateral, reticular infiltrates. **B, C, D:** 1.5-cm collimated, retrospectively targeted CT sections obtained through the mid- and lower lung fields sequentially in a patient with bronchoscopically diagnosed PCP, prior to the initiation of therapy. Scattered foci of poorly defined air-space disease are easily defined, primarily involving the peripheral lung fields (*arrows* in B, C, D). Note the near complete sparing of the medial basilar segment of the right lower lobe (*curved arrow* in C).

possible utilizing targeted reconstructions. These images should be obtained through preselected portions of the lung, determined either from routine 10-mm thick sections or from the initial scout view.

Despite significant differences in both the clinical presentation and incidence of adverse drug reactions in AIDS patients as compared with patients with other immunodeficiencies, to date no significant statistical differences have been documented to occur in the spectrum of radiographic findings, although meaningful comparisons between published series is limited by a failure to standardize radiographic descriptions (Table 1), (10–21). Atypical patterns have been described in both groups; some of these may be more common in patients with AIDS (Table 1).

In a review of 30 proven cases of PCP diagnosed in the

TABLE 1. *P. carinii:* radiographic findings

| Author | No. of patients | Diffuse interstitial/ alveolar infiltrates | Parenchymal findings | | Normal | Associated findings | |
|---|---|---|---|---|---|---|---|
| | | | Unilateral focal infiltrates | Cystic disease | | Hilar/ mediastinal adenopathy* | Pleural effusions* |
| DeLorenzo et al. (21) | 104 | 99 | 5 | 7 | — | 4 | — |
| Kovacs et al. (11) | 49 | 46 | 1 | — | 2 | — | — |
| Suster et al. (20) | 59 | 53 | 2 | 1 | 4 | 2 | — |
| Cohen et al. (18) | 34 | 23 | 2 | 1 | 8 | — | 1 |
| Garay et al. (Unpublished data) | 205 | 147 | 24 | — | 8 | — | — |
| Stover et al. (10) | 36 | 31 | — | 2 | 5 | 2 | 4 |
| Total | 487 | 399 (81.9%) | 34 (6.9%) | 11 (2%) | 34 (7%) | 8 (1.6%) | 5 (1%) |

* Unconfirmed histologically.

preAIDS era, Doppman et al. (15) reported a 56% incidence of atypical radiographic findings, including unilateral distribution, lobar involvement, nodularity, abscess formation with cavitation, and linear atelectasis. A similar spectrum of radiographic changes has been noted in patients with AIDS, including asymmetrical pulmonary disease (Fig. 4), as well as predominant upper lobe involvement simulating tuberculosis (Fig. 5) (22). Of particular interest is the finding of air-filled, cystic parenchymal changes complicating otherwise unremarkable PCP (Fig. 6) (21,23). In the series reported by DeLorenzo et al. (21), cystic changes were noted to occur radiographically in 7 of 104 (6.7%) documented cases. The mechanism by which these cysts develop is unknown. While concurrent bacterial, fungal, or viral infection may play a role in select cases, as documented in several series, the failure of serial laboratory studies to reveal other sources of infection makes this explanation unlikely. It is possible that cystic changes represent focal areas of pulmonary emphysema, possibly related to obstruction of distal airways, as distinct from honeycombing, which results from interstitial fibrosis or actual cavitation, as may occur with infection, especially in i.v. drug abusers with septic emboli (Figs. 7, 8, and 9). Regardless of their etiology, the presence of these cysts poses a significant potential risk for the development of

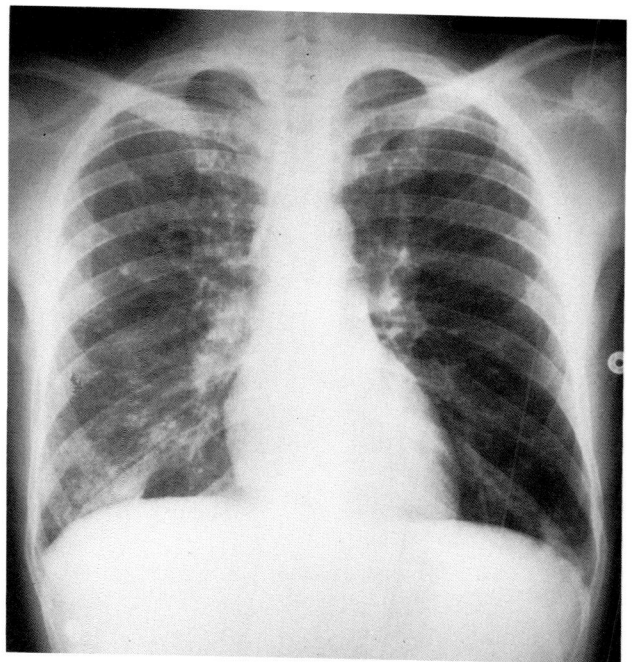
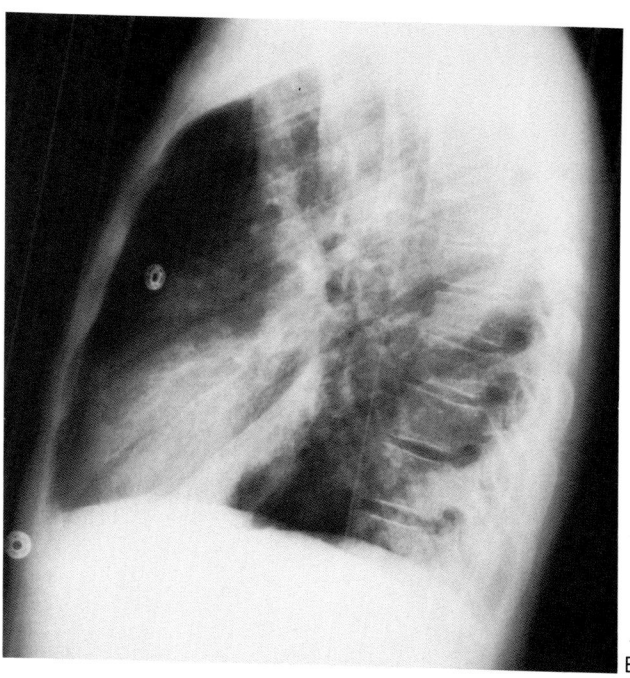

**FIG. 4.** PCP: Asymmetric disease. **A, B:** PA and lateral chest radiographs, respectively, show asymmetric pulmonary consolidation, especially prominent in the right lower lobe. TBB-documented PCP.

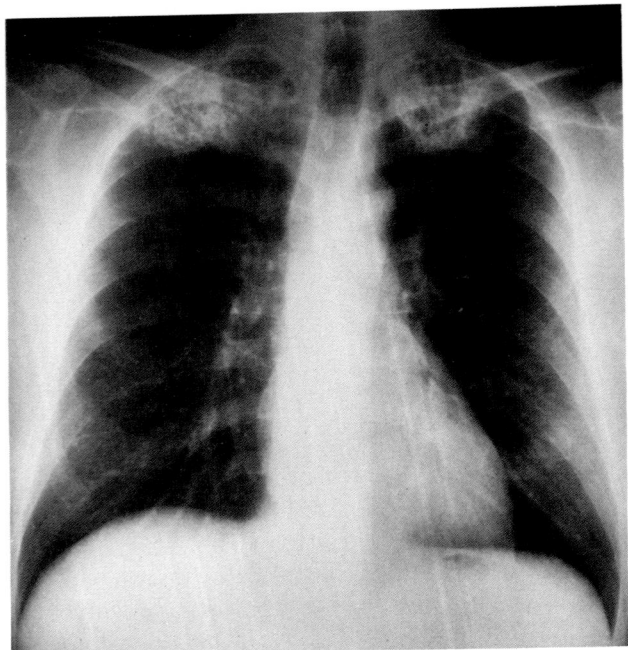

**FIG. 5.** PCP: Apical disease. PA radiograph shows atypical pattern of bilateral lung disease restricted to the apices, initially suggestive of mycobacterial infection. TBB-proven PCP. All subsequent cultures for TB proved negative.

pneumothoraces, both spontaneous or following transbronchial or percutaneous biopsy (Fig. 10) (23,24). As already illustrated, CT may be of value in detecting cysts in select, high-risk patients, (Figs. 6 and 7). While enlarged hilar and mediastinal nodes have been described in patients with documented PCP (as have pleural effusions), in our experience these findings are uncharacteristic and warrant suspicion of associated secondary infections such as mycobacterial disease, Kaposi's sarcoma (KS), lymphoma, or fungi. Significantly, although enlarged nodes have been reported in select series, pathologic documentation is conspicuously lacking (10,18,20,21). PCP may present rarely as miliary disease, or simulate masses or solitary nodules, both parenchymal and extrapleural (Figs. 11, 12, and 13) (25).

Radiographically significant clearing of infiltrates usually can be demonstrated 13 to 15 days following initiation of therapy in adequately treated patients with uncomplicated PCP (9). This may be somewhat longer than time intervals previously established for other immunosuppressed populations (11). Occasionally there is significant worsening in the appearance of the chest approximately three to five days following initiation of therapy. While this may be due to rapid progression of disease, more often this results from alterations in fluid balance consequent to the large volume of fluid required for administration of trimethoprim-sulfamethoxazol. Improvement usually is noted following fluid restriction or diuresis. Acceleration of radiographic resolution has been documented to occur in response to steroid therapy (26,26a), although its use is controversial.

In a percentage of cases, there is radiographic and pathologic evidence of residual disease, usually indistinguishable from other causes of pulmonary interstitial disease. This finding does not necessarily correlate clinically with residual infection (27–29), but may be associated with the continued presence of Pneumocystis organisms (documented either with alveolar lavage or transbronchial biopsy), and recurrence of PCP. Unfor-

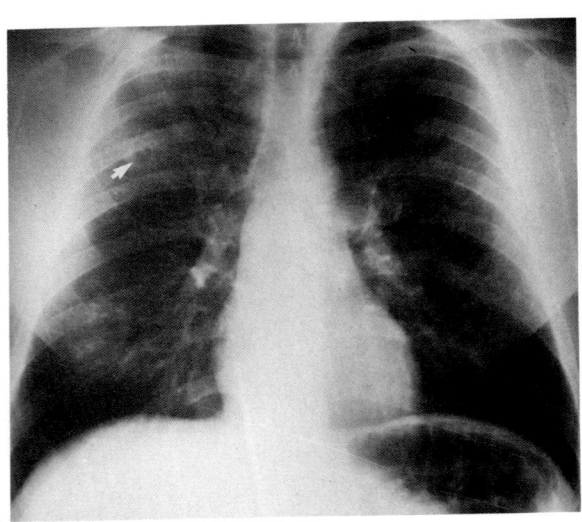
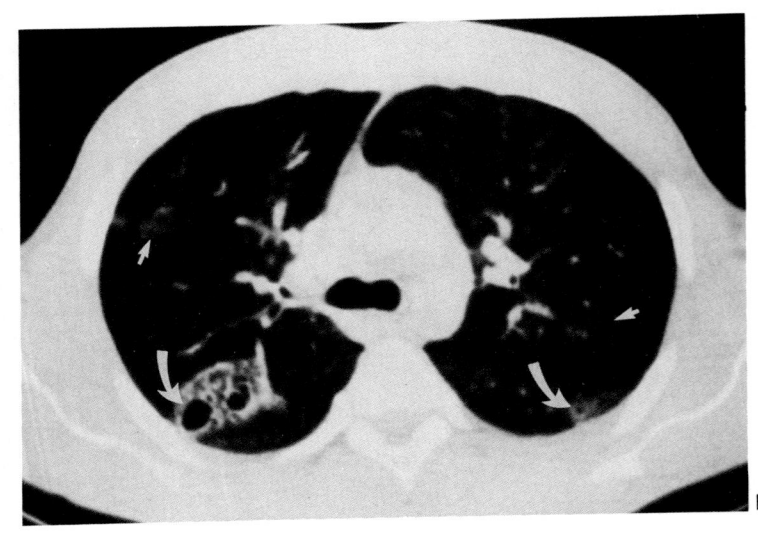

**FIG. 6.** PCP: Cavitary/cystic disease. **A:** PA radiograph shows subtle, bilateral infiltrates, slightly more obvious on the right side. There is a suggestion of cavitation in the right upper lobe (*arrow*). **B:** CT section at the level of the carina shows scattered foci of poorly defined air-space disease characteristic of PCP (*arrows*). Numerous cavities in varying stages of development can be identified (*curved arrows*). TBB-proven PCP (compare with Fig. 3).

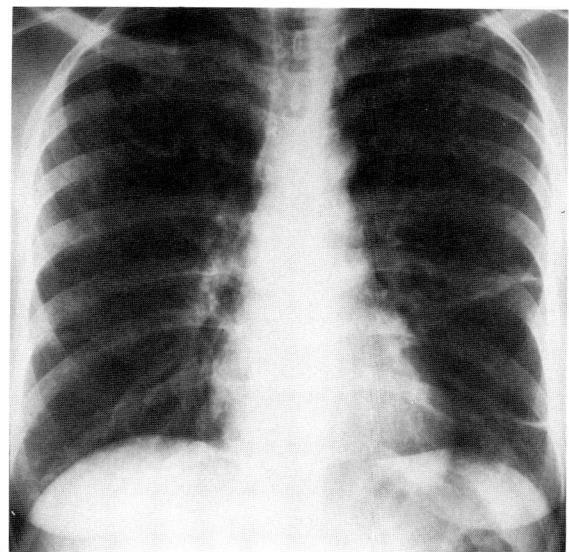
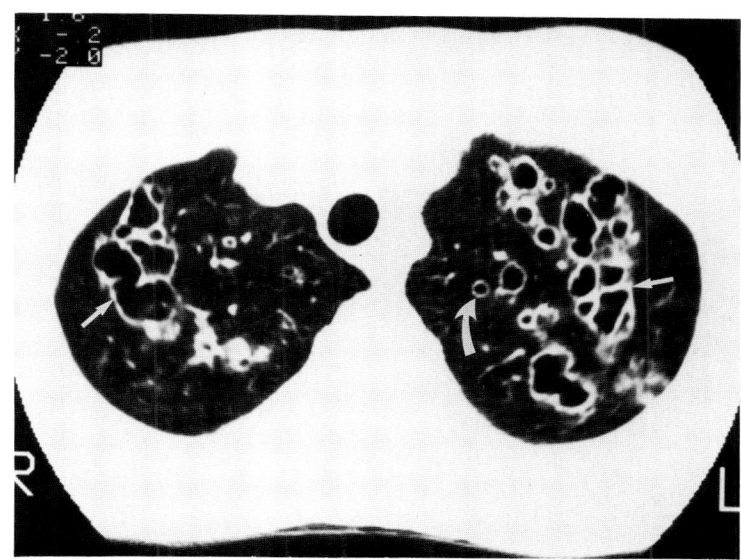

**FIG. 7.** PCP: Cavitary/cystic disease. **A:** PA radiograph shows diffuse cystic disease in a patient with biopsy-proven PCP. **B:** CT section obtained through the upper lobes shows scattered thin-walled cysts of various sizes, some of which appear to have coalesced (*arrows*). Significantly, there is a paucity of parenchymal disease surrounding most of these cavities (*curved arrow*), most of which are considerably larger and better delineated than those illustrated in Fig. 6.

tunately, recurrent infection occurs in 20 to 40% of all cases.

Chest radiography, especially in conjunction with arterial blood gas evaluation, can be of value in the follow-up and management of patients with potentially recurrent disease. Lipper et al. (29), in their study of 45 cases of patients previously diagnosed and successfully treated with PCP re-presenting at least 3 months after recovery with pulmonary symptoms, found that of 27 patients with simultaneous worsening in the appearance of their chest radiographs and arterial blood gases, 23 (86%) had recurrent PCP. Significantly, of 14 patients presenting with a change in just one parameter, either a worsening chest radiograph or arterial blood gases, only eight (56%) had recurrent disease; of the four patients without change, none had evidence or recurrence. These

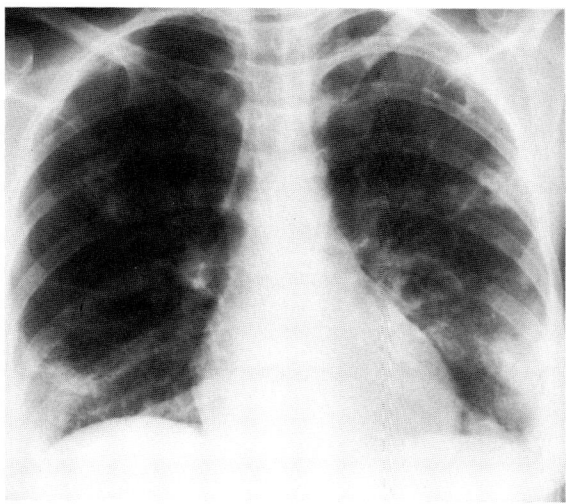
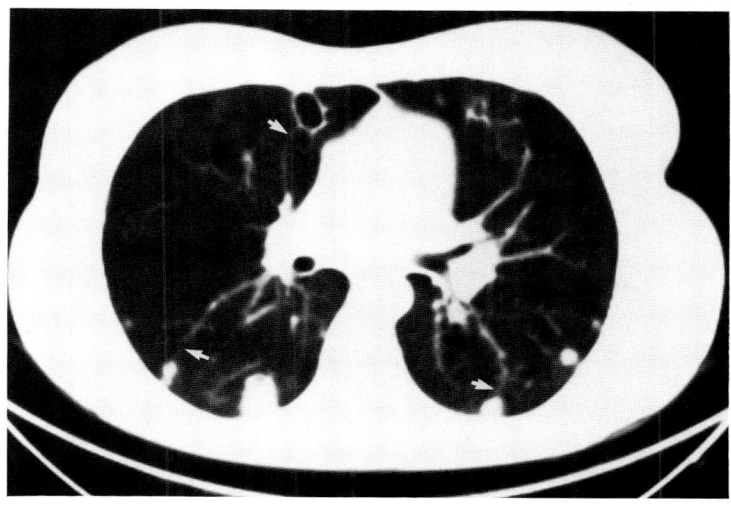

**FIG. 8.** Septic Emboli. **A:** PA radiograph shows scattered infiltrates and cavities in both lung fields in a known i.v. drug addict, an appearance easily confused with the cystic/cavitary changes that can develop in select cases of PCP (compare with Figs. 6 and 7). **B:** CT section through the mid-lung fields shows the typical cross-sectional appearance of septic emboli, including the presence of numerous peripheral masses and cavities in varying stages of evolution, many of which have clearly definable feeding vessels (arrows).

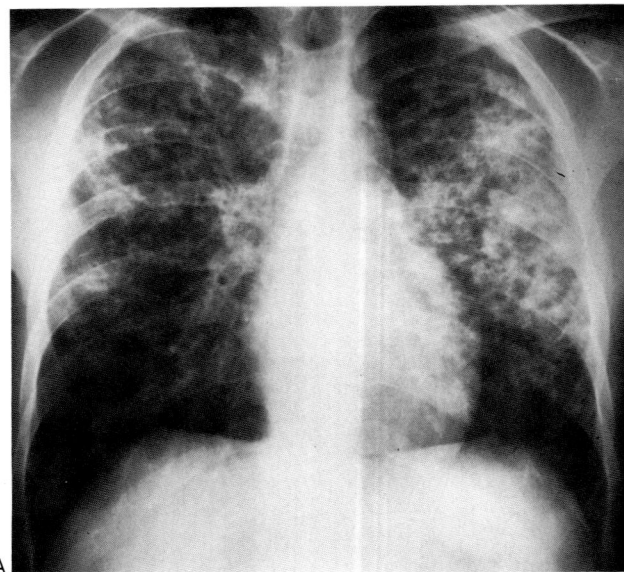 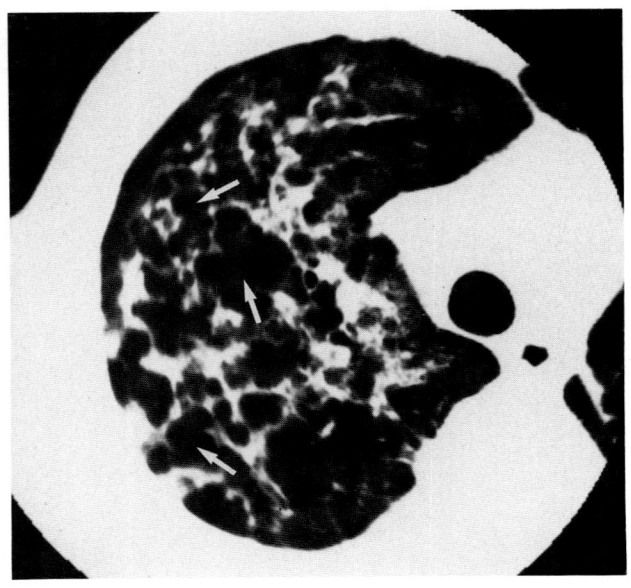

**FIG. 9.** PCP: Interstitial fibrosis. **A:** PA radiograph in a patient with documented PCP, several months following conventional therapy. Extensive, bilateral parenchymal disease is apparent, especially in the mid-lung fields. The presence of cavities cannot be excluded. **B:** Enlargement of a retrospectively targeted CT section through the right upper lobe shows marked reticulation compatible with the clinical diagnosis of residual interstitial fibrosis. Residual hyperinflated parenchyma can be identified intervening between areas of thickened interstitium, accounting for the apparent cystic changes identified on the PA radiograph (*arrows*), (compare with Figs. 6, 7, and 8).

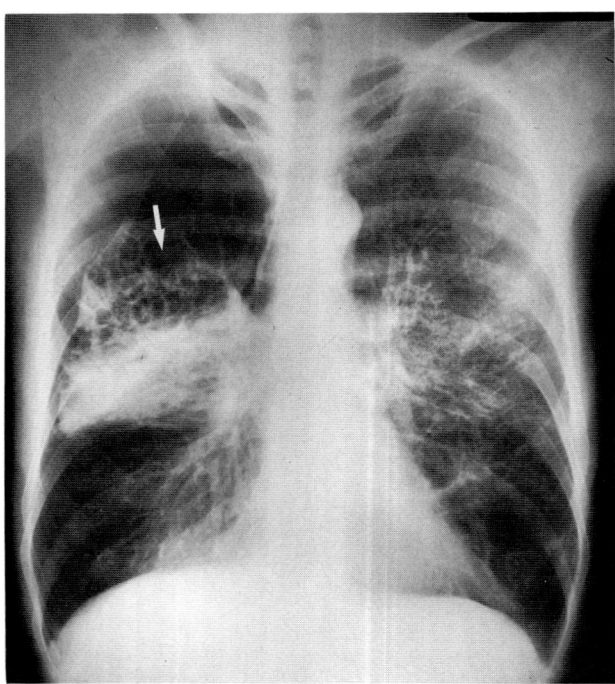

**FIG. 10.** PCP: Spontaneous pneumothorax. PA radiograph shows extensive cystic changes in both upper lung fields, especially on the right (*arrow*). While nonspecific, cystic changes are seen in patients with PCP and clearly pose an increased threat of pneumothorax following TBB.

data suggest that a change in the radiographic appearance of the chest, especially when coupled with corresponding alterations in the arterial blood gases, may allow initiation of empiric therapy in select patients without the need of additional invasive diagnostic procedures.

Schinella et al. (30) recently documented that PCP itself may cause fibrosis, unassociated with antibiotic or oxygen therapy (Fig. 14). While the true incidence of pulmonary fibrosis developing in patients with AIDS has yet to be determined, there is considerable evidence that this is a frequent occurrence (29–31). Simmons et al. (33), in their review of 105 patients with AIDS and clinical evidence of pneumonitis, found that nonspecific interstitial pneumonitis occurring in the absence of an identifiable infection could be documented histologically in 36 cases (34%). Of these, 20 (56%) had an abnormal chest radiograph otherwise indistinguishable from the 52 patients (50%) with documented PCP. In our experience, the incidence of non-specific interstitial pneumonitis is significantly less than that reported by Simmons et al. (about 10% of cases).

Unfortunately, despite a good initial response in patients with PCP, relapse and/or recurrence is frequent. In approximately 20 to 25% of patients, respiratory failure, indistinguishable from other forms of the Acute Respiratory Distress Syndrome (ARDS), develops de-

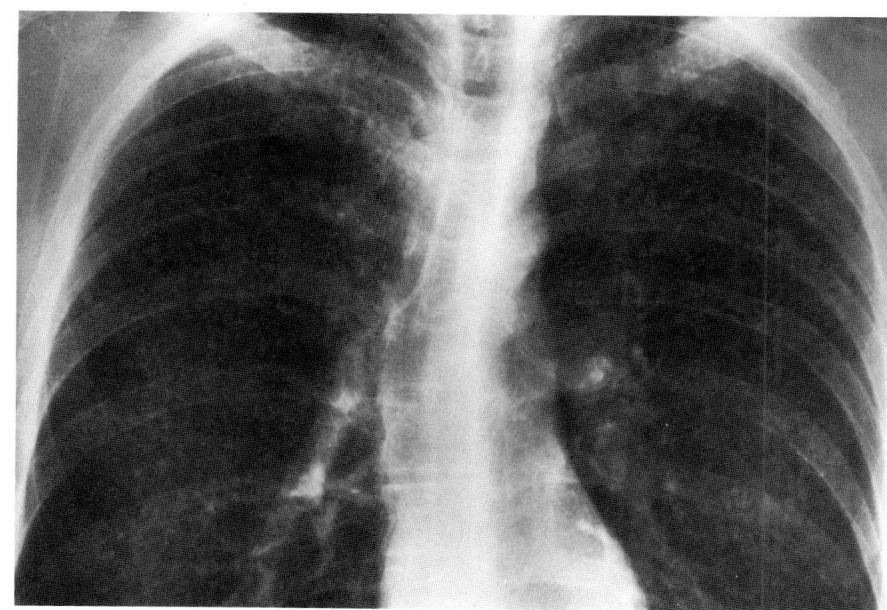

FIG. 11. PCP: Atypical appearance. PA radiograph shows a pattern of typical miliary disease. While more characteristic of fungal disease, as documented in this case by TBB, this pattern rarely may be caused by PCP.

spite adequate initial therapy (Fig. 15). Mortality approximates 90% for those patients requiring endotracheal intubation and mechanically assisted ventilation (9,10,34).

## MYCOBACTERIAL INFECTIONS

Infection with Mycobacterial tuberculosis (MTB) occurs in approximately 10% of AIDS patients (3,4,35). In a significant percentage of cases infection may precede the diagnosis of AIDS, sometimes by several months. As reported by Louie et al. (35), in 15 of 24 patients (62%), TB was diagnosed prior to or concomitant with the diagnosis of AIDS (35). The incidence of MTB may be more common in intravenous drug abusers and Haitians as compared to homosexual or bisexual men (see Chapter 1). Pitchenik et al. (36), in their prospective evaluation of 71 consecutive patients confirmed to have TB at the Dade County Florida Public Health Department—Tuberculosis Clinic found that 22 (31%) were seropositive. This group had a significantly higher proportion of young, black, and Haitian patients. Importantly, the seropositive group also had higher than average false-negative tuberculin skin tests, more frequent extrapulmonary, lymphatic disease, and a significantly lower proportion of positive sputum cultures when compared to seronegative patients. At the time of diagnosis only six (27%) of the seropositive patients with TB had clinical evidence of AIDS or AIDS-related complex.

While evidence suggests reactivation as the primary mechanism of infection, chest radiographs usually show a pattern more consistent with primary infection, including hilar and mediastinal adenopathy and noncavitary pulmonary infiltrates distributed equally in both the upper and lower lung fields (Fig. 16) (36–38). In the absence of adenopathy, differentiation from other infections, such as PCP, may be difficult. Apical and/or cavitary disease is unusual, as is tuberculous pleuritis. These manifestations presumably require a relatively intact immune system, as may occur in those cases developing prior to the onset of documented AIDS. While typical granulomatous tissue reaction and hence necrosis is rare, in our experience mycobacterial lymph nodes typically have low density when evaluated by contrast-en-

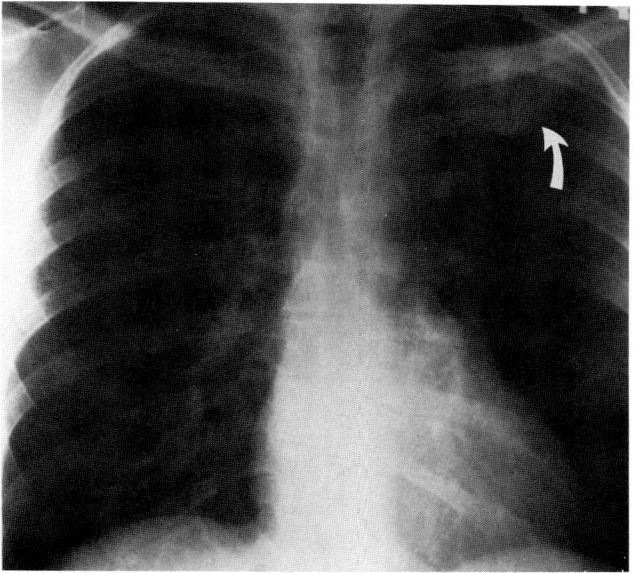

FIG. 12. PCP: Atypical appearance. PA radiograph shows focal, masslike area of consolidation in the left upper lobe, an appearance more typically associated with fungal or even neoplastic disease (arrow). Biopsy-proven PCP.

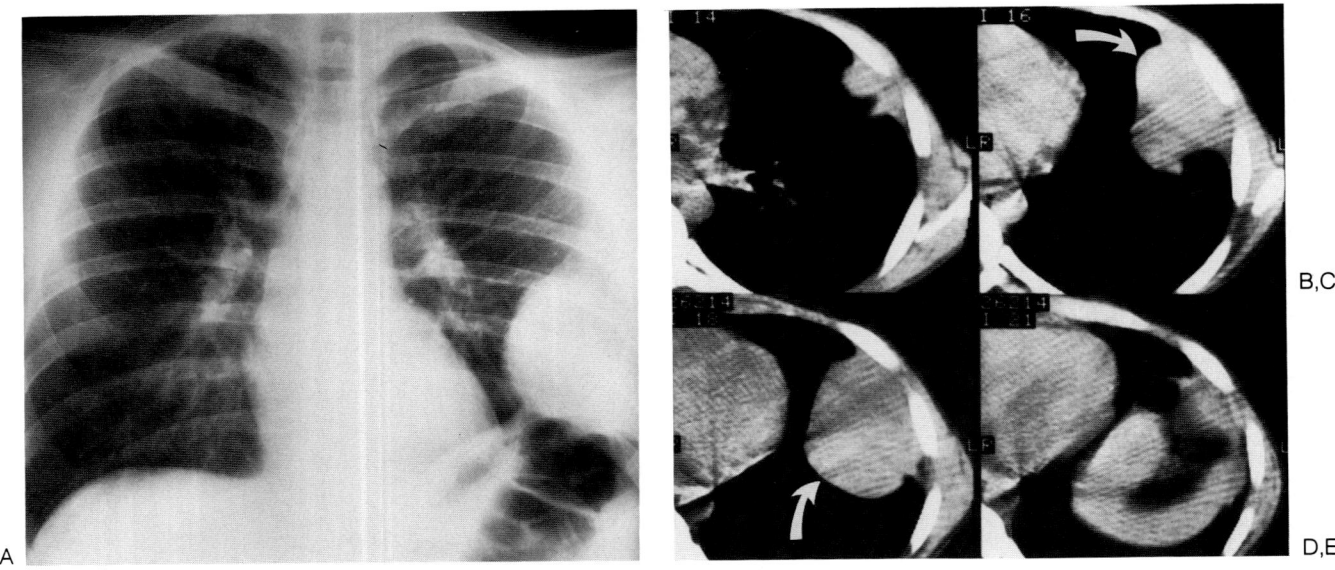

**FIG. 13.** PCP: Atypical appearance. **A:** PA radiograph shows a discrete, apparent extrapleural mass at the left costophrenic angle. The remainder of the chest is normal. **B, C, D, E:** Sequential magnified CT sections through the left lung base and diaphragm respectively document the presence of a well-defined, homogeneous extrapleural mass (*arrows* in B and C). At surgery an inflammatory mass was discovered which proved on biopsy to be secondary to P. carinii.

hanced CT (Fig. 17). The significance of this finding is still to be determined. Diagnosis generally is made from sputum culture; histologic examination usually does not reveal acid-fast organisms or granulomata (35). Adequate therapy necessitates a culture-confirmed diagnosis. In nearly 50% of cases, MTB can be documented from at least one extrapulmonary site; as a consequence, in suspected cases specimens should be obtained not only from respiratory secretions, but from urine, blood, lymph nodes, bone marrow, or even the liver. Evaluation with abdominal CT is of clear efficacy in determining dissemination (see Chapter 5). As recommended by the CDC, initial therapy for MTB is conventional triple drug therapy, usually including isoniazid and rifampin,

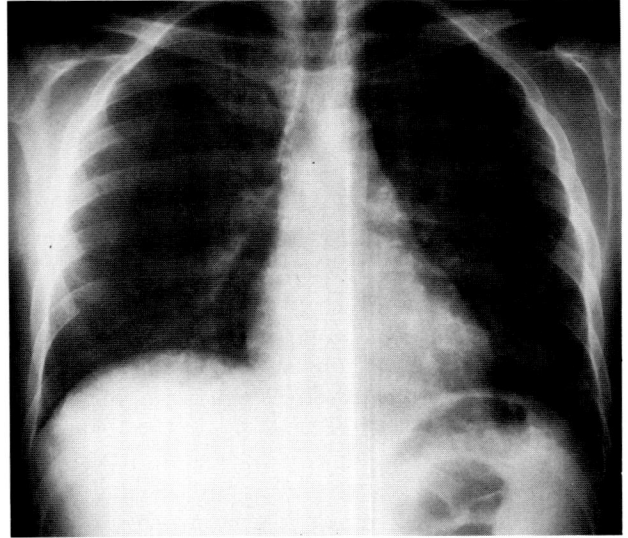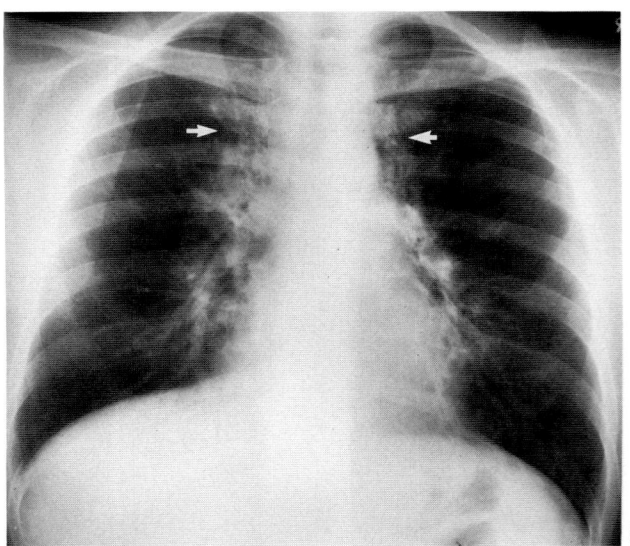

**FIG. 14.** PCP: Atypical interstitial fibrosis. **A:** PA radiograph shows subtle bilateral parenchymal infiltrates subsequently proven secondary to PCP. **B:** PA radiograph obtained 3 months after a course of standard antibiotic therapy. Coarse interstitial markings can be identified paralleling the mediastinum bilaterally, a pattern otherwise indistinguishable from that caused by mediastinal irradiation (*arrows*).

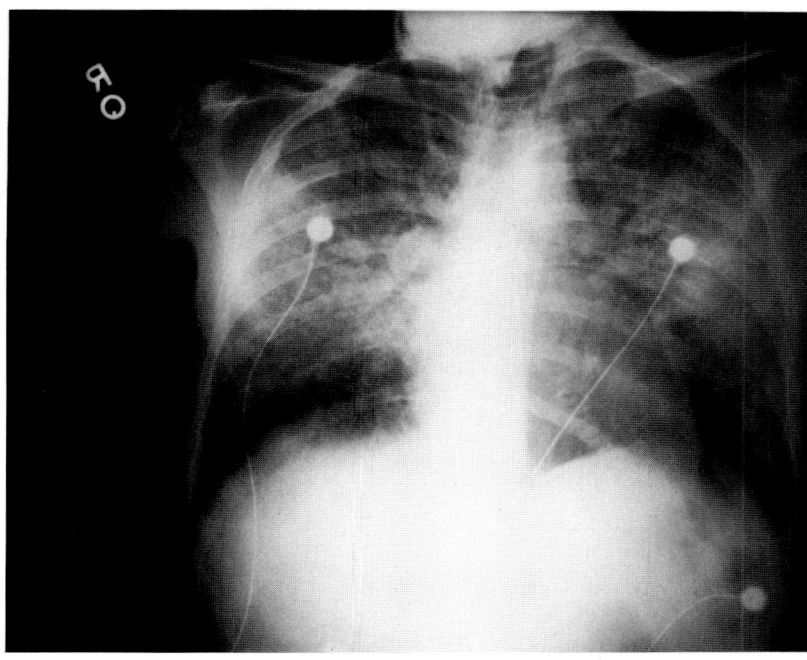

FIG. 15. PCP/ARDS. PA radiograph shows diffuse air-space disease in a patient with respiratory failure, indistinguishable from other forms of ARDS.

and should be continued for a minimum of nine months (39). It has been recommended that HIV-positive patients should be tuberculin skin tested, and treated prophylactically if positive. Unlike many other infections seen in AIDS patients, there is generally a good clinical response to appropriate chemotherapy (Fig. 18).

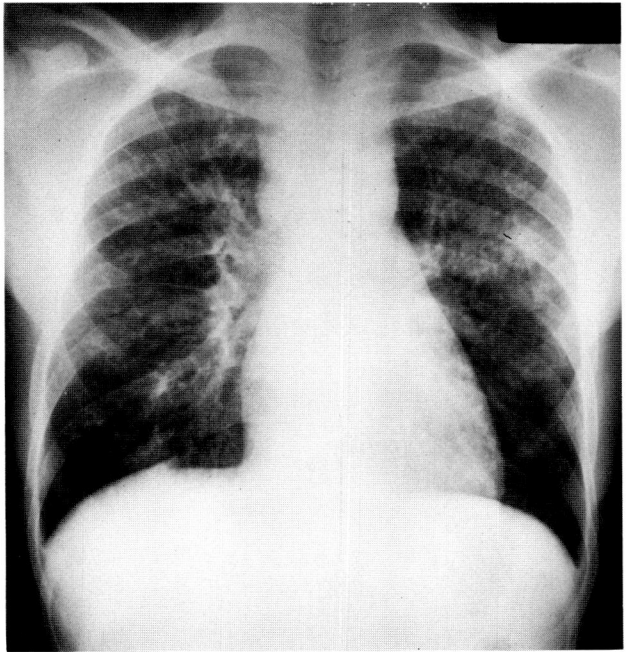

FIG. 16. MTB. PA radiograph shows evidence of diffuse mediastinal and hilar adenopathy associated with ill-defined densities in both lungs. These findings are most consistent with primary infection despite epidemiologic evidence suggesting reactivation as the primary mechanism of disease.

M. avium-intracellulare (MAI) infection in AIDS patients is also common, isolated with greater frequency than MTB in all patients except intravenous drug abusers and Haitians, and varies considerably from its manifestations in nonimmunocompromised patients (40–42). In normal hosts, MAI is primarily a pulmonary process, characterized by slowly progressing focal lesions with frequent cavitation, usually in patients between 50 and 60 years of age, especially those with emphysema. In contrast, in patients with AIDS, MAI usually is widely disseminated at the time of diagnosis (42). Although chest radiographic findings may be present, including mediastinal and hilar lymphadenopathy, diffuse patchy alveolar infiltrates, pulmonary nodules, and even miliary disease, the most important clinical involvement often is nonpulmonary. MAI often is diagnosed from lymph nodes, liver, bone marrow, stool, blood, and urine even when corresponding chest radiographs are normal (40–42). Treatment of disseminated disease requires a four drug regimen, including two experimental drugs—rifabutine (ansamycin), and clofazamine (39). Unlike the response to therapy of patients with MTB, treatment for MAI frequently is ineffective.

## CYTOMEGALOVIRUS

While cytomegalovirus (CMV) is the most frequent infectious organism found in autopsied AIDS patients, the clinical significance of this finding is unclear (43–45). Disseminated disease frequently occurs, especially terminally, with infarction and necrosis of the adrenal glands noted in particular. CMV pneumonitis is

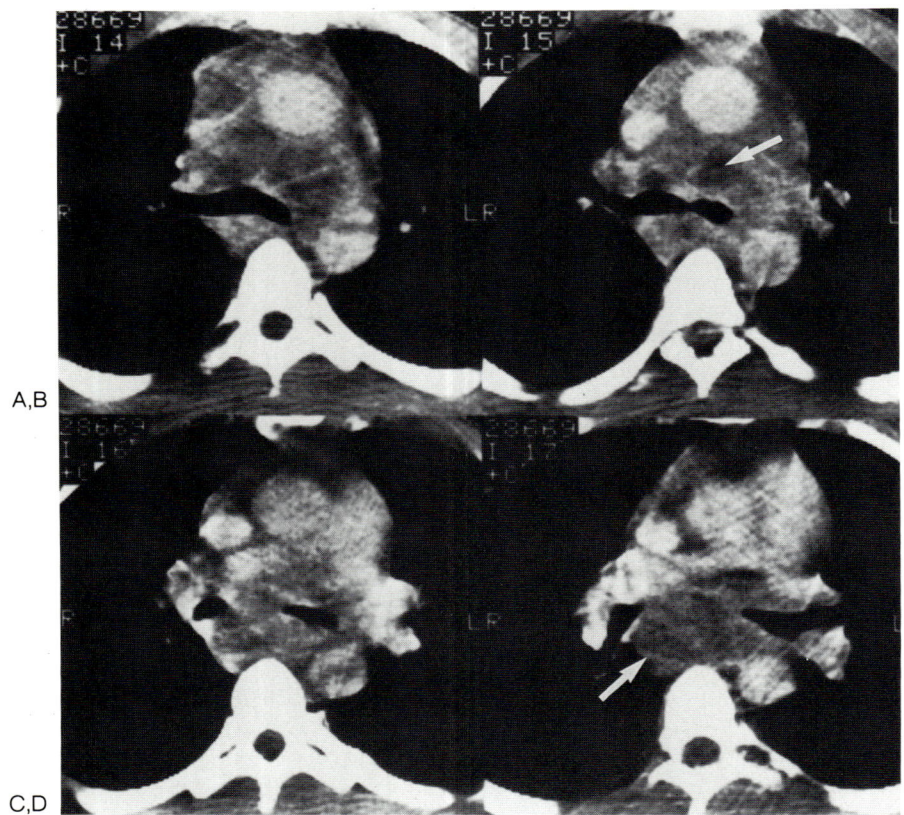

**FIG. 17.** MTB. **A, B, C, D:** Enlargements of CT sections obtained through the carina following a bolus of i.v. contrast demonstrate the presence of extensive, low-density, enlarged lymph nodes (*arrows* in B and D); while nonspecific, in our experience this finding is highly suggestive of granulomatous infection.

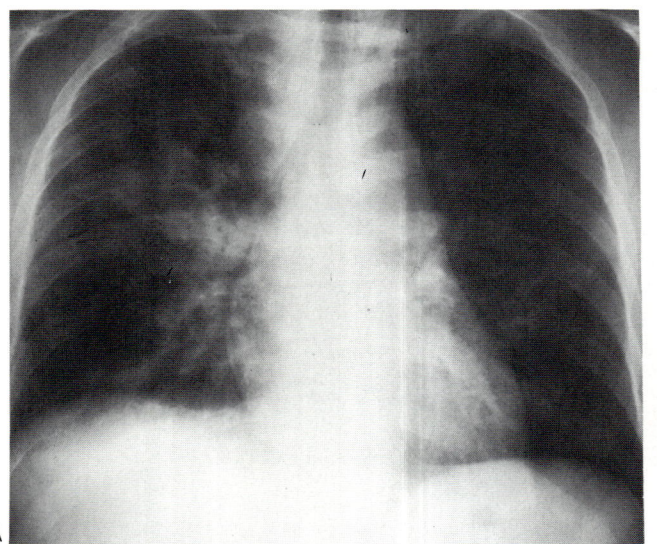 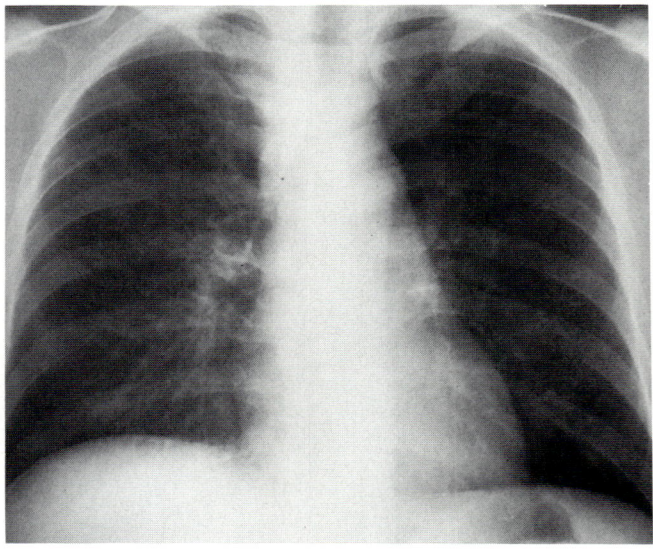

**FIG. 18.** M. kansasii. **A:** PA radiograph shows diffuse mediastinal and hilar adenopathy with diffuse pulmonary infiltrates, somewhat more prominent on the right. Diagnosis is established by sputum culture. **B:** PA radiograph obtained 16 days after that illustrated in A, following initiation of triple drug chemotherapy. Significant interval improvement is apparent, reinforcing the need to establish an accurate diagnosis. Cultures subsequently grew M. kansasii. (Courtesy of Dr. Clement Marks, New York University Medical Center, N.Y.).

a common postmortem finding. In a study of 39 patients with autopsy-documented CMV infection, pneumonitis was found in 31 (80%), although, significantly, CMV was found to be the sole causative pathogen in only two cases (45). Radiographically, CMV pneumonia is associated with bilateral infiltrates indistinguishable from those caused by PCP or fibrosis (Fig. 1).

Although often recovered from bronchoscopic lavage specimens, evidence of disease requires histologic demonstration of typical viral inclusion bodies. In an attempt to improve premortem diagnosis, immunofluorescence with CMV-specific monoclonal antibodies has been used to examine bronchoalveolar lavage (BAL) material (46). Emanuel et al. (46) have reported 100% sensitivity of this assay compared with other diagnostic tests; furthermore, there appears to be a correlation between the number of fluorescent cells identified and the presence of CMV pneumonia. Despite recent advances, there is no effective treatment for CMV pneumonia (47).

## MISCELLANEOUS PULMONARY INFECTIONS

### Fungi

Compared with the incidence of other opportunistic infections, fungal pneumonias are unusual, occurring in less than 5% of AIDS patients (3). The prevalence of these diseases is geographically influenced. When identified they usually accompany disseminated infection. Cryptococcus neoformans is most common, found usually in association with either brain or meningeal involvement (48). In noncompromised hosts, cryptococcal infection is associated most often with peripheral pulmonary nodules, whereas immunocompromised hosts demonstrate a wider variety of radiographic abnormalities (49). These include single and/or multiple nodules that may progress to confluence or cavitation, mediastinal adenopathy, segmental consolidation, or bilateral foci of bronchopneumonia (Figs. 19 and 20). With dissemination, usually to involve the meninges,

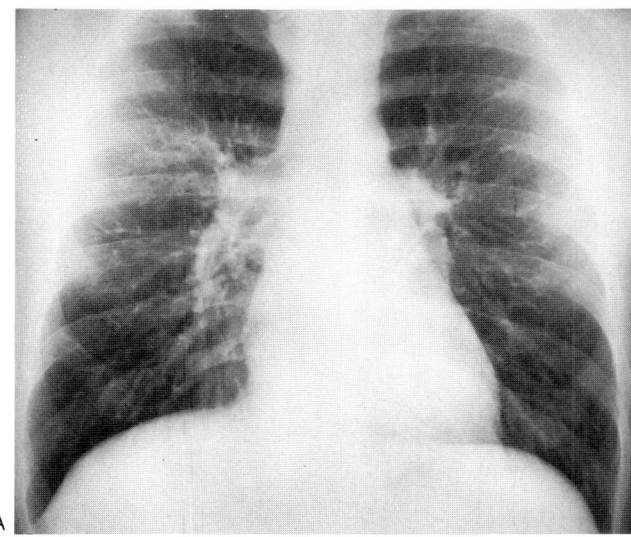

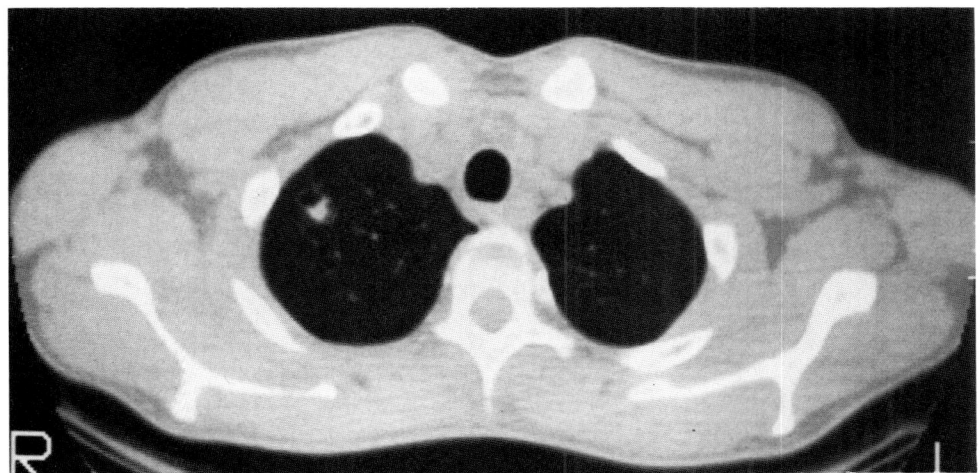

FIG. 19. Cryptococcus neoformans. A: PA radiograph, initially interpreted as normal. B: CT section through the upper lobes documents the presence of a cavity on the right side. Retrospectively, there is an ill-defined density in the right lung apex, although cavitation cannot be seen.

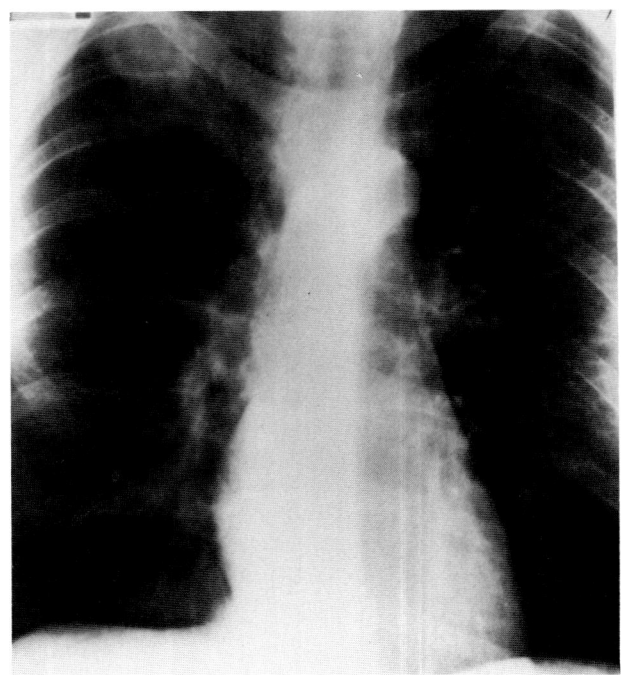

FIG. 20. Cryptococcus neoformans. PA radiograph shows a large, thick-walled cavity in the right upper lobe, associated with subtle mediastinal widening. Diagnosis established by TBB.

diffuse interstitial or miliary disease may be observed (Fig. 21) (50,51). Rarely, cryptococcal infection may cause isolated pleural effusions (52). C. neoformans may be recovered from BAL fluid; histologic confirmation is variable but has been shown both with transbronchial and open lung biopsy specimens (Fig. 21). Amphotericin B generally is recommended, usually as a prolonged course due to the frequency of relapse (50,51).

Disseminated histoplasmosis is an indicator disease for the diagnosis of AIDS in patients with laboratory evidence of HIV infection. While not necessarily confined to endemic regions, the prevalence of infection does tend to be geographical, with the highest rates of infection reported from the Midwest (53–56). As reviewed by Johnson et al. (56) occurrence ranges from 2.7% of cases in Houston to as high as 53% in Indianapolis. At New York University Medical Center, 15 patients with pulmonary histoplasmosis have been diagnosed, representing 0.2% of AIDS patients with documented pulmonary disease. Like patients with MAI, chest radiographs have been reported to be normal in up to 35% of cases with disseminated disease, as documented by culture of either blood or bone marrow. Recognition of disseminated histoplasmosis is significant because this may be the initial manifestation of AIDS, especially in patients from endemic regions (56).

Associated infections, including PCP, esophageal candidiasis, recurrent mucocutaneous herpes simplex, and disseminated MAI also are common. When abnormal, chest radiographs reveal diffuse interstitial infiltrates, or less commonly, evidence of miliary disease (Fig. 22) (53–56). Lung biopsy usually is diagnostic, given radiographic abnormalities; care must be exercised, however, not to misinterpret the typical configuration of H. capsulatum from cysts of P. carinii. Confirmation of disseminated disease usually is made by bone marrow aspiration and biopsy. Initial therapy with Amphotericin B can be effective, although relapses are common.

In addition to C. neoformans and H. capsulatum, various other fungi may present in patients with AIDS, especially C. immitis. Infection typically occurs in pa-

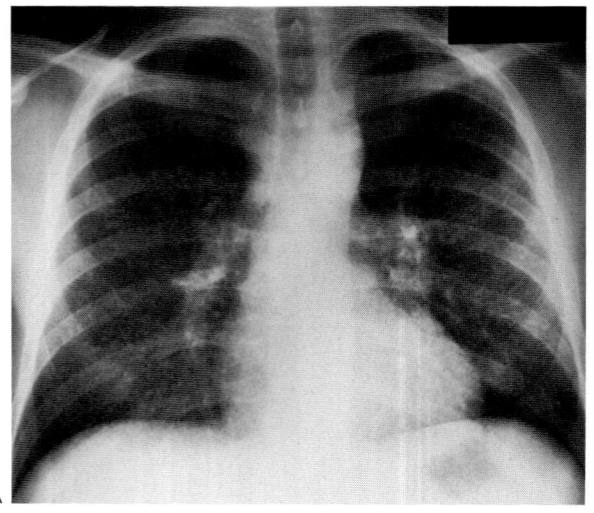 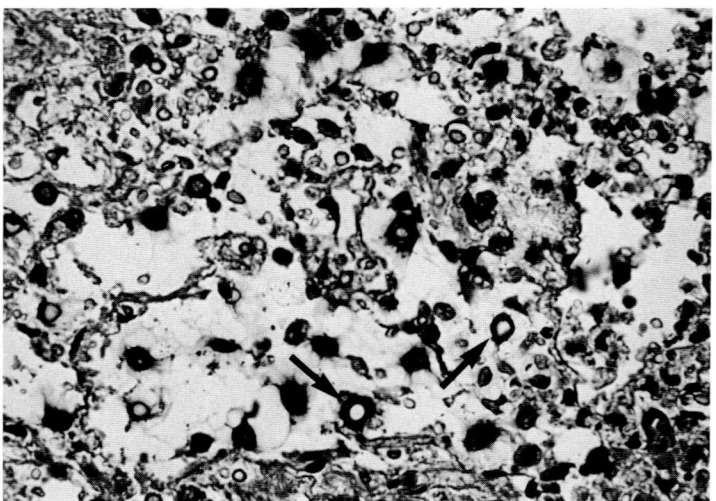

FIG. 21. Disseminated cryptococcosis. A: PA radiograph shows diffuse miliary disease associated with mediastinal and hilar lymphadenopathy. B: Histologic section from a different patient. TBB shows extensive alveolar exudates within which are numerous cryptococci identifiable by their characteristically mucicarmin stained capsules (arrows), as well as numerous cysts of P. carinii.

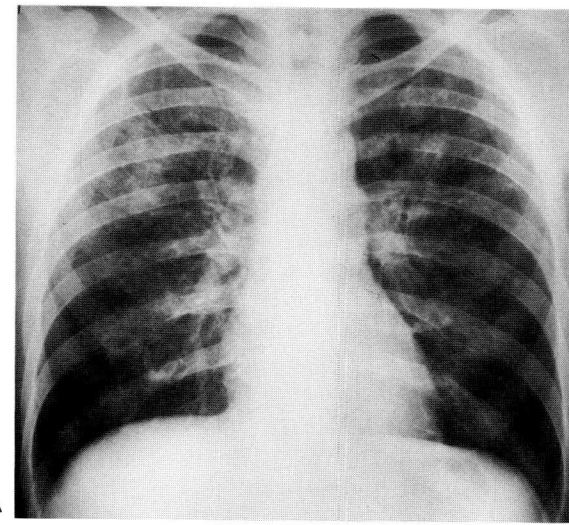
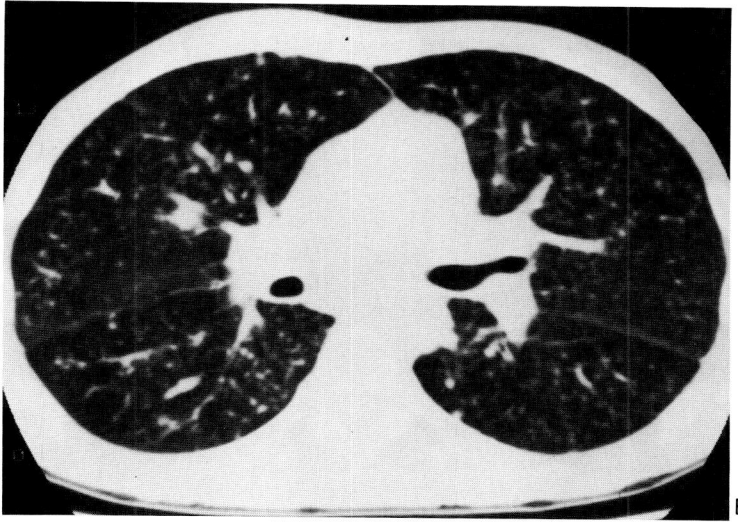

**FIG. 22.** Disseminated histoplasmosis. **A:** PA radiograph. While ill-defined densities are present bilaterally, the pattern is not typically miliary. **B:** CT section through the mid-lung fields documents the presence of innumerable small nodules with evidence of early confluence apparent near the right hilum. This appearance is nonspecific; in drug addicts, miliary nodules may be the result of foreign-body granulomas as well as the usual gamut of granulomatous diseases. H. capsulatum was documented both by TBB and bone marrow biopsy and culture.

tients from endemic regions; of 27 patients with AIDS reported from Tucson, Arizona, 7 had evidence of coccidiomycosis (57). Like other fungal infections, hematogenous dissemination is characteristic. Chest radiographs usually demonstrate diffuse interstitial infiltrates and thin-walled cavities, although with dissemination, a miliary pattern may be seen (Fig. 23). Lung biopsy generally shows poorly formed granulomas, with numerous thickwalled, 30- to 60-micron spherules containing numerous endospores. Lavage fluid cultures typically are positive. As with other fungal infections, treatment typically is with Amphotericin B (57).

Surprisingly, other infections typically associated with immune dysfunction are not commonly seen in patients with AIDS. Nocardiosis, invasive candidiasis, and aspergillus are rarely documented pulmonary pathogens. Nocardia most commonly presents as a unilateral segmental or lobar cavitary infiltrate, often associated with mycobacterial disease (Fig. 24). Aspergillosis is rare in AIDS patients, especially invasive disease, although a form of pseudomembranous necrotizing bronchial aspergillosis has been described (58). More commonly, aspergillus presents as a saprophyte that colonizes previously formed cavities, almost always in association with some other pulmonary infection (Fig. 25). Spores and pseudohyphae of Candida spp. also may invade bronchial walls and even the pulmonary parenchyma without inciting significant inflammation. The significance of this finding histologically is questionable.

### Bacteria

Although initially thought to be a rare manifestation of pulmonary disease, the incidence of bacterial infections in patients with AIDS is increasing (59,60). Streptococcus pneumonia and Hemophilus influenza are most commonly cited as causing focal parenchymal disease; other bacteria, including Legionella pneumonia, have been observed either in isolation or associated with other infections, most notably PCP (Fig. 26 and 27) (59,60). When properly identified, most bacterial infections respond to appropriate antibiotic therapy, hence the need for prompt and accurate diagnosis.

Rarely, other pulmonary pathogens, including toxoplasmosis, cryptosporidiosis, adenovirus, and varicella may occur; diagnosis almost always depends on histologic and/or microbacteriologic confirmation, often in a patient with documented extrathoracic disease (Fig. 28).

## NEOPLASMS

### Kaposi's Sarcoma

Approximately 25% of AIDS patients have proven KS, although recently a statistical downturn in the prevalence of this tumor has been noted. Most cases have been documented to occur in either homosexual or bisexual men (3,4,61).

Pulmonary involvement has been documented to occur in approximately 20% of patients with epidemic KS, almost always preceded by documented cutaneous and/or visceral involvement, (Table 2). Clinically, pulmonary manifestations may be indistinguishable from disease caused by opportunistic infections (61–67).

The premortem diagnosis of KS is difficult. Fiberoptic bronchoscopy can provide a presumptive diagnosis by

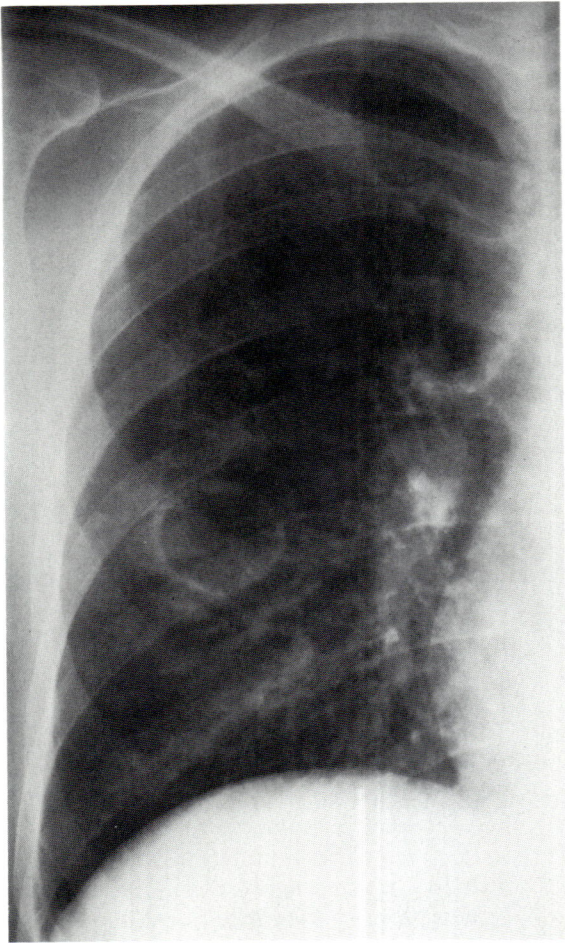

**FIG. 23.** Coccidiomycosis/PCP. Coned-down view of the right lung shows a well-defined, thin-walled cavity in the right lower lobe, associated with faintly definable perihilar interstitial infiltrates. TBB and lavage documented the presence of pneumocystitis. While initially felt to be consistent with PCP, a repeat biopsy specifically directed to the region of the cavity confirmed the diagnosis of coccidomycosis.

allowing visualization of endobronchial tumors (61,63). These appear as multiple red or violaceous lesions which are slightly raised and vascular in appearance (Color plate 3, Fig. 29). While the diagnosis may be difficult to confirm with transbronchial biopsy (TBB), especially when parenchymal involvement is suspected, recent reports have documented the safety and feasibility of obtaining tissue confirmation in this manner (67a,67b). Histologically, the tumor consists of spindle cells often containing atypical nuclei and occasional mitoses, and vascular slits and hemosiderin deposits are characteristically present (Color plate 4, Fig. 30). Significantly, tumor tends to surround small bronchi and blood vessels within the interstitium (Color plate 5, Fig. 31; Fig. 32) (61). Pulmonary involvement tends to be focal, relatively acellular, and is generally randomly scattered throughout the pulmonary parenchyma. This may make the diagnosis problematic, even with open-lung biopsy, especially if limited thoracotomies with lingular or middle lobe biopsies only are obtained. Effusions are common, and typically are exudative and serosanguinous; cytological examination, however, is nondiagnostic, as is pleural biopsy.

In the preAIDS era, radiographic descriptions of KS included hilar and mediastinal adenopathy, nodular infiltrates, and pleural effusions. These same findings have been reported to occur in AIDS patients, as well as the finding of diffuse interstitial disease otherwise indistinguishable from PCP (61–67), (Table 2). Parenchymal disease most commonly appears as diffuse interstitial/alveolar infiltrates, although unilateral disease or multifocal disease have been reported (see Figs. 33 and 34). While the reported frequency of nodular parenchymal disease varies, the appearance of poorly defined angio- and bronchocentric nodules and infiltrates, in our experience, is characteristic, especially when seen with CT (Figs. 31–34).

An important limitation in characterization of the pulmonary manifestations of KS is the frequent presence of concurrent infection (Table 2). As discussed by Davis et al. (62) in their series of 24 patients with AIDS and autopsy-proved intrathoracic KS, findings with a high positive predictive value included parenchymal nodules, pleural effusions, and mediastinal and hilar adenopathy, features distinctly unusual in most cases of PCP (Table 1). These findings are significant given the degree of difficulty in making a premortem diagnosis. While controversial, a high degree of suspicion is warranted despite the progressive nature of pulmonary KS, as short-lived palliation has been reported with combination chemotherapy (68,69).

## LYMPHOPROLIFERATIVE DISEASES

### Lymphocytic Interstitial Pneumonitis

Lymphocytic interstitial pneumonitis (LIP) is a diffuse pulmonary disorder characterized by the interstitial accummulation of mature lymphocytes, plasma cells, and reticuloendothelial cells. Frequently idiopathic, LIP also is associated with a wide variety of immunologic disorders such as Sjoren syndrome, systemic lupus erythematosis, myasthenia gravis, pernicious anemia, and chronic active hepatitis. This disorder is also considered diagnostic of AIDS when confirmed histologically in a child under 13 years of age, or if documented in serologically positive adults (5,6,70).

LIP may be indistinguishable clinically and radiographically from other opportunistic infections (Fig. 35). Diagnosis usually requires open-lung biopsy, although the diagnosis has been made by TBB (71). Histologically there is evidence of diffuse infiltration of the alveolar septa and peribronchial areas with a variable

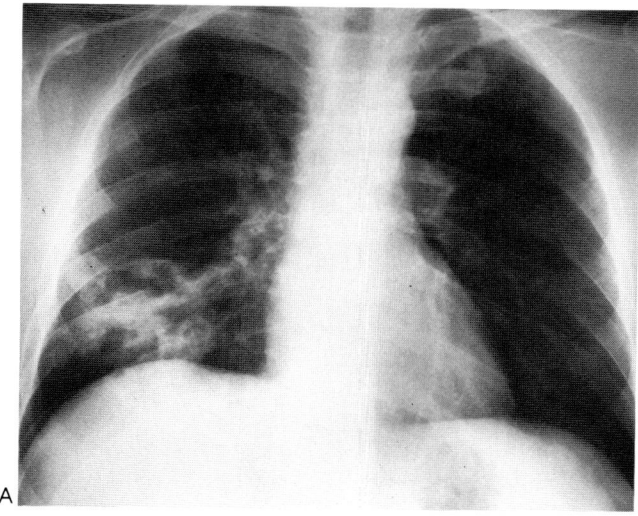
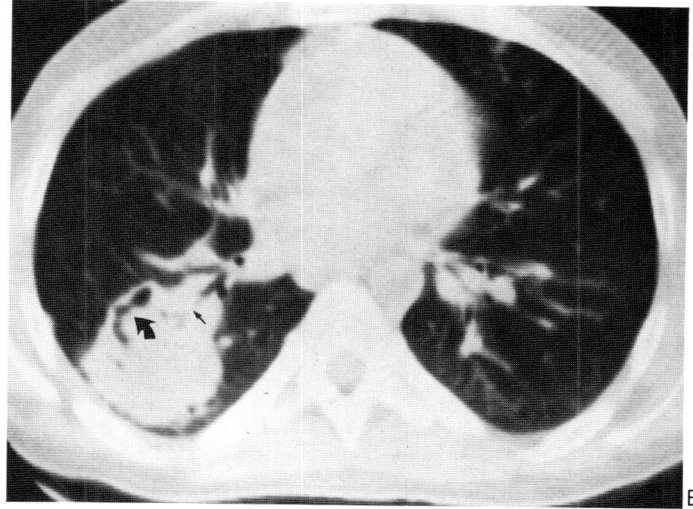

**FIG. 24.** Nocardia asteroides. **A:** PA radiograph. There are focal, bilateral cavitary infiltrates in both lungs. Note the absence of effusions and adenopathy. These findings are characteristic of necrotizing bacterial infections. **B:** Corresponding CT scan shows an ill-defined mass in the right lower lobe within which a crescentic-appearing area of cavitation can be identified (*curved arrow*). The basilar segmental bronchi are patent, although there is some attenuation of the lateral basilar segmental bronchus (*arrow*). Diagnosis confirmed by TBB in the region of the right lower lobe.

admixture of inflammatory cells, frequently associated with nodular aggregates of lymphoid cells with germinal centers. Isolation of HIV in bronchoalveolar lavage fluid has been documented in select cases, as well as significantly elevated concentrations of HIV-specific antibodies (72,73). These findings are consistent with the idea that LIP may represent a direct and specific immune response to HIV pulmonary infection. In support of this hypothesis, Chayt et al. (74) have documented the presence of cells in the lung infected with HIV in a patient with LIP by the technique of *in situ* molecular hybridization. Whatever the etiology, clinical response has

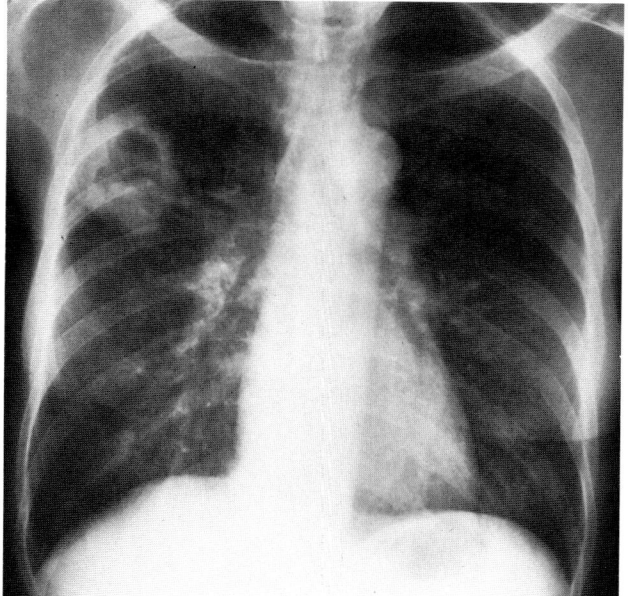
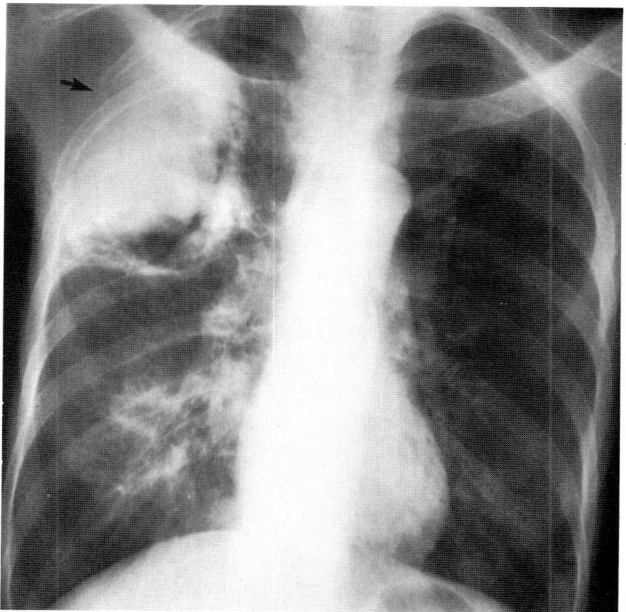

**FIG. 25.** P. carinii/MTB/Aspergillus fumigatus/Squamous cell carcinoma. **A:** PA radiograph demonstrates an irregular cavity in the right upper lobe within which there is a well-defined filling defect. In addition, there are subtle, bilateral perihilar infiltrates. Initial TBB confirmed all three infections. The cavity was of uncertain age. **B:** PA radiograph obtained several months later documents the presence of a large mass in the right upper lobe which has eroded several adjacent ribs (*arrow*). Sputum proved positive for malignant squamous cells.

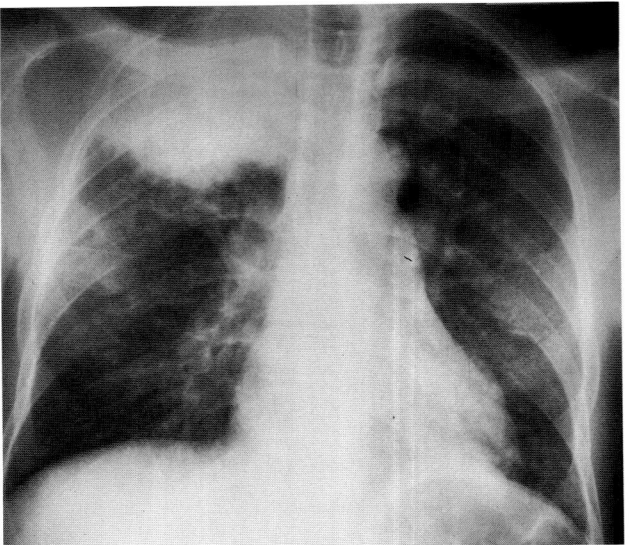

FIG. 26. Legionella pneumonia. PA radiograph shows an area of dense consolidation in the right upper lobe. The diagnosis was confirmed by direct fluorescent antibody (DFA) stains. While focal consolidation occasionally may be caused by PCP, especially when dense or cavitary, consolidation should raise a suspicion of bacterial infection, including staphylococcal or gram-negative pneumonia.

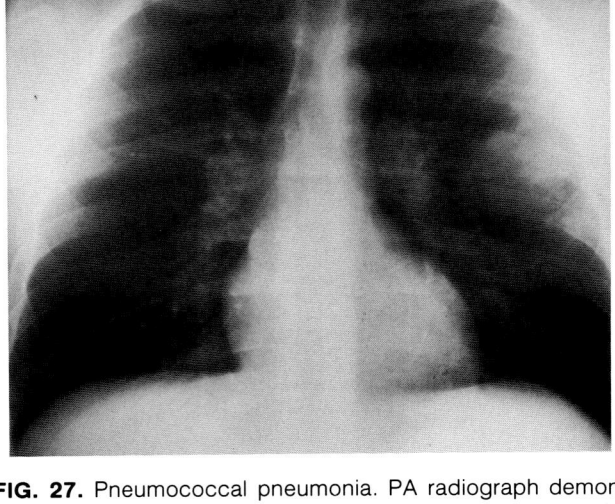

FIG. 27. Pneumococcal pneumonia. PA radiograph demonstrates focal, poorly defined air-space consolidation in the lingula. Diagnosis established by sputum culture and response to appropriate antibiotic therapy.

been documented following appropriate immunosuppressive therapy, making histologic confirmation mandatory in suspected cases (68).

## AIDS-RELATED LYMPHOMA

Primary central nervous system (CNS) lymphomas and undifferentiated lymphomas are now recognized by the CDC as critera for the diagnosis of AIDS (5,6) (see Appendix A). Most are non-Hodgkin's lymphomas (NHLs), primarily of B-cell phenotype, although an increased incidence of all lymphomas, including Hodgkin's disease, has been noted (75–85). Similar to lymphomas that arise in immunosuppressed patients from other causes, such as renal transplant recipients, AIDS-related lymphomas (ARLs) have in common a tendency

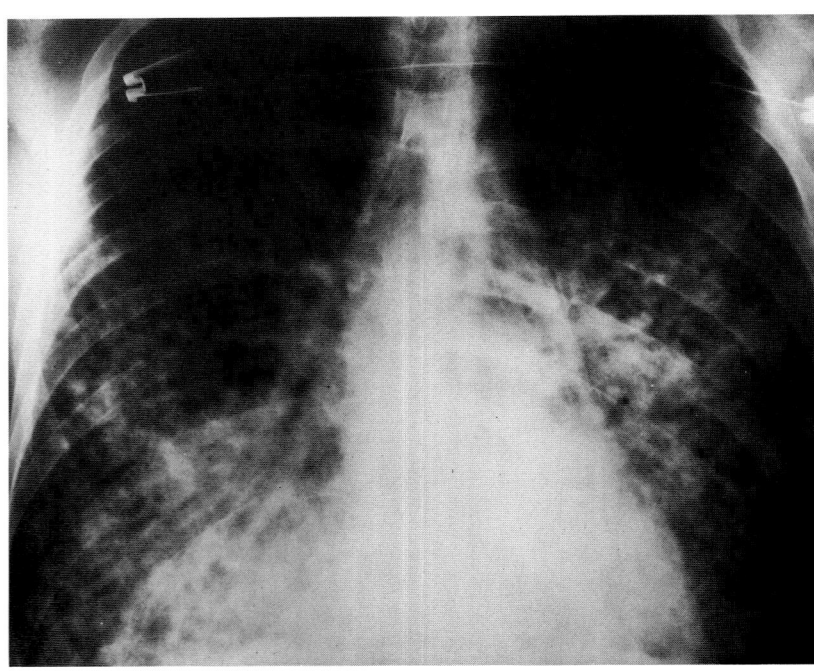

FIG. 28. Disseminated toxoplasmosis. PA radiograph shows diffuse, nonspecific infiltrates in both lungs. The mediastinal contour is grossly normal. TBB-proven toxoplasmosis.

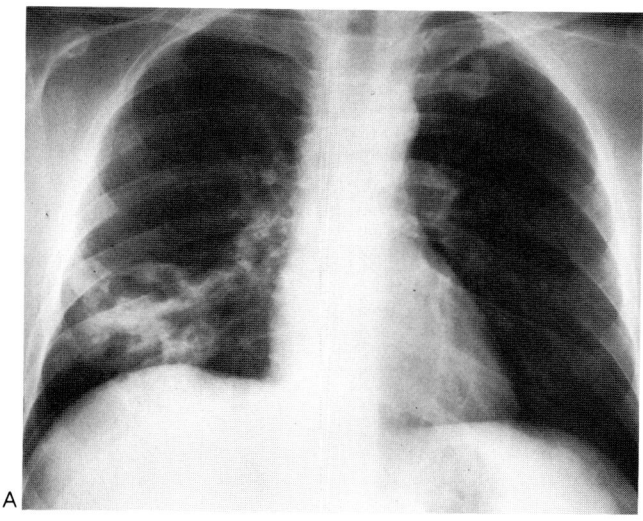
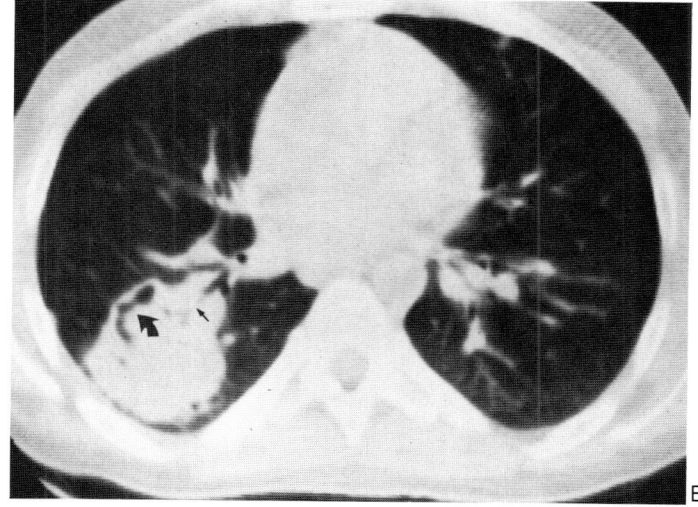

**FIG. 24.** Nocardia asteroides. **A:** PA radiograph. There are focal, bilateral cavitary infiltrates in both lungs. Note the absence of effusions and adenopathy. These findings are characteristic of necrotizing bacterial infections. **B:** Corresponding CT scan shows an ill-defined mass in the right lower lobe within which a crescentic-appearing area of cavitation can be identified (*curved arrow*). The basilar segmental bronchi are patent, although there is some attenuation of the lateral basilar segmental bronchus (*arrow*). Diagnosis confirmed by TBB in the region of the right lower lobe.

admixture of inflammatory cells, frequently associated with nodular aggregates of lymphoid cells with germinal centers. Isolation of HIV in bronchoalveolar lavage fluid has been documented in select cases, as well as significantly elevated concentrations of HIV-specific antibodies (72,73). These findings are consistent with the idea that LIP may represent a direct and specific immune response to HIV pulmonary infection. In support of this hypothesis, Chayt et al. (74) have documented the presence of cells in the lung infected with HIV in a patient with LIP by the technique of *in situ* molecular hybridization. Whatever the etiology, clinical response has

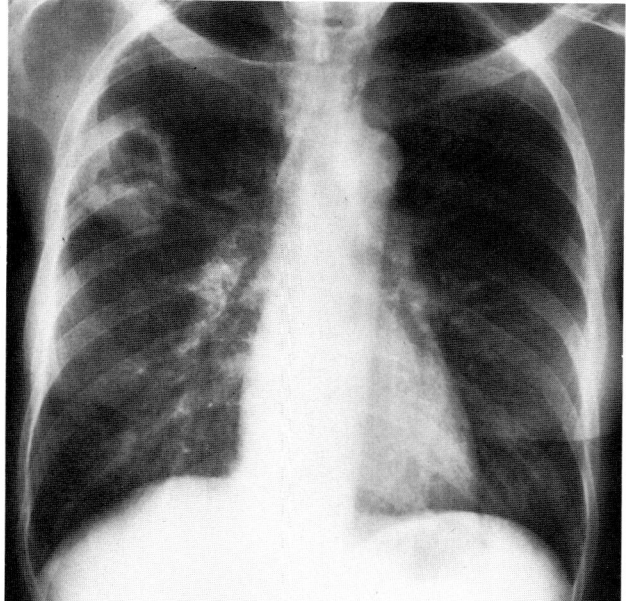
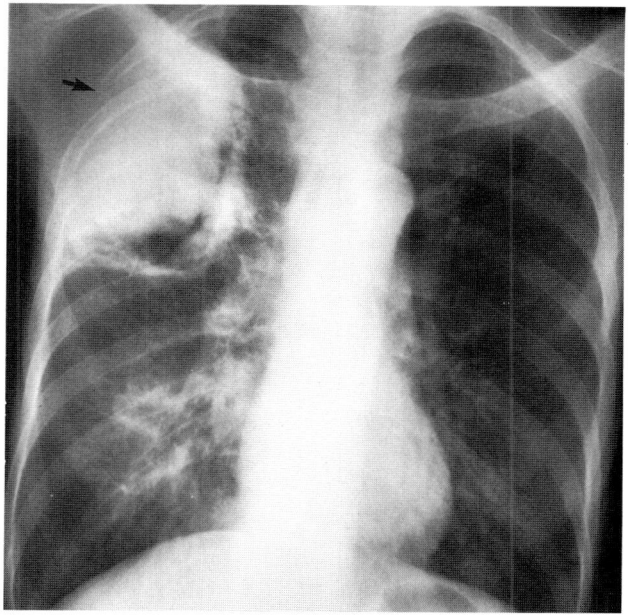

**FIG. 25.** P. carinii/MTB/Aspergillus fumigatus/Squamous cell carcinoma. **A:** PA radiograph demonstrates an irregular cavity in the right upper lobe within which there is a well-defined filling defect. In addition, there are subtle, bilateral perihilar infiltrates. Initial TBB confirmed all three infections. The cavity was of uncertain age. **B:** PA radiograph obtained several months later documents the presence of a large mass in the right upper lobe which has eroded several adjacent ribs (*arrow*). Sputum proved positive for malignant squamous cells.

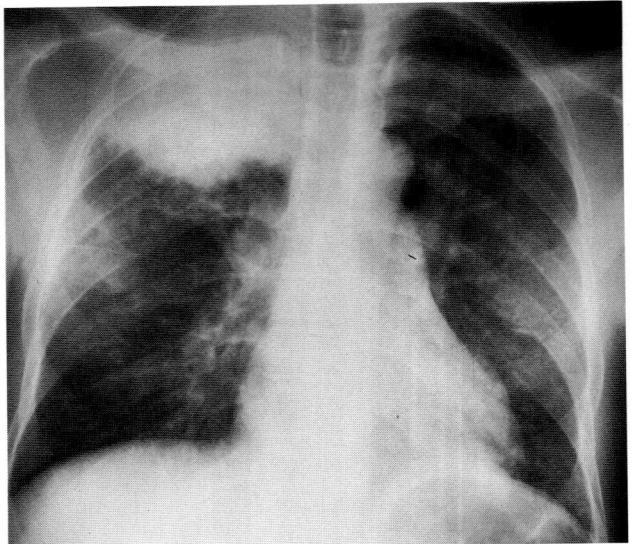

**FIG. 26.** Legionella pneumonia. PA radiograph shows an area of dense consolidation in the right upper lobe. The diagnosis was confirmed by direct fluorescent antibody (DFA) stains. While focal consolidation occasionally may be caused by PCP, especially when dense or cavitary, consolidation should raise a suspicion of bacterial infection, including staphylococcal or gram-negative pneumonia.

**FIG. 27.** Pneumococcal pneumonia. PA radiograph demonstrates focal, poorly defined air-space consolidation in the lingula. Diagnosis established by sputum culture and response to appropriate antibiotic therapy.

been documented following appropriate immunosuppressive therapy, making histologic confirmation mandatory in suspected cases (68).

## AIDS-RELATED LYMPHOMA

Primary central nervous system (CNS) lymphomas and undifferentiated lymphomas are now recognized by the CDC as critera for the diagnosis of AIDS (5,6) (see Appendix A). Most are non-Hodgkin's lymphomas (NHLs), primarily of B-cell phenotype, although an increased incidence of all lymphomas, including Hodgkin's disease, has been noted (75–85). Similar to lymphomas that arise in immunosuppressed patients from other causes, such as renal transplant recipients, AIDS-related lymphomas (ARLs) have in common a tendency

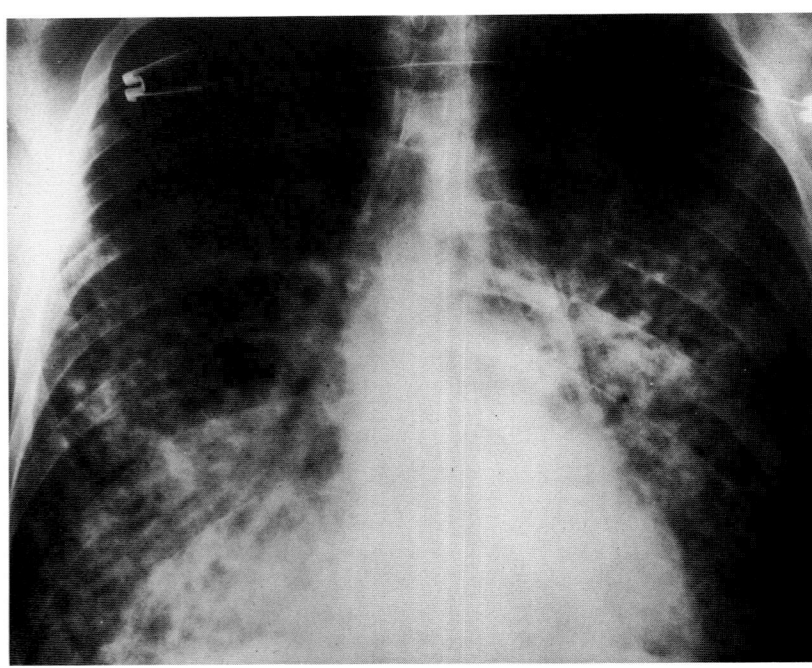

**FIG. 28.** Disseminated toxoplasmosis. PA radiograph shows diffuse, nonspecific infiltrates in both lungs. The mediastinal contour is grossly normal. TBB-proven toxoplasmosis.

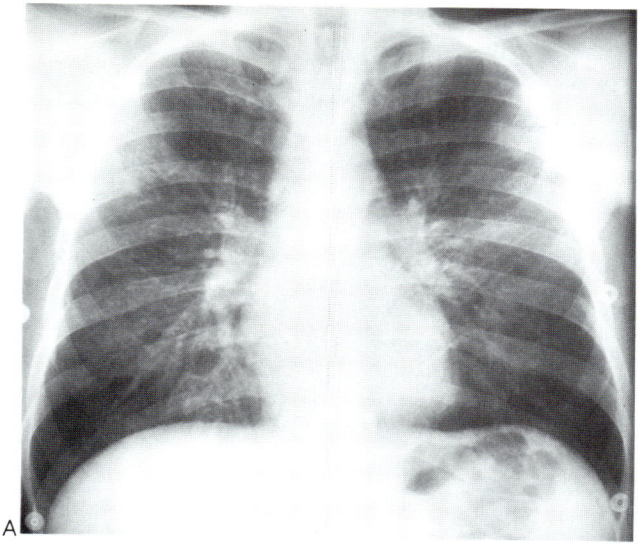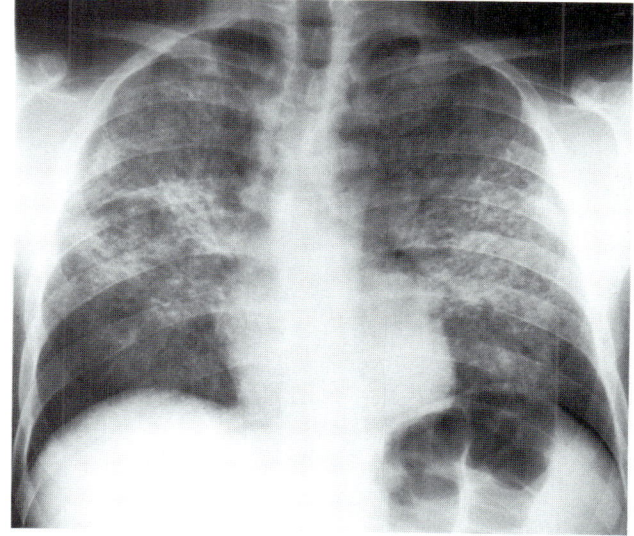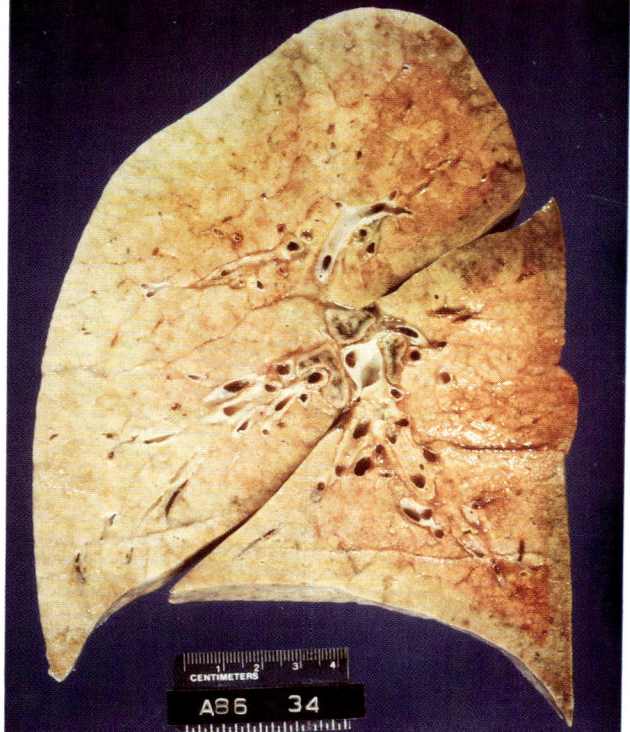

**Color Plate 1 (FIG. 1).** Pneumocystis carinii pneumonia. **A:** PA radiograph shows usual appearance of bilateral, perihilar infiltrates, without adenopathy or evidence of effusions. **B:** Follow-up PA radiograph shows typical appearance of rapidly progressive disease. **C:** Section of fixed lung specimen demonstrates grayish, diffusely consolidated parenchyma with focal areas of hemorrhage. Histologically verified PCP.

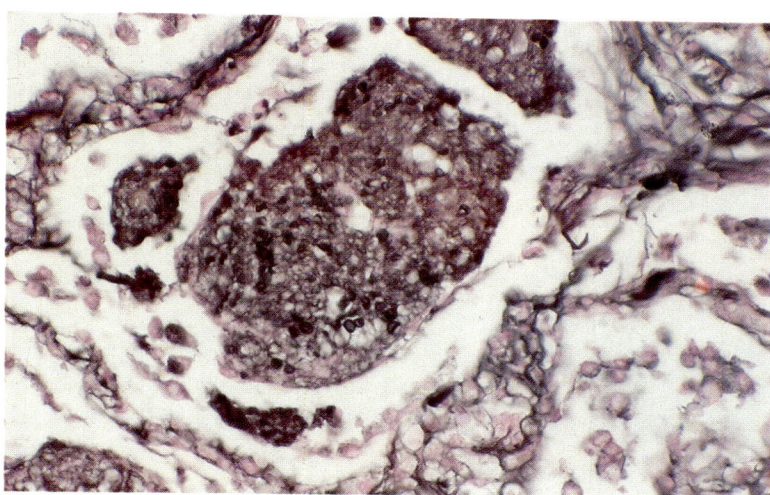

**Color Plate 2 (FIG. 2).** Pneumocystis carinii pneumonia. Histologic section from a TBB. PCP is characterized predominantly by intraalveolar foamy exudates within which individual round cysts can be identified (silver methenamine stain)

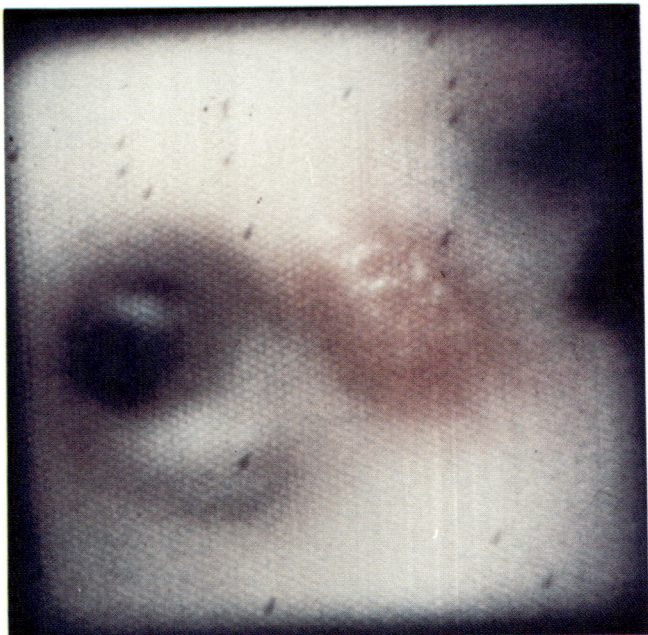

**Color Plate 3 (FIG. 29).** KS. Image of the carina obtained at bronchoscopy shows a discrete, slightly raised, violacious lesion, characteristic endoscopically of endobronchial KS.

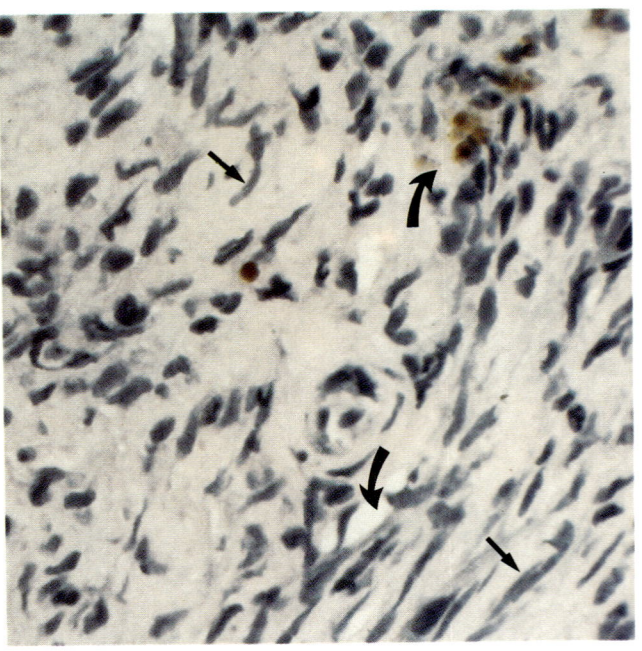

**Color Plate 4 (FIG. 30).** KS. Histologic section from an open-lung biopsy showing characteristic features of KS. This tumor consists of aggregated spindle cells (*arrows*) often containing atypical nuclei and occasional mitoses that tend to surround small bronchi and blood vessels. Vascular slits and hemosiderin deposits are characteristically present as well (*curved arrows*).

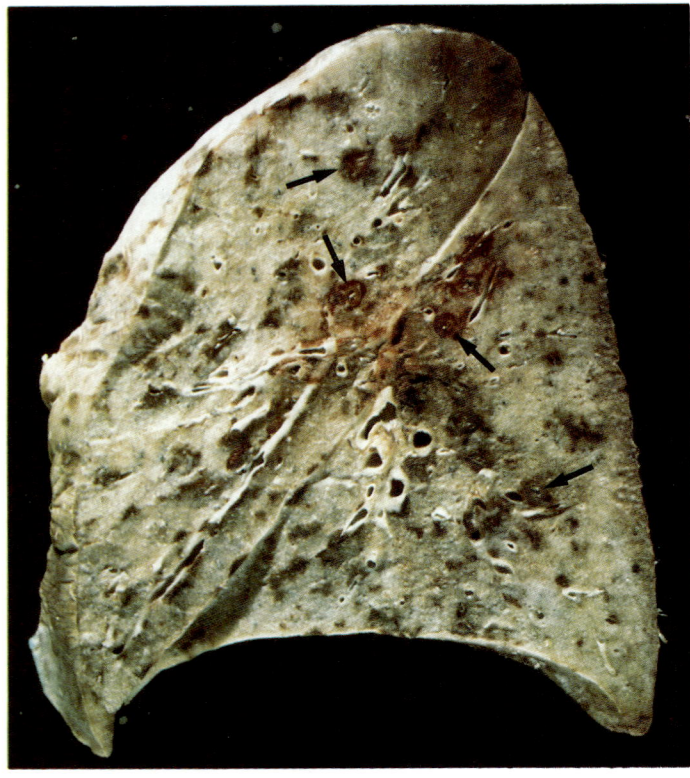

**Color Plate 5 (FIG. 31).** KS. Section of fixed lung shows innumerable, scattered foci of tumor in a characteristically perivascular and peribronchial distribution (*arrows*).

**TABLE 2.** *KS: Radiographic findings*

| | | | Parenchymal findings | | | | Associated findings | | |
|---|---|---|---|---|---|---|---|---|---|
| Author | No. of patients | Perihilar/ diffuse infiltrates | Nodules/ nodular infiltrates | Focal disease | Normal | Pleural effusions | Hilar/ mediastinal adenopathy | History of previous or concurrent infection | Evidence of concurrent or prior cutaneous/ visceral KS |
| Garay et al. (61) | 19 | 11 | 5 | 1 | 1 | 3 | 5 | 15 | 18 |
| Zibrak et al. (63) | 8 | 6 | 2 | — | — | 4 | 5 | 2 | 8 |
| Sivit et al. (64) | 9 | 4 | 2 | 2 | 1 | 3 | 3 | — | 7 |
| Meduri et al. (65) | 11 | 2 | 6 | 3 | — | 6 | — | 5 | 11 |
| Ognibene et al. (66) | 12 | 12 | — | — | — | 4 | — | 6 | 12 |
| Davis et al. (62) | 24 | 16 | 3 | — | 4 | 16 | 12 | 21 | 22 |
| Total | 83 | 51 (61%) | 18 (22%) | 6 (7%) | 6 (7%) | 36 (43%) | 25 (30%) | 49 (59%) | 78 (94%) |

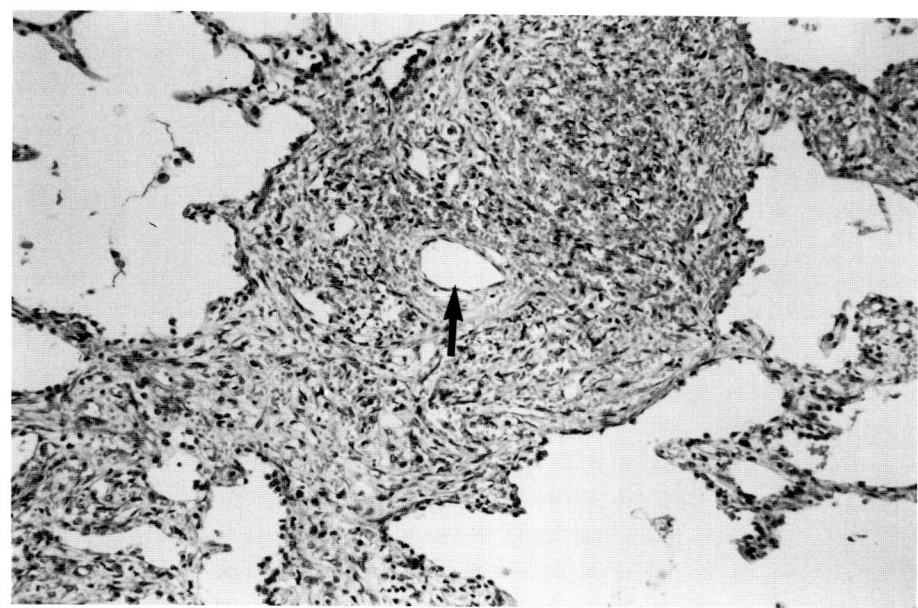

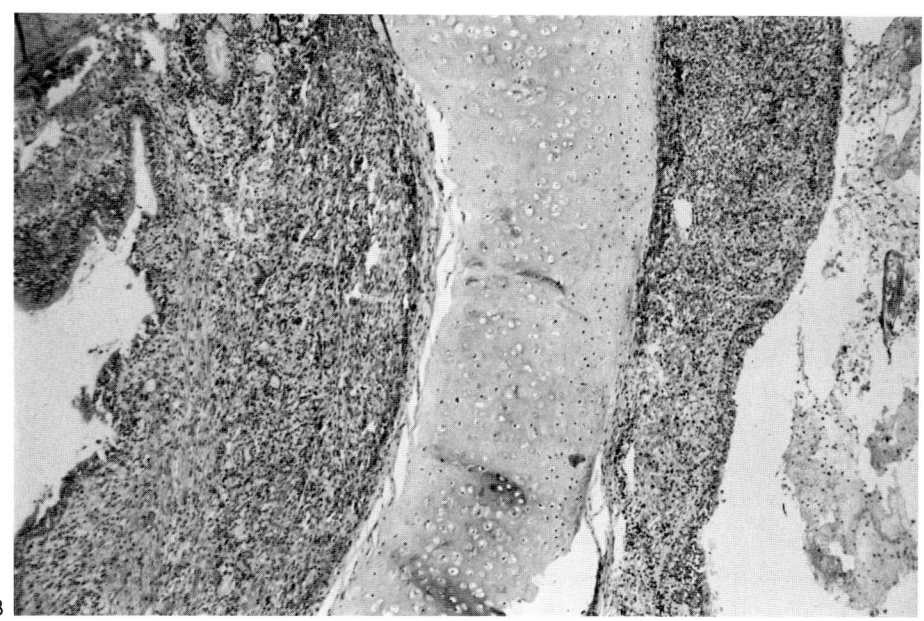

**FIG. 32.** KS. **A:** Histologic section obtained at autopsy shows aggregated spindle cells and vascular slits distinctly perivascular in distribution, characteristic of KS (*arrow*). The tumor forms a poorly defined nodular mass that extends peripherally along interstitial pathways (compare with Fig. 31). **B:** Histologic section in the same patient as shown in A through a central airway demonstrates typical peribronchial distribution with tumor identifiable on both sides of the bronchial cartilage.

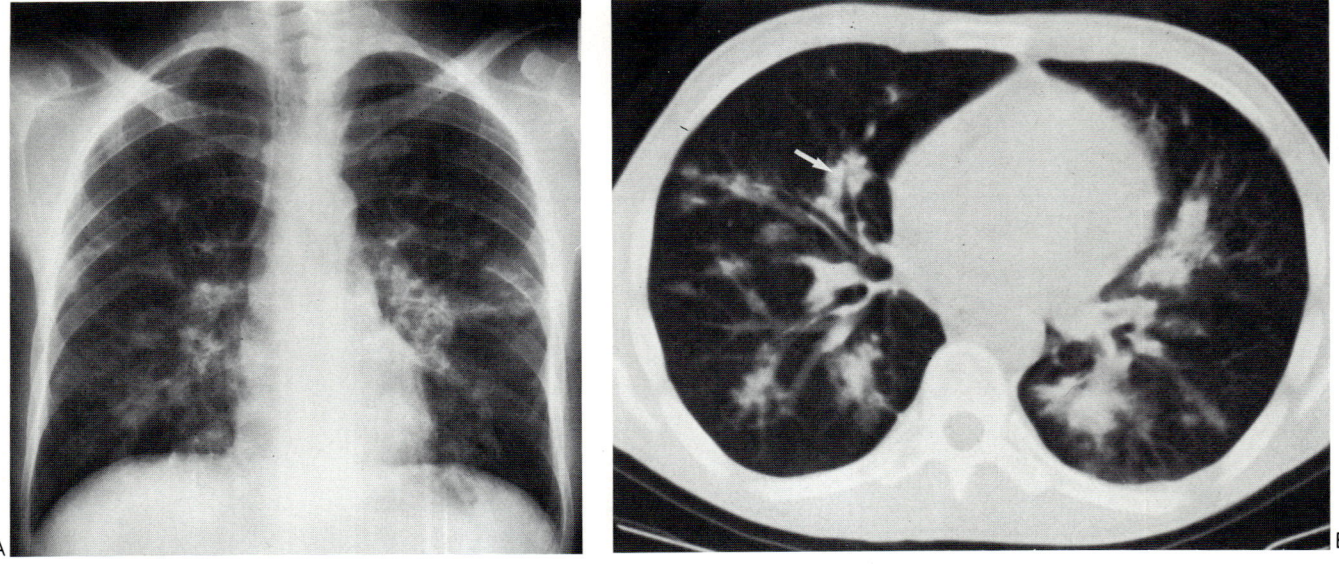

**FIG. 33.** KS. **A:** PA radiograph shows ill-defined, bilateral nodular densities. **B:** CT section documents the presence of poorly marginated parenchymal opacities scattered throughout the lungs, some of which are clearly peribronchial in distribution (*arrow*). Open-lung biopsy documented KS.

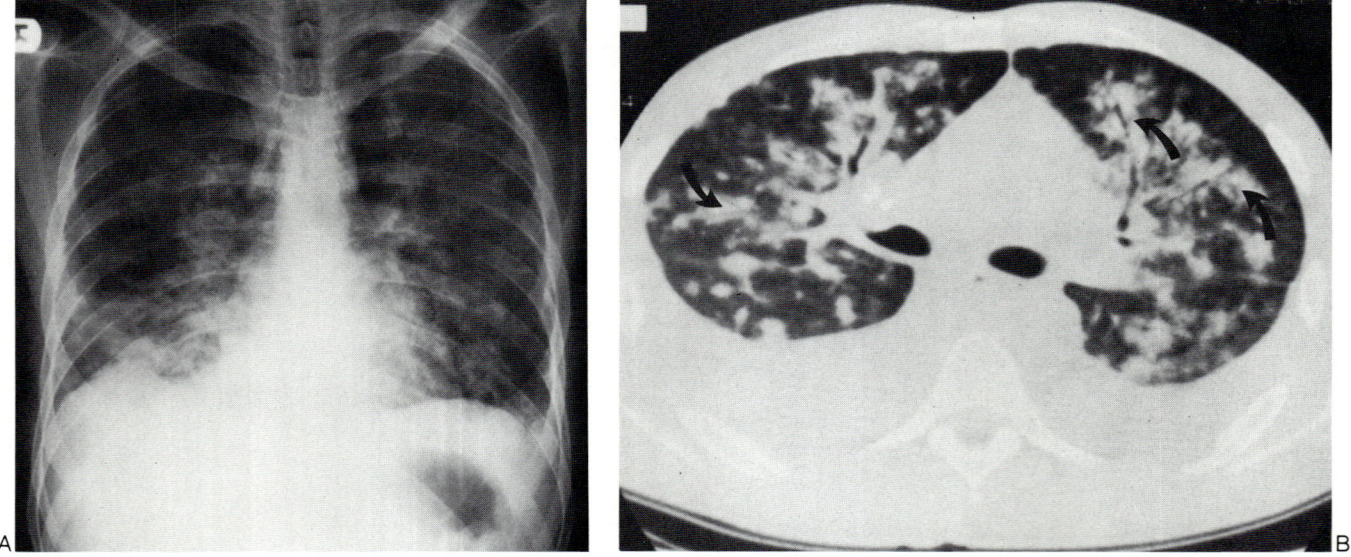

**FIG. 34.** KS. **A:** PA radiograph shows diffuse parenchymal infiltrates with a suggestion of nodularity, associated with a moderate bilateral pleural effusions and subtle mediastinal widening. **B:** CT section shows extensive nodular infiltrates throughout the lungs, many of which have a distinctly peribronchial distribution (*arrows*).

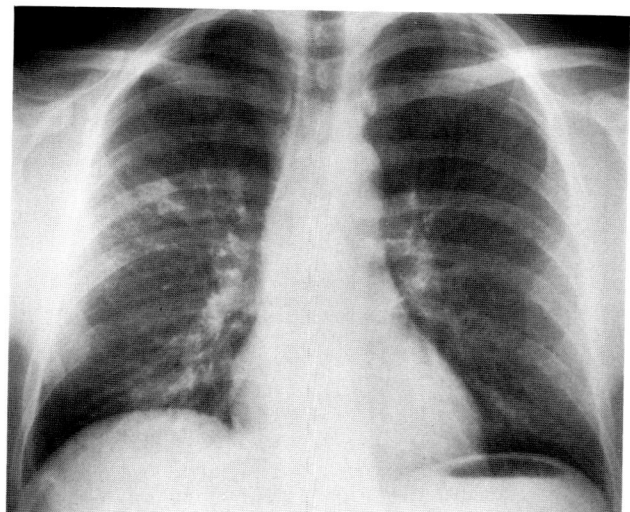

**FIG. 35.** LIP. PA radiograph shows evidence of very subtle, increased linear parenchymal markings bilaterally; a nodular density is present in the right upper lobe. These findings, including the presence of a nodular density, are nondescript. Open-lung biopsy documented LIP.

to be highly aggressive tumors with poorly differentiated histologic subtypes associated with a poor prognosis. Typically, disease is in an advanced stage at the time of diagnosis.

ARLs are primarily extranodal in distribution (76–78). Pathologically, involvement is most frequently noted in the CNS, the gastrointestinal system, and the liver, spleen, and bone marrow. Thoracic involvement is relatively rare and often difficult to document. Significantly, in a series of 70 patients reported by Marchevsky et al. (86), only two patients were documented to have pulmonary lymphoma; both cases were associated only with bilateral interstitial changes, and in one case, an associated left pleural effusion. Isolated mediastinal and hilar lymphadenopathy may occur, although pulmonary parenchymal involvement may predominate, with parenchymal disease presenting as extensive, rapidly progressive tumor infiltration, or even as isolated, focal pulmonary nodules or masses (Figs. 36–39). While nonspecific, adenopathy is significant; as emphasized by Stern et al. (85), enlarged hilar and mediastinal nodes are not present in patients with lymphadenopathy syndrome.

### Other Neoplasms

Other malignancies associated with AIDS are rare, and no clear association has been established, although this possibility has not been excluded. In a recent report of 29 AIDS patients who developed malignancies, four nonlymphomatous, solid tumors were noted, each in patients over 50 years of age (78). While the authors concluded that these may represent the chance occurrence of age-appropriate tumors, we recently have seen solid tumors develop in relatively younger patients as well (Figs. 25 and 40; see also Chapter 1). While suggestive, at present, any potential association between nonlymphomatous tumors and AIDS remains speculative.

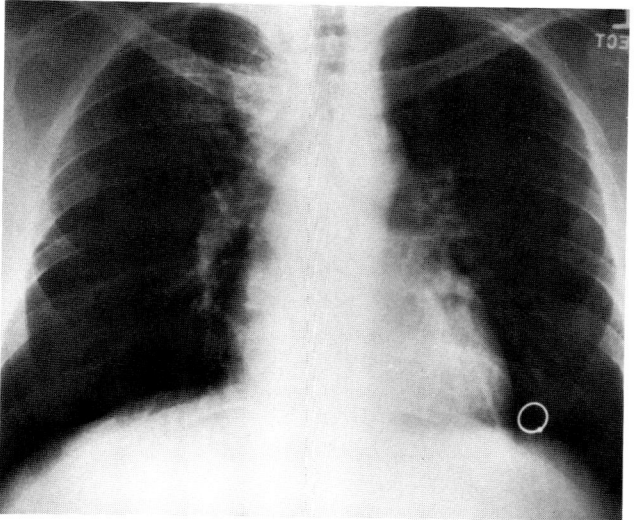
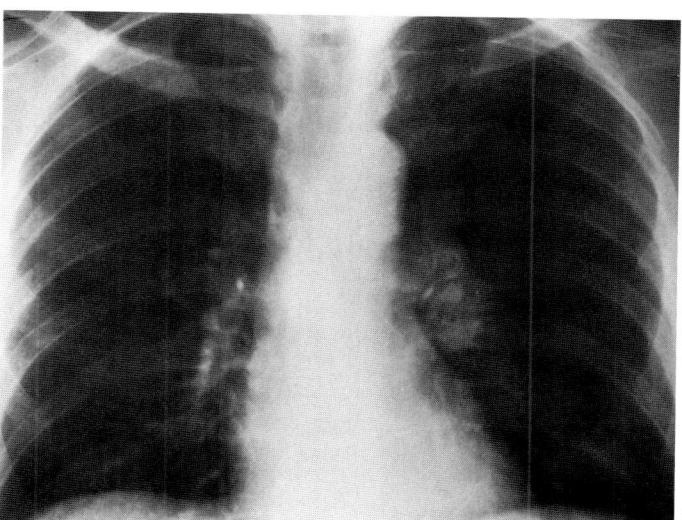

**FIG. 36.** NHL. **A:** PA radiograph shows mediastinal and bilateral hilar enlargement compatible with extensive adenopathy. Ill-defined parenchymal changes can be identified in the right upper lobe. A nipple ring is present on the left. NHL diagnosed by percutaneous biopsy of enlarged retroperitoneal lymph nodes. Mediastinal nodes subsequently responded to appropriate therapy. **B:** PA radiograph in another patient demonstrates a markedly enlarged, nodular left hilum. NHL established at thoracotomy.

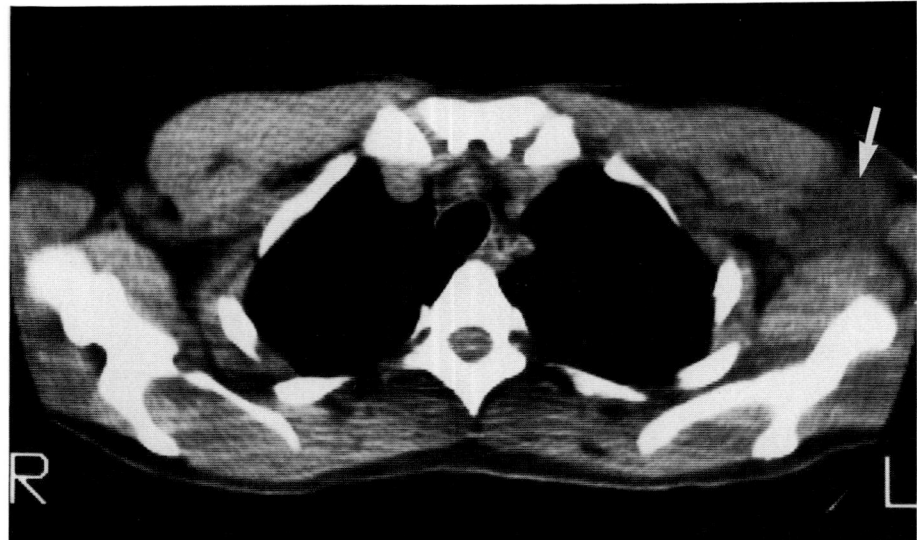

**FIG. 37.** Burkitt lymphoma. CT section through the great vessels demonstrates an ill-defined soft tissue mass in the left axilla (*arrow*), the only evidence of thoracic disease in this patient. Axillary lymph node biopsy confirmed Burkitt lymphoma.

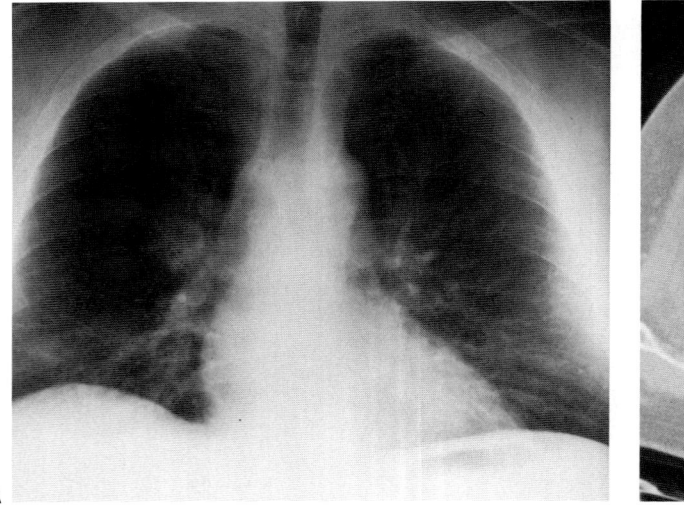
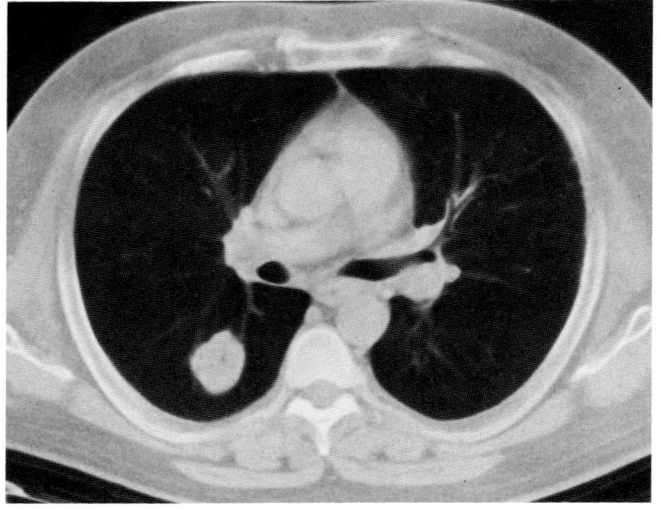

**FIG. 38.** NHL. **A:** PA radiograph demonstrates a well-defined mass near the right hilum. **B:** CT section through the mid-lung field demonstrates a well-defined soft tissue mass in the superior segment of the right lower lobe. No other abnormalities are present. Open-lung biopsy documented NHL.

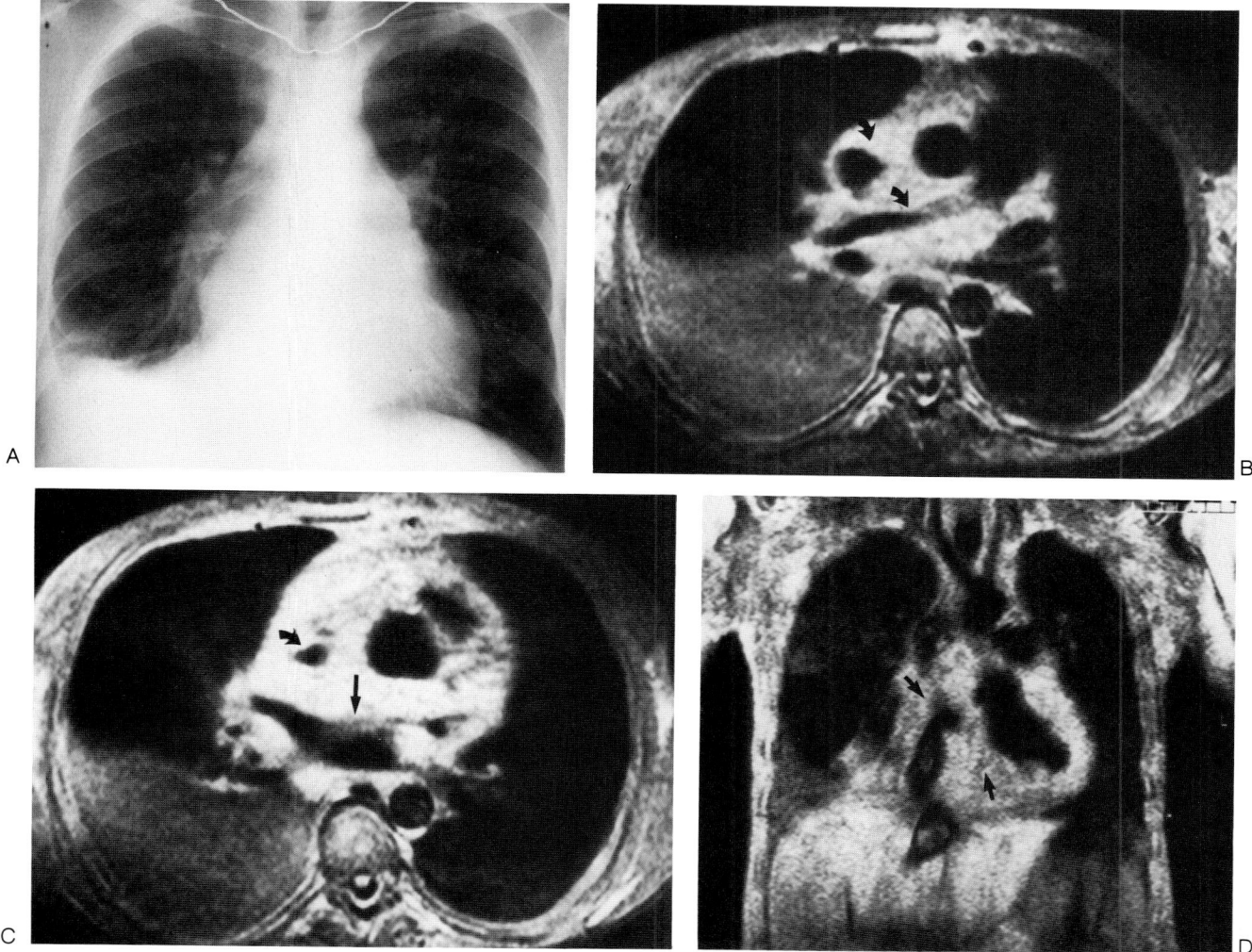

**FIG. 39.** NHL's—Cardiac involvement. **A:** PA radiograph demonstrates enlargement of both the mediastinum and cardiac silhouette, with increased density identifiable in the retrocardiac region on the left. A moderate-sized right pleural effusion is also present. **B, C:** Transaxial, gated, T1-weighted, MRIs obtained at the level of the right main pulmonary artery and the left atrium, respectively. There is extensive tumor infiltration of the entire mediastinum, identifiable as areas of intermediate signal intensity surrounding and narrowing all of the great vessels (*curved arrows* in B and C), as well as the left atrium (*straight arrow* in C). A large pleural effusion is easily identified on the right side. **D:** Coronal, gated, T1-weighted MRI obtained through the mid-thorax further confirms the extensive, infiltrating nature of this tumor (*arrows*). Histologic confirmation obtained by mediastinoscopy.

## CARDIAC DISEASE

A number of reports have documented a growing awareness of cardiac disease in AIDS patients (87–92). The clinical spectrum of disease includes congestive cardiomyopathy, nonbacterial thrombotic endocarditis, KS, and pericarditis, caused by a wide variety of fungal and viral etiologies. In an autopsy study of 41 patients with AIDS, 10 patients were found to have cardiac disease, including four patients with KS involving coronary arteries, myocardium and pericardium, three with culture-negative thrombotic endocarditis, two with nonspecific pericarditis, and one with cryptococcal myocarditis (87). Generalized cardiomyopathy with focal myocarditis also has been described in the absence of bacterial or parasitic infection, findings suggestive of a viral pathogenesis (88). Myocarditis may lead to the diffuse uptake of gallium, (Fig. 41). In addition to KS, lymphomatous infiltration of the heart may occur, usually in association with signs and symptoms of cardiac dysfunction (Fig. 39) (91,92).

### Gallium Scintigraphy

Numerous reports have documented the utility of gallium-67 citrate scanning in AIDS patients (93–98).

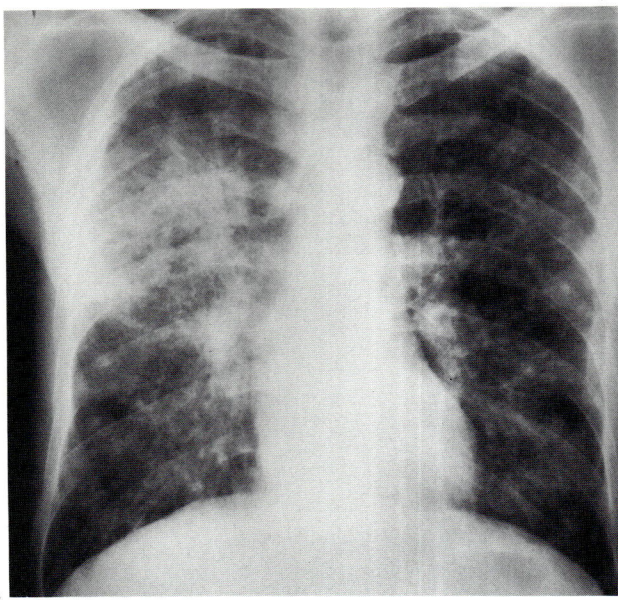 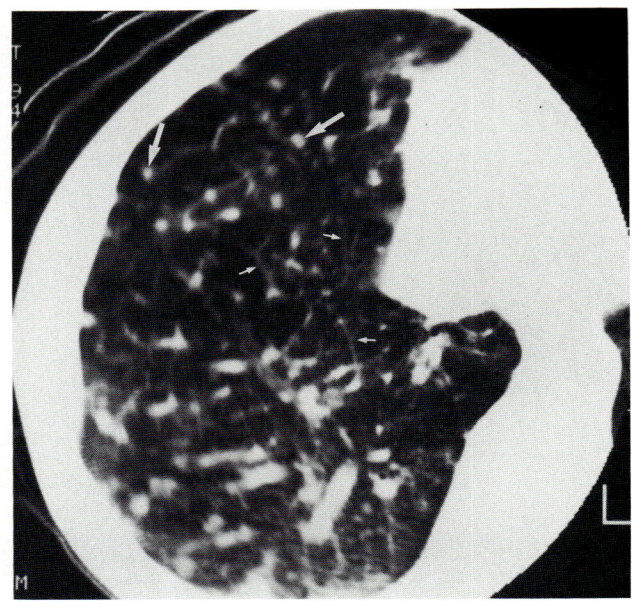

**FIG. 40.** Adenocarcinoma. **A:** PA radiograph shows diffuse nodules in both lungs, associated with mediastinal adenopathy. Coalescent densities are present in the right upper lobe. **B:** Magnified CT section through the right lower lobe. There are numerous scattered nodules throughout the right lower lobe, many of which are associated with adjacent vessels (*large arrows*). In addition, there is marked accentuation of the interstitial markings, especially apparent centrally (*small arrows*). While nonspecific, these findings highly suggest lymphangitic carcinomatosis. TBB-proven adenocarcinoma. Subsequent evaluation revealed diffuse liver metastases, but no obvious primary source of tumor.

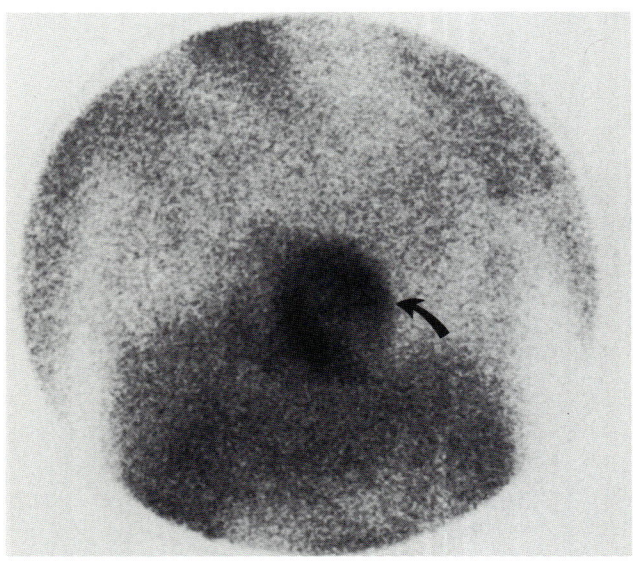

**FIG. 41.** Viral myocarditis. Anterior view of the thorax from a gallium scan obtained at 48 hr. Diffuse myocardial uptake is apparent (*arrow*), significantly greater than that identifiable in the liver and spleen. Little uptake can be identified in the lungs. CMV was subsequently identified from numerous sources, including the bone marrow. The cause of myocardial uptake is presumed secondary to viral myocarditis in the absence of other identified pathogens.

Gallium scanning has played a particularly important role in the detection of PCP, especially when chest radiographs and arterial blood gases are equivocal or normal. Reported sensitivities range from 95 to 100% (93–98) (Table 3). Typically PCP is associated with diffuse pulmonary uptake. Less frequently, localized or perihilar uptake may be identified (Fig. 42). Diffuse uptake is nonspecific; in addition to PCP, this pattern has been identified in patients with a wide range of pulmonary pathogens, as well as in patients with documented, nonspecific interstitial pneumonitis (93,98). Apparent limitations in specificity may be obviated to some degree by use of more selective interpretive criteria. As documented by Coleman et al. (94) use of a grading system based on intensity of uptake increases specificity in the detection of PCP to greater than 90%. A negative correlative radiograph also increases the specificity of a positive scan for PCP (96). Similar specificities have been documented for the value of a negative gallium scan in excluding PCP (93–98), further enhancing the potential role of gallium scintigraphy as a screening test.

Several scan patterns other than diffuse uptake occur, and as noted by Kramer et al. (93), the diagnostic significance of these varies. Focal uptake corresponding to regional lymph nodes commonly is seen with mycobacterial infections and lymphomas (Fig. 43). Significantly,

TABLE 3. Gallium-67 scanning: Results in patients with P. carinii pneumonia

| Author | No. of patients | # of patients with P. carinii pneumonia | Sensitivity* | Specificity* | NL chest x-rays |
|---|---|---|---|---|---|
| Coleman et al. (94) | 22 | 12 | 100%; graded | 20%; nongraded | 4 (33%) |
| Tuazon et al. (95) | 20 | 20 | 100%; graded | 50%; graded | 1 (4%) |
| Barron et al. (96) | 34 | 18 | 93%; nongraded (86%; patients with nl CXR's) | 74%; nongraded (85%; patients with nl CXR's) | 7 (39%) |
| Woolfenden et al. (97) | 33 | 20 | 95%; graded | NA 51%; all patterns nongraded | 3 (18%) |
| Kramer et al. (93) | 71 | 30 | 100%; nongraded | 83%; (diffuse uptake only) | 14 (48%) |

* Grading system as per Coleman et al. (94).
NA, Not applicable.

gallium rarely localizes in patients with KS. In select cases, differential localization may have diagnostic implications (Fig. 44). Localized parenchymal uptake usually correlates with bacterial infection, although this pattern may be seen with PCP (Fig. 44).

## DIAGNOSIS

In October 1983, the National Heart, Lung and Blood Institute (NHLBI) convened a workshop to assess the diagnosis and treatment of pulmonary complications in AIDS patients (3). Of 1,067 patients with the diagnosis of AIDS evaluated by the six participating medical centers, 441 patients (41%) were found to have pulmonary disorders, (Table 4). To facilitate diagnostic evaluation, the following guidelines were adopted by the NHLBI workshop which, with some variations, are still widely accepted.

While other procedures have been proposed as alternate methods for identifying opportunistic infections, including sputum induction and transthoracic needle biopsy, symptomatic patients with diffuse abnormalities noted on chest roentgenograms should have diagnostic fiberoptic bronchoscopy (FOB) (99–103). This should include both BAL and TBB, preferably in combination. As reported by Broaddus et al. (101), in their series of 276 bronchoscopic examinations done on 171 patients

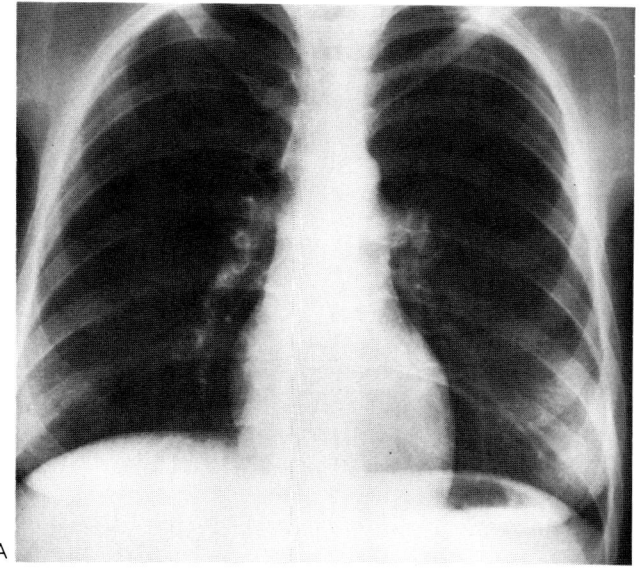 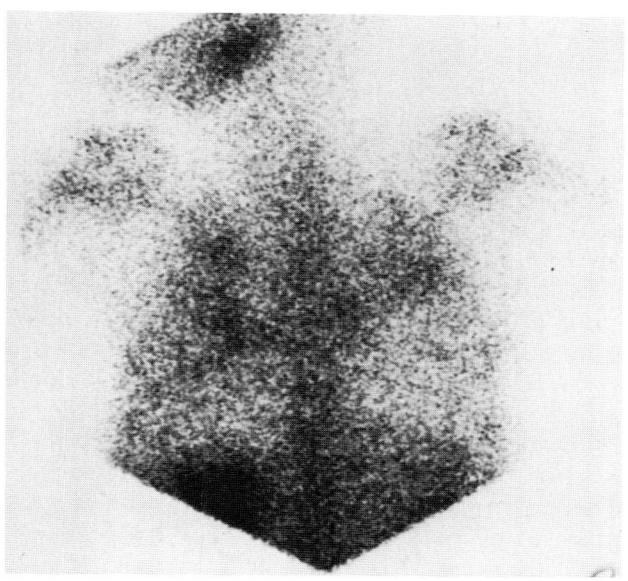

FIG. 42. PCP—Gallium scintigraphy. **A:** Normal chest radiograph. **B:** Gallium scan of the thorax obtained at the same time as the radiograph shown above. There is considerable activity identifiable throughout the lungs bilaterally. Bronchoalveolar lavage documented PCP. (Courtesy of Dr. Howard Banner, Department of Nuclear Medicine, Bellevue Hospital, New York, N.Y.)

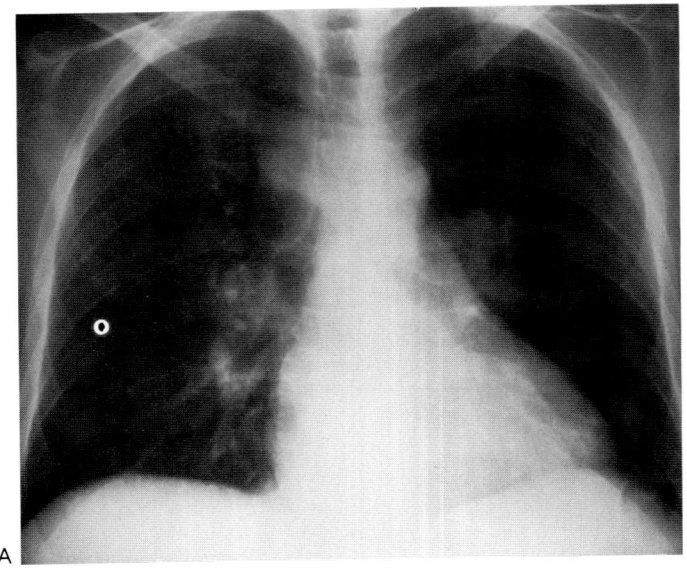
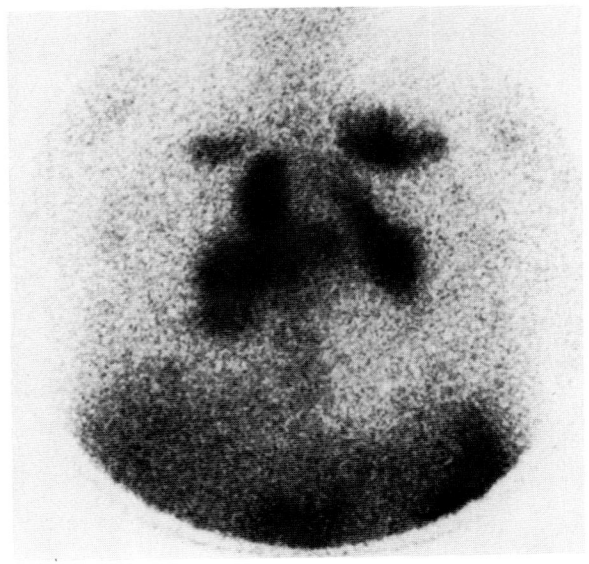
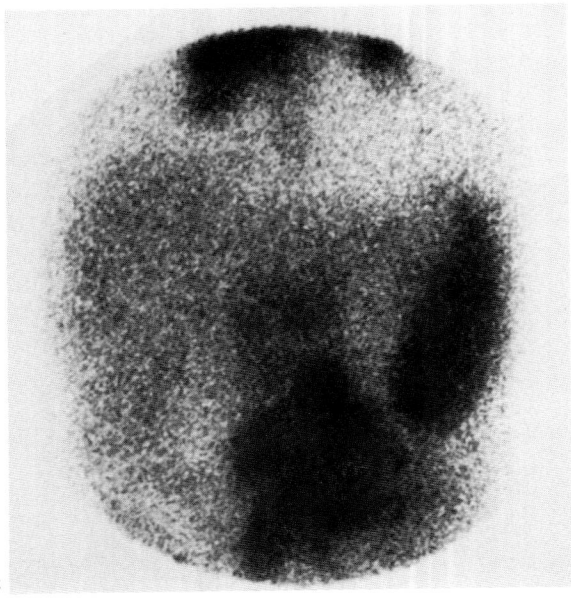

**FIG. 43.** MAI—Gallium scintigraphy. **A:** PA radiograph shows diffuse mediastinal and hilar adenopathy. **B:** Anterior view of the thorax from a gallium study demonstrates focal nodal accumulation in the mediastinum and hila, as well as the supraclavicular fossa, especially on the left. While nonspecific, nodal accumulation is usually due to mycobacterial infection or lymphoma; significantly, gallium accumulation is only rarely associated with KS (compare with Fig. 44). **C:** Anterior view of the abdomen confirms the presence of widely scattered mesenteric and retroperitoneal nodes in this patient with documented disseminated TB.

with known or suspected AIDS, BAL and TBB proved to have sensitivities of 86 and 87% respectively, in the detection of all pathogens combined. When BAL and TBB were combined, the yield for all pathogens was 98%; the sensitivity for P. carinii alone was 100%. Similar results have been reported in the diagnosis of PCP using only BAL. Golden et al. (102) prospectively evaluated 40 consecutive potential AIDS patients presenting with respiratory complaints; in this series, P. carinii was documented in 36 of 37 patients (97%) (102). Because of its low complication rate, BAL alone has been advocated in particular for patients with bleeding diatheses or for those requiring mechanical ventilation. Because the organism load appears overwhelming, induction of sputum has proved effective. Initial reports of induced sputum suggests a diagnostic sensitivity ranging from 57 to 78% for PCP.

The role of open-lung biopsy in AIDS patients is more controversial (68,69). Fitzgerald et al. (68), in their retrospective review of 42 patients, found open-lung biopsy to be of value specifically for patients in whom bronchoscopy proved nondiagnostic, or for whom the procedure was contraindicated. Open-lung biopsy was significantly less beneficial when used to evaluate patients because of progressive deterioration, despite treatment for diseases initially diagnosed bronchoscopically.

Despite limitations, radiographic interpretation plays an important role in the initial work-up and management of patients suspected of having AIDS. While there is considerable overlap in the radiographic appearances

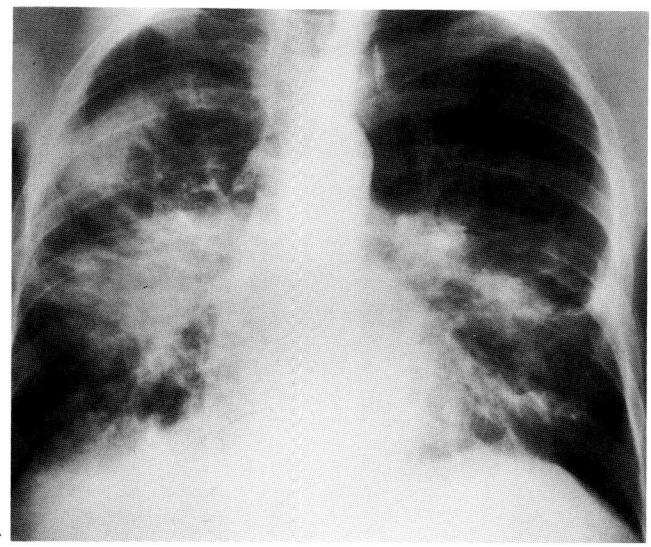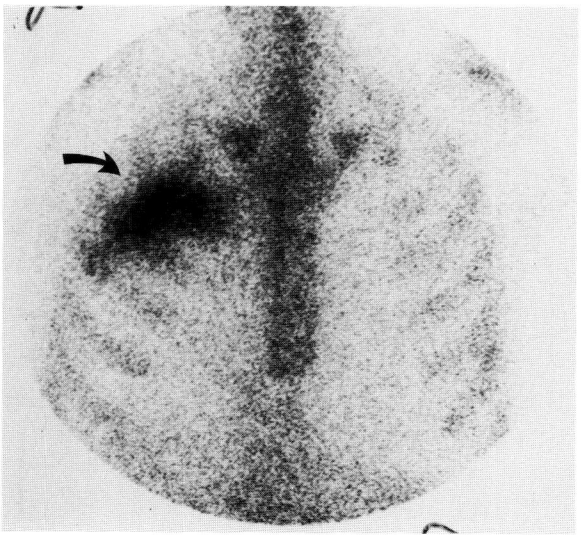

FIG. 44. KS/Klebsiella pneumonia—Gallium scintigraphy. **A:** PA radiograph shows diffuse, asymmetric pulmonary infiltrates in a patient with known cutaneous KS. **B:** Anterior view from a gallium scan obtained at 48 hours shows intense uptake, largely limited to the right upper lobe (*arrow*). TBB directed to the right upper lobe revealed Klebsiella pneumonia. Subsequent biopsies of the right lower lobe revealed KS. This case illustrates the potential value of gallium scintigraphy to enhance bronchoscopic evaluation.

of many of the most common AIDS-related pulmonary disorders, it is possible to establish diagnostic priorities (Table 5). The following interpretative guidelines are suggested:

**TABLE 4.** *Types and frequency of pulmonary disorders in 441 patients with AIDS\**

| Pulmonary disorder | No. of patients | % |
|---|---|---|
| PCP | 373 | 84.6 |
|   Without coexisting infection | 255 | 57.8 |
|   With coexisting infection | 118 | 26.8 |
|     CMV | 50 | 11.3 |
|     MAI | 37 | 8.4 |
|     MTB | 15 | 3.5 |
|     Legionella | 9 | 2.0 |
|     Cryptococcus | 8 | 1.8 |
|     Other | 3 | 0.6 |
| Other pulmonary infections | 93 | 21.1 |
|   MAI | 37 | 8.4 |
|   CMV | 18 | 4.0 |
|   CMV/MAI | 5 | 1.1 |
|   CMV/cryptococcus | 1 | 0.2 |
|   Pyogenic bacteria | 11 | 2.5 |
|   Legionella | 10 | 2.3 |
|   Fungi | 6 | 1.4 |
|   MTB | 4 | 0.9 |
|   Herpes simplex | 2 | 0.5 |
|   Toxoplasmosis | 1 | 0.2 |
| KS | 36 | 8.2 |

\* (Modified from ref. 3)

1. There are no pathognomonic radiographic abnormalities; histologic or bacteriologic confirmation needs to be obtained whenever possible in order to maximize therapy and limit unnecessary adverse drug reactions.

2. Opportunistic infection and tumor may be present despite a normal-appearing chest radiograph. When symptomatic, in the presence of borderline arterial blood gases (especially following exercise), or diffusing capacity, patients should be evaluated further with a Gallium scan.

3. Mediastinal and hilar adenopathy always should be interpreted as indicative of serious intrathoracic disease. Adenopathy should not be interpreted as a manifestation of the diffuse lymphadenopathy syndrome, or AIDS-related complex (ARC). In our experience, adenopathy is a distinctly unusual manifestation of PCP, and instead is most frequently caused by myobacterial infections, fungi, KS, and lymphoma. Similar diagnostic considerations apply to the identification of both unilateral and bilateral pleural disease.

4. While focal parenchymal disease may be a manifestation of PCP, the increasing incidence of serious bacterial infections in patients with AIDS justifies an aggressive diagnostic approach in order to identify potentially treatable infections.

5. CT may be of value in select cases in which TBB or transthoracic biopsy is planned for precise localization, or to exclude the presence of parenchymal cysts in high-risk patients. Similarly, CT can be used to map the extent and precise location of intrathoracic lymph nodes. While suggestive, CT characterization of nodal disease is

**TABLE 5.** *Radiographic signs: Differential diagnosis*

Diffuse infiltrates
- Common:
  - PCP
  - PCP plus other infections (CMV, MAI, MTB, candida, toxoplasma, fungi)
  - PCP plus KS
  - Idiopathic interstitial fibrosis
  - TB
  - KS
- Uncommon: Lymphocytic interstitial pneumonitis

Focal infiltrates
- Common:
  - Pyogenic bacterial pneumonia
  - PCP
  - MTB
- Uncommon:
  - NHL
  - KS
- Rare:
  - Legionella
  - Nocardia

Cavitation
- Common:
  - Septic emboli (addicts)
  - PCP
- Uncommon: Fungi
- Rare:
  - MTB/MAI
  - Nocardia

Nodules
- Common:
  - KS
  - Fungi
  - Septic emboli
- Uncommon: Lymphoma
- Rare: PCP

Adenopathy
- Common:
  - MTB/MAI
  - Fungi
  - KS
  - Lymphoma
- Rare: PCP

Miliary disease
- Common:
  - Histoplasmosis
  - Cryptococcosis
  - MTB
- Uncommon: Foreign body granulomas (addicts)
- Rare: PCP

Pleural disease
- Common:
  - KS
  - Pyogenic bacterial pneumonia
- Uncommon:
  - Lymphoma
  - Cryptococcus
  - MTB
- Rare: PCP

not established. CT also may be helpful to characterize further otherwise confusing radiographic patterns, such as differentiating cavitating infarcts from cystic changes identified with PCP, or in identifying the typical pattern of peribronchial and vascular KS. CT has no role in the initial evaluation of patients suspected of having PCP.

# REFERENCES

1. Centers for Disease Control (1981): Pneumocystis pneumonia—Los Angeles. *M.M.W.R.*, 30:250–252.
2. Centers for Disease Control (1981): Kaposi's sarcoma and pneumocystis pneumonia among homosexual men—New York City and California. *M.M.W.R.*, 30:305–308.
3. Murray, J. F., Felton, C. P., Garay, S. M., et al. (1984): Pulmonary complications of the acquired immunodeficiency syndrome. *N. Engl. J. Med.*, 310:1682–1688.
4. Hopewell, P. C., and Luce, J. M. (1985): Pulmonary involvement in the Acquired Immunodeficiency Syndrome. *Chest*, 87:104–112.
5. Centers for Disease Control (1987): Revision of the CDC surveillance case definition for acquired immunodeficiency syndrome. *M.M.W.R.*, 365:3–14.
6. Solomon, S. L., and Curran, J. W. (1987): Editorial: Public health applications of a classification system for human immunodeficiency virus infection. *Ann. Int. Med.*, 106:319–321.
7. Naidich, D. P., Garay, S. M., Leitman, B. S., and McCauley, D. I. (1987): Radiographic manifestations of pulmonary disease in the aquired immunodeficiency syndrome (AIDS). *Semin. Roentgenol.*, 22:14–30.
8. Goodman, P. C., and Gamsu, G. (1987): Radiographic findings in the aquired immunodeficiency syndrome. *Postgrad. Rad.*, 7:3–15.
9. Garay, S. M., Belenko, M., Schwiep, F., and Greene, J.: The initial episode of Pneumocystis carinii pneumonia in the acquired immunodeficiency syndrome. *Chest (in press)*.
10. Stover, D. E., White, D. A., Romano, P. A., Gellene, R. A., and Robeson, W. A. (1985): Spectrum of pulmonary diseases associated with the acquired immunodeficiency syndrome. *Am. J. Med.*, 78:429–437.
11. Kovacs, J. A., Hiemenz, J. W., and Macher, A. M. (1984): Pneumocystis carinii pneumonia. A comparison between patients with the acquired immunodeficiency syndrome and patients with other immunodeficiencies. *Ann. Intern. Med.*, 100:663–671.
12. Forrest, J. V. (1972): Radiographic findings in Pneumocystis carinii pneumonia. *Diag. Radiol.*, 103:539–544.
13. Dee, P., Winn, W., and McKee, K. (1979): Pneumocystis carinii infection of the lung: Radiologic and pathologic correlation. *A.J.R.*, 132:741–746.
14. Seigel, R., and Wolson, A. H. (1977): The radiographic manifestations of chronic pneumocystis carinii pneumonia. *Am. J. Roentgenol.*, 128:150–152.
15. Doppman, J. L., Geelhoed, G. W., and De Vita, V. T. (1975): Atypical radiographic features in Pneumocystis carinii pneumonia. *Radiology*, 114:39–44.
16. McCauley, D. I., Naidich, D. P., Leitman, B. S., and Reede, D. L., Laubenstein, L. (1982): Radiographic patterns of opportunistic lung infections and Kaposi saroma in homosexual men. *A.J.R.*, 139:653–658.
17. Gamsu, G., Hecht, S. T., Birnberg, F. A., Coleman, D. L., and Golden, J. A. (1982): Pneumocystis carinii pneumonia in homosexual men. *A.J.R.*, 139:647–651.
18. Cohen, B. A., Pomeranz, S., Rabinowitz, J. G., et al. (1984): Pulmonary complications of AIDS: Radiologic features. *A.J.R.*, 143:115–122.
19. Goodman, P. C., Broaddus, V. C., and Hopewell, P. C. (1984): Chest radiographic patterns in the acquired immunodeficiency syndrome. *Am. Rev. Respir. Dis.*, 129:36.
20. Suster, B., Akerman, M., Orenstein, M., and Wax, M. R. (1986): Pulmonary manifestations of AIDS: Review of 106 episodes. *Radiology*, 161:87–93.
21. DeLorenzo, L. J., Huang, C. T., Maguire, G. P., and Stone, D. J. (1987): Roentgenographic patterns of Pneumocystis carinii pneumonia in 104 patients with AIDS. *Chest*, 91:323–327.
22. Milligan, S. A., Stulbarg, M. S., Gamsu, G., and Golden, J. A. (1985): Pneumocystis carinii pneumonia radiographically simulating tuberculosis. *Am. Rev. Respir. Dis.*, 132:1124–1126.
23. Goodman, P. C., Daley, C., and Minagi, H. (1986): Spontaneous

pneumothorax in AIDS patients with pneumocystis carinii pneumona. *A.J.R.,* 147:29-31.
24. Sherman, M., Levin, D., and Breidbart, D. (1986): Pneumocystis carinii pneumonia with spontaneous pneumothorax: A report of three cases. *Chest,* 90:609-610.
25. Barrio, J. L., Suarez, M., Rodriguez, J. L., Saldana, M. J., and Pitchenik, A. E. (1986): Case report. Pneumocystis carinii pneumonia presenting as cavitating and noncavitating solitary pulmonary nodules in patients with the acquired immunodeficiency syndrome. *Am. Rev. Respir. Dis.,* 134:1094-1096.
26. Rankin, J. A., and Pella, J. A. (1987): Radiographic resolution of Pneumocystis carinii pneumonia in response to corticosteroid therapy. *Am. Rev. Respir. Dis.,* 136:182-183.
26a. McFadden, D. K., Hyland, R. H., Inouye, T., Edelson, J. D., Rodriguez, C. H., and Rebuck, A. S. (1987): Corticosteroids as adjunctive therapy in treatment of PCP in patients with AIDS. *Lancet,* 1:1477-1479.
27. DeLorenzo, L. J., Maguire, G. P., Wormser, G. P., Davidian, M. M., and Stone, D. J. (1985): Persistence of Pneumocystis carinii pneumonia in the acquired immunodeficiency syndrome. Evaluation of therapy of follow-up transbronchial lung biopsy. *Chest,* 88:79-82.
28. Shelhamer, J. H., Ognibene, F. P., Macher, A. M., et al. (1984): Persistence of Pneumocystis carinii in lung tissue of acquired immunodeficiency syndrome patients treated for Pneumocystis pneumonia. *Am. Rev. Respir. Dis.,* 130:1161-1165.
29. Lipper, B., Garay, S. M., and Aranda, C. P. (1987): Diagnosis of recurrent Pneumocystis pneumonia in patients with the acquired immunodeficiency syndrome. *Chest* (Submitted).
30. Schinella, R. A., Clancey, C., Fazzini, E., and Garay, S. (1986): Pneumocystis carinii as a cause of pulmonary fibrosis. *Am. Rev. Respir. Dis.,* 133(Abstr.):180.
31. Ramaswamy, G., Jagadha, V., and Tchertkoff, V. (1985): Diffuse alveolar damage and interstitial fibrosis in acquired immunodeficiency syndrome patients without concurrent pulmonary infection. *Arch. Pathol. Lab. Med.,* 109:408-412.
32. Suffredini, A. F., Ognibene, F. P., Lack, E. E., et al. (1987): Nonspecific interstitial pneumonitis: A common cause of pulmonary disease in the acquired immunodeficiency syndrome. *Ann. Intern. Med.,* 107:7-13.
33. Simmons, J. T., Suffredini, A. F., Lack, E. E., et al. (1987): Nonspecific interstitial pneumonitis in patients with AIDS: Radiologic features. *A. J. R.,* 149:265-268.
34. Rosen, M. J., Cucco, R. A., and Teirstein, A. S. (1986): Outcome of intensive care in patients with the acquired immunodeficiency syndrome. *J. Intens. Care Med.,* 1:55-60.
35. Louie, E., Rice, L. B., and Holzman, R. S. (1986): Tuberculosis in non-Haitian patients with acquired immunodeficiency syndrome. *Chest,* 90:542-545.
36. Pitchenik, A. E., Cole, C., Russell, B. W., Fischl, M. A., Spira, T. J., and Snider, Jr., D. E. (1984): Tuberculosis, atypical mycobacteriosis, and the acquired immunodeficiency syndrome among Haitian and non-Haitian patients in South Florida. *Ann. Intern. Med.,* 101:641-646.
37. Pitchenik, A. E., and Rubinson, H. A. (1985): The radiographic appearance of tuberculosis in patients with the acquired immune deficiency syndrome (AIDS) and Pre-Aids. *Am. Rev. Respir. Dis.* 131:393-396.
38. Pitchenik, A. E., Burr, J., Suarez, M., et al. (1987): Human T-cell lymphotropic virus III (HTLV-III) seropositivity and related disease among 71 consecutive patients in whom tuberculosis was diagnosed. *Am. Rev. Respir. Dis.,* 135:875-879.
39. Centers for Disease Control (1987): Diagnosis and management of mycobacterial infection and disease in persons with human immunodeficiency virus infection. *Ann. Intern. Med.,* 106:254-256.
40. Marinelli, D. L., Albelda, S. M., Williams, T. M., Kern, J. A., Iozzo, R. V., and Miller, W. T. (1986): Nontuberculous mycobacterial infection in AIDS: Clinical, pathologic, and radiographic features. *Radiology,* 160:77-82.
41. Macher, A. M., Kovacs, J. A., Vee, G., et al. (1983): Bacteremia due to Mycobacterium avium-intracellulare in the acquired immunodeficiency syndrome. *Ann. Intern. Med.,* 99:782-785.
42. Hulnick, D. H., Megibow, A. J., Naidich, D. P., Hilton, S., Cho, K. C., and Balthazar, E. J. (1985): CT in abdominal tuberculosis. *Radiology,* 157:199-204.
43. Niedt, G. W., and Schinella, R. A. (1985): Acquired immunodeficiency syndrome: Clinicopathologic study of 56 patients. *Arch. Pathol. Lab. Med.,* 109:727-734.
44. Brodie, H. R., Broaddus, C., Hopewell, A., et al.: Is cytomegalovirus (CMV) a cause of lung disease in patients with AIDS. *Am. Rev. Respir. Dis.,* 131(Abstr.):227.
45. Wallace, J. M., and Hannah, J. (1987): Cytomegalovirus pneumonitis in patients with AIDS. *Chest,* 92:198-203.
46. Emanuel, D., Peppard, J., Stover, D., et al. (1986): Rapid immunodiagnosis of cytomegalovirus pneumonia by bronchoalveolar lavage using human and murine monoclonal antibodies. *Ann. Intern. Med.,* 104:476-481.
47. Collaborative DHPG Treatment Study Group (1986): Treatment of serious cytomegalovirus infections with 9-(1,3-dihydroxy-2-propoxy-methyl) guanine in patients with AIDS and other immunodeficiencies. *N. Engl. J. Med.,* 314:801-805.
48. Zuger, A., Louie, E., Holzman, R. S., Simberkoff, M. S., and Rahal, J. J. (1986): Cryptococcal disease in patients with the acquired immunodeficiency syndrome. *Ann. Intern. Med.,* 104:234-240.
49. Khoury, M. B., Godwin, J. D., Ravin, C. E., Gallis, H. A., Halvorsen, R. A., and Putman, C. E. (1984): Thoracic cryptococcosis: Immunologic competence and radiologic appearance. *A. J. R.,* 141:893-896.
50. Eng, R. H. K., Bishburg, E., and Smith, S. M. (1986): Cryptococcal infections in patients with acquired immune deficiency syndrome. *Am. J. Med.,* 81:19-23.
51. Witt, D., McKay, D., Schwam, L., Goldstein, D., and Gold, J. (1987): Acquired immune deficiency syndrome presenting as bone marrow and mediastinal cryptococosis. *Am. J. Med.,* 82:149-150.
52. Newman, T. G., Soni, A., Acaron, S., and Huang, C. T. (1987): Pleural cryptococosis in the acquired immunodeficiency syndrome. *Chest,* 91:459-461.
53. Wheat, L. J., Slama, T. G., and Zeckel, M. L. (1985): Histomosis in the acquired immune deficiency syndrome. *Am. J. Med.,* 78:203-210.
54. Wheat, L. J., and Small, C. B. (1984): Disseminated histoplasmosis in the acquired immune deficiency syndrome. *Arch. Intern. Med.,* 144:2147-2149.
55. Mandell, W., Goldberg, D. M., and Neu, H. C. (1986): Histoplasmosis in patients with the acquired immune deficiency syndrome. *Am. J. Med.,* 81:974-978.
56. Johnson, P. C., Sarosi, G. A., Septimus, E. J., and Satterwhite, T. K. (1986): Progressive disseminated histoplasmosis in patients with the acquired immune deficiency syndrome: A review of 12 cases and a literature review. *Semin. Resp. Infect.,* 1:1-8.
57. Bronnimann, D. A., Adam, R. D., Galgiani, J. N., et al. (1987): Coccidiomycosis in the acquired immunodeficiency syndrome. *Ann. Intern. Med.,* 106:372-379.
58. Pervez, N. K., Kleinerman, J., Kattan, M., et al. (1985): Pseudomembranous necrotizing bronchial aspergillosis. *Am. Rev. Respir. Dis.,* 131:961-963.
59. Polsky, B., Gold, J. W. M., Whimbey, E., et al. (1986): Bacterial pneumonia in patients with the acquired immunodeficiency syndrome. *Ann. Intern. Med.,* 104:38-41.
60. Simberkoff, M. S., Sadr, W. E., and Rahal, Jr., J. J. (1984): Streptococcus pneumoniae infections and bacteremia in patients with acquired immune deficiency syndrome, with report of a pneumococcal vaccine failure. *Am. Rev. Respir. Dis.,* 130:1174-1176.
61. Garay, S. M., Belenko, M., Fazzini, E., and Schinella, R. (1987): Pulmonary manifestations of Kaposi's saroma. *Chest,* 91:39-43.
62. Davis, S. D., Henschke, C. I., Chamides, B. K., and Westcott, J. L. (1987): Intrathoracic Kaposi sarcoma in AIDS patients: Radiographic-pathologic correlation. *Radiology,* 163:495-500.
63. Zibrak, J. D., Silvestri, R. C., Costello, P., et al. (1986): Bron-

choscopic and radiologic features of Kaposi's sarcoma involving the respiratory system. *Chest,* 90:476–479.
64. Sivit, C. J., Schwartz, A. M., and Rockoff, S. D. (1987): Kaposi's sarcoma of the lung in AIDS: Radiologic-pathologic analysis. *A. J. R.,* 148:25–28.
65. Meduri, G. U., Stover, D. E., Lee, M., et al. (1986): Pulmonary Kaposi's sarcoma in the acquired immune deficiency syndrome: Clinical, radiographic, and pathologic manifestations. *Am. J. Med.,* 81:11–18.
66. Ognibene, F. P., Steis, R. G., Macher, A. M., et al. (1985): Kaposi's sarcoma causing pulmonary infiltrates and respiratory failure in the acquired immunodeficiency syndrome. *Ann. Intern. Med.* 102:471–475.
67. Lau, K. Y., Av, J., Rubin, A., Littner, M., and Krauthammer, M. (1986): Letter to the Editor: Kaposi's sarcoma of the tracheobronchial tree. *Chest,* 89:158–159.
67a. Hanson, P. J. V., Harcourt-Webster, J. N., Gazzard, B. G., and Collins, J. V. (1987): Fiberoptic bronchoscopy in diagnosis of bronchopulmonary Kaposi's sarcoma. *Thorax,* 42: 269–271.
67b. Fouret, P. J., Touboul, J. Z., Mayaud, C. M., Akoun, G. M., and Roland, J. (1987): Pulmonary Kaposi's sarcoma in patients with AIDS: A clinicopathological study. *Thorax,* 42:262–268.
68. Fitzgerald, W., Bevelaqua, F. A., Garay, S. M., and Aranda, C. P. (1987): The role of open lung biopsy in patients with the acquired immunodeficiency syndrome. *Chest,* 91:659–661.
69. Stulbarg, M. S., and Golden, J. A. (1987): Editorial: Open lung biopsy in the acquired immunodeficiency syndrome (AIDS). *Chest,* 91:639–640.
70. Solal-Celigny, P., Couderc, L. J., Herman, D., et al. (1985): Lymphoid interstitial pneumonitis in acquired immunodeficiency syndrome-related complex. *Am. Rev. Respir. Dis.,* 131:956–960.
71. Morris, J. C., Rosen, M. J., Marchevsky, A., and Teirstein, A. S. (1987): Lymphocytic interstitial pneumonia in patients at risk for the acquired immune deficiency syndrome. *Chest,* 91:63–67.
72. Resnick, L., Pitchenik, A. E., Fisher, E., and Croney, R. (1987): Detection of HTLV-III/LAV-specific IgG and antigen in bronchoalveolar lavage fluid from two patients with lymphocytic interstitial pneumonitis associated with AIDS-related complex. *Am. J. Med.,* 82:553–556.
73. Ziza, J. M., Brun-Vezinet, F., Venet, A., et al. (1985): Letter: Lymphadenopathy-associated virus isolated from bronchoalveolar lavage fluid in AIDS-related complex with lymphoid interstitial pneumonitis. *N. Engl. J. Med.,* 313:183.
74. Chayt, K. J., Harper, M. E., Marselle, L. M., et al. (1986): Detection of HTLV-III RNA in lungs of patients with AIDS and pulmonary involvement. *J. A. M. A.,* 256:2356–2359.
75. Zeigler, J. L., Beckstead, J. A., Volberding, P. A., et al. (1984): Non-Hodgkin's lymphoma in 90 homosexual men: Relation to generalized lymphadenopathy and the acquired immunodeficiency syndrome. *N. Engl. J. Med.,* 311:565–570.
76. Ioachim, H. L., Cooper, M. C., and Hellman, G. C. (1985): Lymphomas in men in high risk for acquired immune deficiency syndrome (AIDS). *Cancer,* 56:2831–2842.
77. Longo, D. L., Steis, R. G., Lane, C., et al. (1985): Malignancies in the AIDS patient: Natural history, treatment strategies, and preliminary results. *Ann. N.Y. Acad. Sci.,* 437:420–430.
78. Kaplan, M. H., Susin, M., Pahwa, S. G., et al. (1987): Neoplastic complications of HTLV-III infection. Lymphomas and solid tumors. *Am. J. Med.,* 82:389–396.
79. Case Records of the Massachusetts General Hospital (1986): Case 51-1986. *N. Engl. J. Med.,* 315:1660–1668.
80. Robert, N. J., and Schneiderman, H. (1984): Letter: Hodgkin's disease and the acquired immunodeficiency syndrome. *Ann. Intern. Med.,* 101:142–143.
81. Schoeppel, S. L., Hoppe, R. T., Dorfman, R. F., et al. (1985): Hodgkin's disease in homosexual men with generalized lymphadenopathy. *Ann. Intern. Med.,* 102:68–70.
82. Baer, D. M., Anderson, E. T., and Wilkinson, L. S. (1986): Acquired immune deficiency syndrome in homosexual men with Hodgkin's disease: Three case reports. *Am. J. Med.,* 80:738–740.
83. Mitsuyasu, R. T., Colman, M. F., and Sun, N. C. (1986): Simultaneous occurrence of Hodgkin's disease and Kaposi's sarcoma in a patient with acquired immune deficiency syndrome. *Am. J. Med.,* 80:954–958.
84. Prior, E., Goldberg, A. F., Conjalka, M. S., et al. (1986): Hodgkin's disease in homosexual men. An AIDS-related phenomena? *Am. J. Med.,* 81:1085–1088.
85. Stern, R. G., Gamsu, G., Golden, J. A., Hirji, M., Webb, W. R., and Abrams, D. I. (1984): Intrathoracic adenopathy: Differential feature of AIDS and diffuse lymphadenopathy syndrome. *A. J. R.,* 142:689–692.
86. Marchevsky, A., Rosen, M. J., Chrystal, G., and Kleinerman, J. (1985): Pulmonary complications of the acquired immunodeficiency syndrome: A clinicopathologic study of 70 cases. *Human Pathol.,* 16:659–670.
87. Cammarosano, C., and Lewis, W. (1985): Cardiac lesions in acquired immune deficiency syndrome (AIDS). *J. Am. Coll. Cardiol.,* 5:703–706.
88. Cohen, I. S., Anderson, D. W., Virmani, R., et al. (1986): Congestive cardiomyopathy in association with the acquired immunodeficiency syndrome. *N. Engl. J. Med.,* 315:628–633.
89. Goldschmidt, R. H., and Mills, J. (1987): Letter: Cardiomyopathy and AIDS. *N. Engl. J. Med.,* 16:1158–1159.
90. Freedberg, R. S., Gindea, A. J., Dieterich, D., and Greene, J. B. (1987): Herpes simplex in AIDS. *N.Y. State. J. Med.,* 87:304–306.
91. Silver, M. A., Macher, A. M., Reichert, C. M., et al. (1984): Cardiac involvement by Kaposi's sarcoma in acquired immune deficiency syndrome (AIDS). *Am. J. Cardiol.,* 53:983–985.
92. Balasubramanyam, A., Waxman, M., Kazal, H. L., and Lee, M. H. (1986): Malignant lymphoma of the heart in acquired immune deficiency syndrome. *Chest,* 90:243–244.
93. Kramer, E. L., Sanger, J. J., Garay, S. M., et al. (1987): Gallium-67 scans of the chest in patients with acquired immunodeficiency syndrome. *J. Nucl. Med.,* 28:1107–1114.
94. Coleman, D. L., Hattner, R. S., Luce, J. M., et al. (1984): Correlation between Gallium lung scans and fiberoptic bronchoscopy in patients with suspected Pneumocystis carinii pneumonia and the acquired immunodeficiency syndrome. *Am. Rev. Respir. Dis.,* 130:1166–1169.
95. Tuazon, C. U., Delaney, M. D., Simon, G. L., Witorsch, P., and Varma, V. M. (1985): Utility of gallium scintigraphy and bronchial washings in the diagnosis and treatment of Pneumocystis carinii pneumonia in patients with the acquired immune deficiency syndrome. *Am. Rev. Respir. Dis.,* 132:1087–1092.
96. Barron, T. F., Birnbaum, N. S., Shane, L. B., et al. (1985): Pneumocystis carinii studied by Gallium-67 scanning. *Radiology,* 154:791–793.
97. Woolfenden, J. M., Carrasquillo, J. A., Larson, S. M., et al. (1987): Acquired immunodeficiency syndrome: Ga-67 citrate imaging. *Radiology,* 162:383–387.
98. Bitran, J., Bekerman, C., Weinstein, R., et al. (1987): Patterns of Gallium-67 scintigraphy in patients with acquired immunodeficiency syndrome and the AIDS related complex. *J. Nucl. Med.,* 28:1103–1106.
99. Bigby, T. D., Margolskee, D., Curtis, J. L., et al. (1986): The usefulness of induced sputum in the diagnosis of Pneumocystis carinii pneumonia in patients with the acquired immunodeficiency syndrome. *Am. Rev. Respir. Dis.,* 133:515–518.
100. Blumfeld, W., Wagar, E., Hadley, W. K. (1984): Use of the transbronchial biopsy for diagnosis of opportunistic pulmonary infections in acquired immunodeficiency syndrome (AIDS). *Am. J. Clin. Pathol.,* 31:1–5.
101. Broaddus, C., Dake, M. D., Stulbarg, M. S., et al. (1985): Bronchoalveolar lavage and transbronchial biopsy for the diagnosis of pulmonary infections in the acquired immunodeficiency syndrome. *Ann. Intern. Med.,* 102:747–752.
102. Golden, J. A., Hollander, H., Stulbarg, M. S., and Gamsu, G. (1986): Bronchoalveolar lavage as the exclusive diagnostic modality for Pneumocystis carinii pneumonia: A prospective study among patients with acquired immunodeficiency syndrome. *Chest,* 90:18–22.
103. Mann, J. M., Altus, C. S., Webber, C. A., et al. (1987): Non-bronchoscopic lung lavage for diagnosis of opportunistic infection in AIDS. *Chest,* 91:319–322.

CHAPTER 4

# Gastrointestinal Radiology in AIDS Patients

Alec J. Megibow, Susan D. Wall, Emil J. Balthazar, and Benito J. Rybak

The gastrointestinal (GI) tract is affected by many AIDS-related disorders. Of the 12 indicator diseases indicative of AIDS without proof of HIV infection, six may directly or exclusively involve the GI tract. GI disease accounts for the second largest overall group of diseases (after Pneumocystis carinii pneumonia) seen in AIDS patients (1).

Candidiasis, cytomegalovirus (CMV), cryptosporidiosis, histoplasmosis, isosporiasis, salmonella (with sepsis), and unusual mycobacteria account for a majority of non-neoplastic disorders. Severe cases of shigella, giardia, or strongyloides, while not considered specific AIDS-related diseases, also may account for significant morbidity in these patients. Many patients may be infected with multiple organisms. Multiple sites are shown to be involved in 64% of patients (2). Neoplasms (Kaposi's sarcoma (KS), and lymphoma) also are seen in the GI tract of AIDS patients.

Many of these entities produce radiographic findings that may suggest a specific diagnosis. Although patients may display radiographic findings caused by several disease processes, the predominant radiographic pattern may suggest the particular entity that is most accountable for clinical symptomatology at the time of examination. As radiologic experience accumulates, further patterns will become more clearly defined, allowing increasing precision in identifying the total extent and etiology of a specific disease.

In this chapter we review the radiographic features of the most common disorders seen in the alimentary tract and biliary tree of AIDS patients. (Chapter 5 details the total imaging spectrum in neoplastic disease in these patients.) The approach is regional rather than disease oriented. The emphasis will be on those features predominantly demonstrated by barium radiography with secondary mention of computed tomography (CT) findings.

## RADIOGRAPHIC TECHNIQUE

Radiographic demonstration of the diagnostic features of GI tract abnormalities in AIDS patients requires meticulous examination techniques, because early disease often produces subtle findings. We recommend the routine use of double-contrast radiographic techniques in the study of the esophagus, stomach, and colon. Wall et al. (3) have shown that double-contrast studies more frequently detected abnormalities (95% of the 40 patients examined) compared with single-contrast studies, which detected abnormalities in 61% of 23 patients examined. Many excellent texts and articles review the methodology by which these studies may be performed (4).

Abdominal CT scans should be performed using sufficient oral contrast material to insure uniform bowel opacification. Air-contrast methodology aids in the detection of gastric, esophagogastric, and colonic lesions. Regardless of the methods used, unopacified bowel loops may be mistaken for mesenteric masses (particularly mesenteric lymph nodes). Therefore, sufficient quantities of oral contrast must be consumed. At least 800 cc, drank evenly over a 30 to 45 min period before the scan begins, generally will provide uniform bowel opacification.

We routinely use intravenous (i.v.) contrast enhancement in all of our cases (unless contraindicated by allergy or renal disease). Intravenous contrast is administered in two phases: a rapid bolus (50 cc) is followed immediately by sustained infusion of the remaining contrast (100–150 cc), which is maintained as the scans are acquired. Scans are obtained using a dynamic sequential protocol that maximizes intravascular contrast levels. This increases the accuracy of detection of intrahepatic masses and discrimination of lymph nodes from vessels in the retroperitoneum and mesentery (5).

We recommend all personnel wear examining gloves during venopuncture, handling of cups, basins, enema tips, and other accessory equipment utilized for GI imaging in these patients. Eye protection is advisable for tableside fluoroscopic procedures. Isolation requirements vary with the specific diagnoses of each particular patient. Chapter 8 details the recommendations for infectious disease protocol followed by departments for the overall handling of patients with AIDS.

## ESOPHAGUS

### Esophagitis

Dysphagia is a common complaint in AIDS patients. Monilial, CMV, and herpes infections account for the significant percentage of cases. Radiographic assessment is useful for several reasons: 1) Candida and CMV infections can be differentiated radiographically; 2) The radiographic pattern may suggest a diagnosis that may necessitate an aggressive endoscopic search and appropriate culture techniques; 3) Therapeutic response can be assessed objectively; 4) Neoplasm can be separated from infection.

Candida infection is the most common cause of esophagitis in AIDS patients (6). Oral thrush may be seen in patients with AIDS-related complex (ARC), but esophageal candida infection is a manifestation of "full-blown" AIDS (7); therefore, careful radiographic examination is critical in these patients. According to recent Centers for Disease Control (CDC) case surveillance criteria, candidiasis of the esophagus may be considered presumptive evidence for the diagnosis of AIDS in patients with laboratory evidence of HIV infection (see Appendix A, Section IIB). Radiologic confirmation of candidal infection will become increasingly important. Frager found candidiasis the most common AIDS related GI infection (12–25 patients) (6). Similarly, Wall et al. encountered candida infection in 15 of 44 patients (3).

Radiographic appearances vary according to the severity of the disease. Classically, candidiasis results in a diffusely ulcerated shaggy esophagus (Fig. 1A) (8). Other forms include cobblestoning, plaques, and thickened folds (Fig. 1B) (9,10). Levine et al. (10) showed that double-contrast esophagography is more sensitive in de-

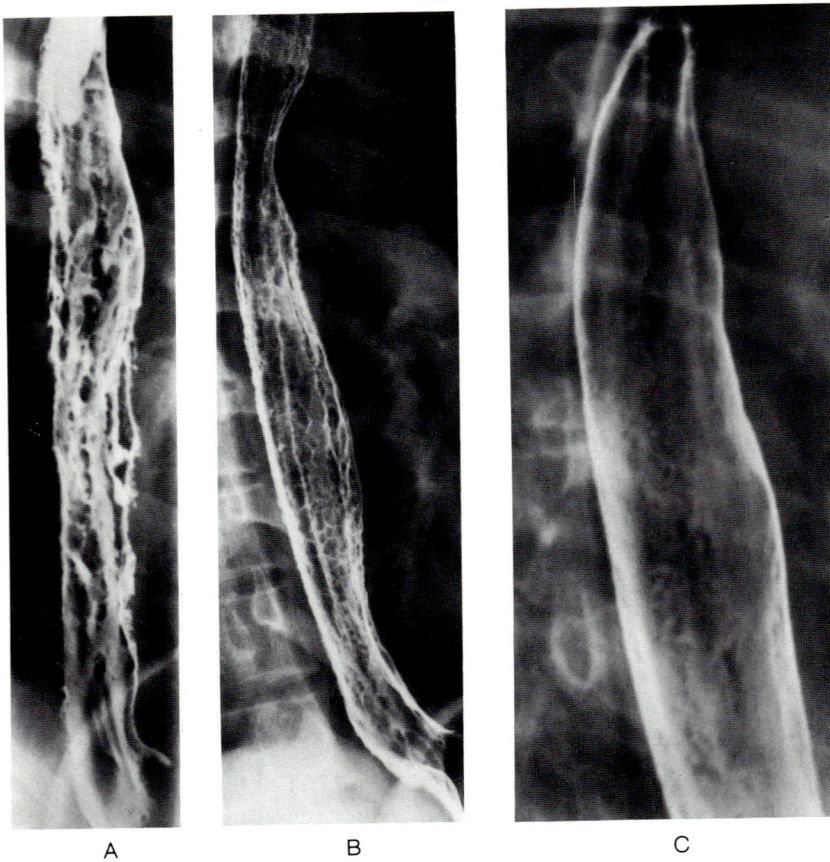

**FIG. 1.** Candidiasis. **A:** Typical monilial infection involving entire esophagus with diffuse ulceration. **B:** "Cobblestoned" esophagus. The pattern is presumably the result of submucosal edema and mucosal plaques. **C:** Minimal disease. Focal filling defects due to localized plaques are scattered throughout the esophagus. Radiologic diagnosis in these cases requires meticulous double-contrast technique.

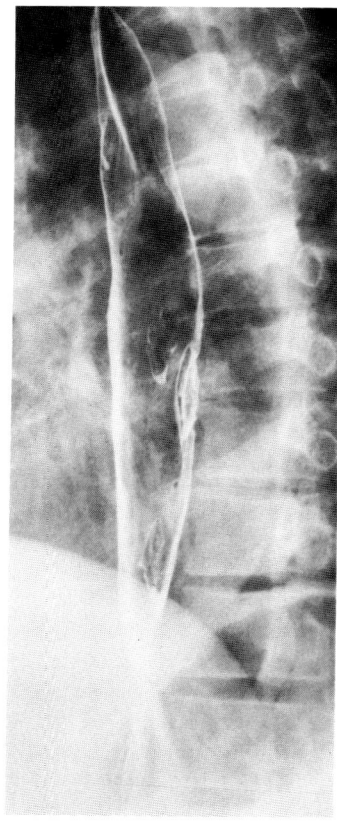
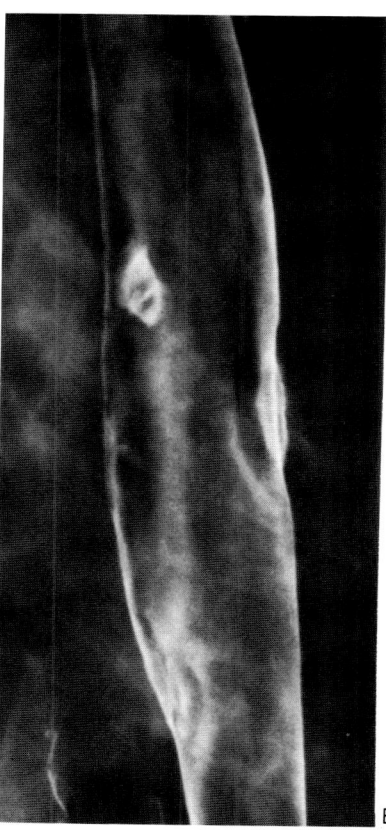

FIG. 2. CMV esophagitis. **A:** Multiple discrete ulcerations of varying sizes. Intervening mucosa is normal. **B:** Magnified view reveals a flat ulcer with a well-defined, peripheral lucent zone presumably due to edema. Note the sharp edges of these somewhat diamond-shaped ulcers.

tecting esophageal candidiasis than single-contrast esophagography, with accuracy of detection approaching 90%. This improved accuracy reflects the ability to detect mucosal plaques that may be focally clustered, producing longitudinally oriented linear filling defects. This pattern accounted for 95% of the candida lesions seen on double-contrast studies (Fig. 1C) (10).

CMV esophagites display several unique appearances that may allow it to be differentiated from candida esophagitis. Focal, discretely marginated diamond-shaped ulcers surrounded by a well-defined peripheral lucency that represents a zone of edema seen against a background of normal esophageal mucosa is commonly seen. Balthazar et al. (11,11a) described radiographic findings in 19 cases of CMV esophagitis. In all, discrete lesions were seen along the length of the esophagus (Fig. 2). Teixidor et al. (12) reported four cases of CMV esophagitis, and in three the diagnoses were missed radiologically but only single-contrast studies were performed. In the fourth, thick, irregular folds with diffuse superficial ulceration of the entire esophagus was seen. This pattern of disease is unusual in our experience although we have seen clustered superficial "apthous" ulcers producing a localized granular appearance (Fig. 3).

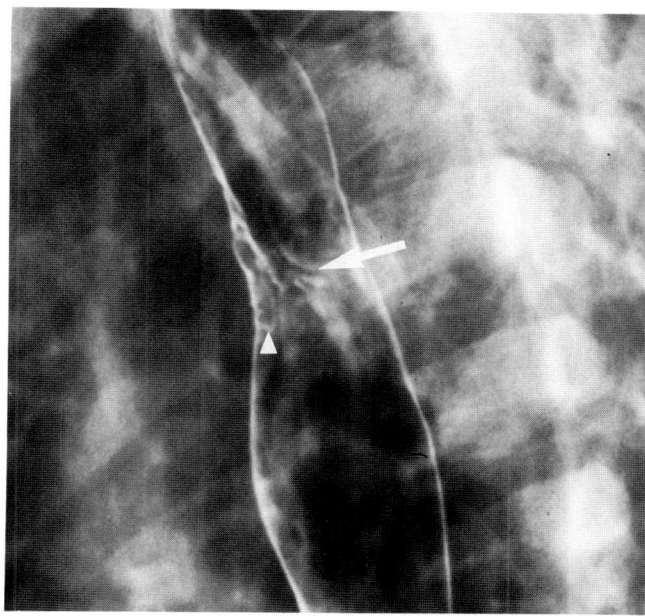

FIG. 3. CMV esophagitis. Film from esophagram in a patient with severe dysphagia. A localized area of mucosal granularity is seen in the mid-esophagus (*arrow*). The edges of a discrete ulcer are beginning to become defined (*arrowhead*). AIDS was unsuspected in this 39-year-old woman.

Two unique manifestations of CMV infections of the esophagus may be radiologically defined. There is a high incidence of ulcerations at the gastroesophageal junction with extension of the process into the proximal stomach (Fig. 4). This may be seen on CT scan as thickening of the abdominal portion of the esophagus and increased density in the lesser omental fat. Large ulcers seen at the lower margin of the esophagus produce thick folds in the gastric fundus. Two of three patients seen in Balthazar's original series had distal gastroesophageal CMV.

The second radiologic feature characteristic of CMV is the formation of giant esophageal ulcers (Fig. 5). This phenomenon, originally described by St. Onge et al. (13), results from a combination of infectious destruction of the mucosa and ischemic necrosis induced by vasculitis. This vasculitis results from CMV infection of the endothelial cells in the submucosal blood vessels. Farman et al. (14) recently described focal candida lesions in 4 of 25 patients resulting in large esophageal ulcers. In our experience it is unusual to see large focal ulcers surrounded by normal mucosa in candidiasis. In their cases, correlation with endoscopy revealed that diffuse lesions as well as the focal ulcer were present. Furthermore, not all of their cases were studied with double-contrast esophagography. This underscores the importance of double-contrast radiography in studying these patients. High quality double-contrast studies often are difficult to obtain in these severely ill and debilitated patients. In our experience, focal giant ulcers with surrounding normal mucosa seen on double-con-

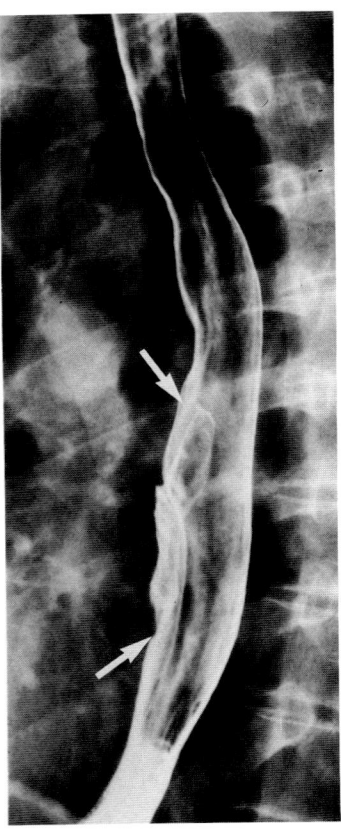

**FIG. 5.** CMV esophagitis, giant ulcer (arrows). This characteristic feature of CMV infection is presumably secondary to both infection and vasculitis resulting in ischemic necrosis of the esophageal wall.

trast esophagography is characteristic of CMV infection (Figs. 5 and 6).

Herpes simplex esophagitis accounts for the other major etiology of esophageal infection in AIDS patients (Fig. 7A). The findings of discrete ulceration are similar to those seen with CMV in contrast to the diffuse ulcerations seen in candida (15). In advanced stages the lesions may be indistinguishable from CMV. We have seen a discrete esophageal ulceration in one patient with proven mycobacterium avium-intracellulare (MAI) infection of the esophagus (Fig. 7B). We have also observed a localized and ulcerating esophagitis in the midportion of the esophagus owing to gram-positive cocci, presumably a group B streptococcal infection (Fig. 7C). Recently, we have encountered three AIDS patients with severe esophagitis manifested by deep ulcers that coalesce into intraluminal sinus tracts paralleling the long axis of the esophagus. In one patient, Actinomycosis was identified as the etiologic agent (Fig. 7D).

### Neoplasm

KS accounts for the majority of AIDS-related neoplasms in the esophagus and hypopharynx. KS lesions

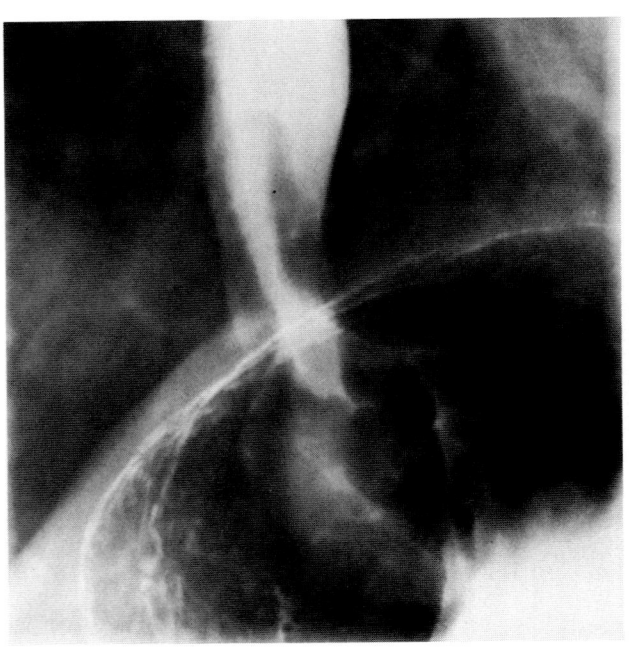

**FIG. 4.** Gastroesophageal CMV. A large, diamond-shaped ulcer straddles the E-G junction. These are thickened folds in the proximal stomach as well as the distal esophagus.

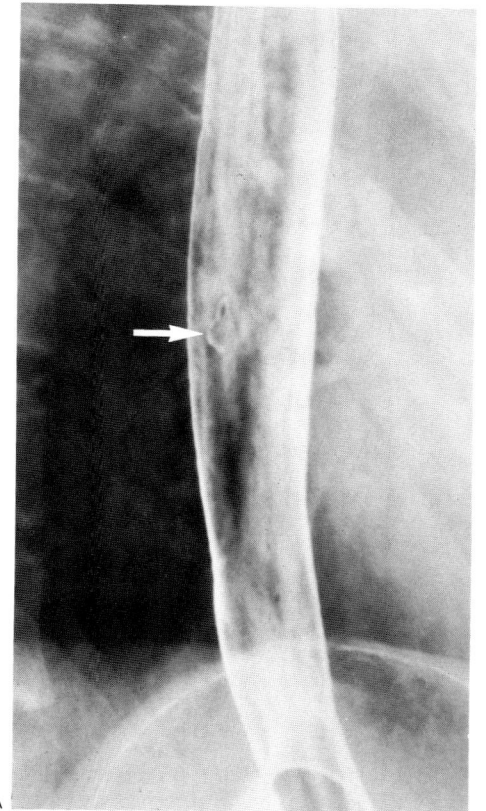 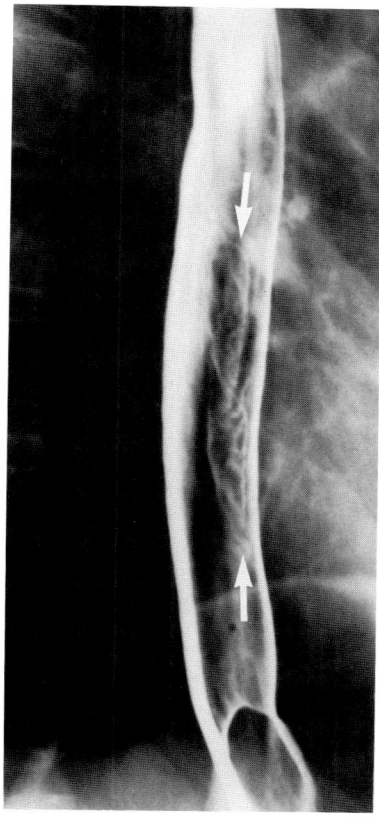

FIG. 6. CMV esophagitis, disease progression. **A:** Film from esophagram in an AIDS patient with odynophagia. A discrete, "apthous" ulcer is seen in the distal esophagus (arrow). **B:** Same patient, 3 months later. A giant ulcer (arrow) has formed.

are discrete, submucosal elevations seen along the length of the esophagus (Fig. 8). Emery and co-workers (16) reported the radiographic findings in hypopharyngeal KS. These lesions may be significant sources of dysphagia due to their location and may be encountered in patients being studied to rule out esophagitis. The lesions may appear as small nodules or infiltrating masses. They can be demonstrated by asking the patient to swallow a high-density barium suspension, and performing a modified valsalva maneuver. On CT scanning one can recognize multiple filling defects distorting the structures of the hypopharynx. Obliteration of parapharyngeal spaces may be appreciated in infiltrating forms of the disease (Figs. 9 and 10).

## STOMACH

AIDS related gastric lesions rarely produce symptoms that direct investigation specifically to the stomach. Many gastric lesions are serendipitously detected during radiographic examination of the esophagus for dysphagia or prior to examinations of the small bowel to evaluate symptoms such as diarrhea or weight loss. The radiologist may be the first to detect gastric diseases in AIDS patients. In Wall et al.'s series (3), gastric lesions were detected in 57% of patients; in Frager et al.'s series (6) gastric pathology was found in 2 of 25 patients.

### Non-neoplastic Lesions

Non-neoplastic lesions are seen most often at the E-G junction and juxtapyloric antrum. In our experience, the major etiology of non-neoplastic gastric pathology is infection due to CMV. Patients with CMV gastritis exhibit symptoms suggestive of malignancy, such as poorly localized abdominal pain and weight loss. Bleeding is rarely encountered. Therefore, barium radiography may not be performed initially, rather, many patients will be examined by CT in search of signs of malignant disease. The radiologist must scrutinize the E-G junction region and antrum for signs of wall thickening (Fig. 11). The CT findings are nonspecific; wall thickening should signal the need for barium radiography and/or endoscopy (Fig. 12).

Barium examination reveals gastroesophageal ulcerations which may result in stricture formation as the disease progresses. The antrum is the most frequent site of involvement (Fig. 13). Submucosal lesions may pro-

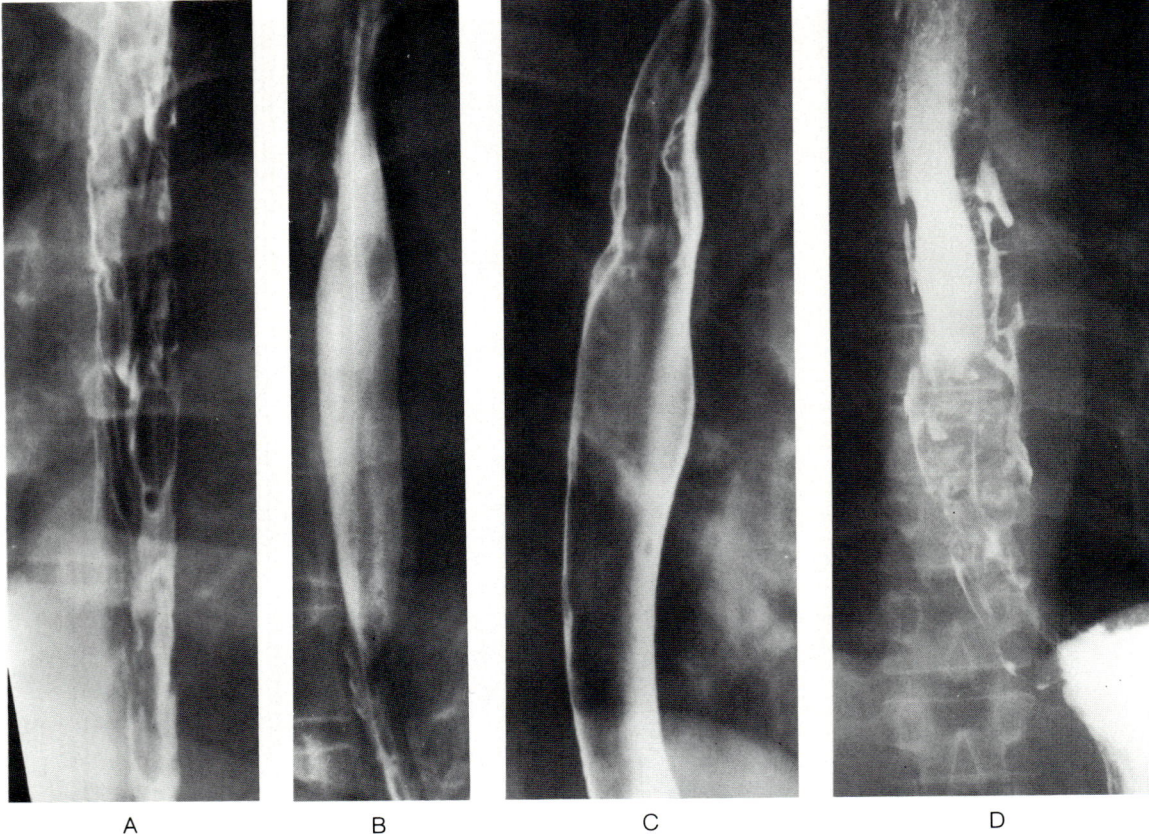

**FIG. 7.** Miscellaneous esophagitis. **A:** Herpes simplex esophagitis. The findings are similar to CMV infection. In our experience, CMV is more commonly seen in AIDS patients. **B:** MAI infection. A discrete ulcer is seen in the proximal esophagus. MAI esophagitis is extremely rare in our experience. **C:** Pyogenic esophagitis. Localized narrowing, fold thickening, and ulceration is seen in the proximal esophagus. Endoscopic biopsy reveals acute suppurative inflammation. Multiple gram-positive cocci (presumably Group B streptococcus) were present. No other organisms were found. **D:** Intramural sinus tracts outlined by barium paralleling the esophagus are noted. Extensive microbiologic study revealed sulfur granules and Actinomycosis.

duce "thumbprinting" along the gastric wall. This may be distinguished from the less regular, more discrete, submucosal masses in KS (11). Biopsy reveals CMV inclusion bodies in the bases of the gastric glands and accompanying inflammation in the surrounding submucosa (Fig. 14). We have seen one case in which multiple nodular elevations were present. This "petechial" appearance has not been reported elsewhere (Fig. 15). Teixidor et al. (12) reported one case based on a single-contrast study in which a granular mucosa was seen endoscopically but not recognized radiographically. Recently, a solitary submucosal antral mass due to CMV infection was reported (17).

CMV may produce ulceration and stenosis in the pyloroantral region. Culture material often is positive for both CMV and cryptosporidial organisms (Fig. 16). CT demonstrates thickening of the antral wall and ulceration (18). Gastric tuberculosis (TB) with lesser omental abscess (19) has been reported. Monilial bezoars have been demonstrated in patients with severe candida of both the stomach and esophagus (Fig. 17).

### Gastric Neoplasms

KS commonly is seen in the stomach of AIDS patients. Most but not all patients will have skin lesions. In one published series, skin lesions were present in 80% of 29 patients with gastrointestinal KS. Gastric lesions were best detected on double-contrast studies (20).

The radiographic finding is discrete, sharply marginated, submucosal nodules that are variable in size, but generally measure between 0.5 and 2 cm. The mucosa overlying the nodule may be breeched. The intervening mucosa is normal. The appearances may vary from small nodules simulating hyperplastic polyps to diffuse nodularity (Fig. 18). Serial examinations may document worsening of disease as the submucosa becomes progres-

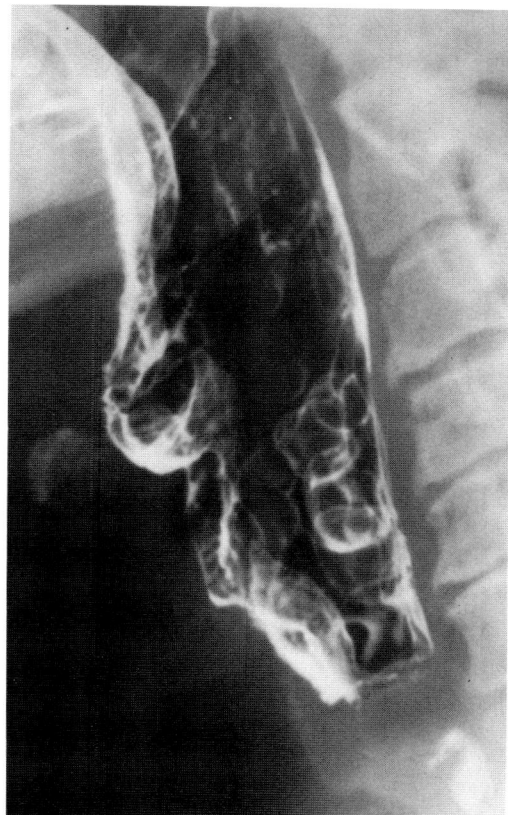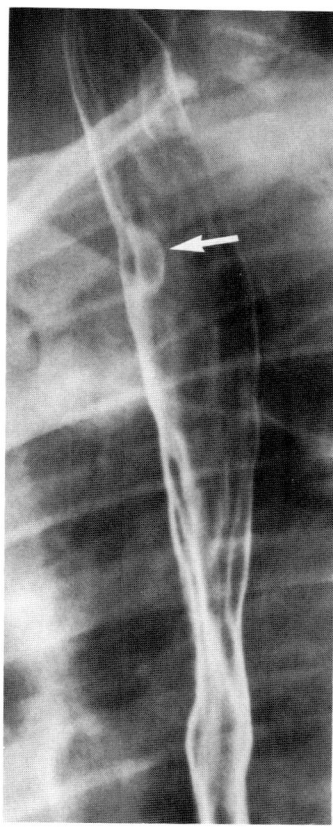

**FIG. 8.** Pharyngoesophageal KS. **A:** Double-contrast pharyngogram (performed routinely on all patients with dysphagia) reveals innumerable discrete nodules in the pharynx and pyriform sinuses. **B:** Esophagram in same patient reveals solitary proximal esophageal KS lesion (*arrow*). Skin lesions were present in this 45-year-old homosexual man.

sively infiltrated (Fig. 19). In advanced cases, CT may reveal gross thickening of the wall of the stomach and hyperrugosity, a nonspecific finding that may be confused with lymphomatous infiltration of the gastric wall. Normal CT examination of the stomach does not exclude the presence of KS in these patients.

Lymphoma may involve any portion of the GI tract, but in our experience the small bowel and colon are involved more frequently in AIDS patients as opposed to the higher incidence of gastric lymphoma in non-AIDS patients. A wide variety of appearances may be expected in lymphoma of the stomach. Focal thickening of the gastric wall with deep ulceration and irregular masses may be seen (Fig. 20). We have not seen discrete submucosal nodules of lymphoma as in KS patients. When KS infiltrates the entire submucosa may be difficult to differentiate from lymphoma.

## DUODENUM AND SMALL BOWEL

Duodenal and small intestinal disease accounts for the greatest percentage of GI abnormalities seen radiographically in AIDS patients. Wall et al. (3) found duodenal abnormality in 82%, jejunal abnormality in 64%, and ileal disease in 46% of 28 AIDS patients with upper GI abnormalities. Frager et al. (6) reported small bowel disease in 13 of 25 patients. Organisms commonly noted to cause enteritis in these patients include CMV and MAI cryptosporidium. KS and lymphoma are commonly seen neoplasms.

Because of the clinical overlap between the symptoms of neoplastic versus infectious disease, the radiologist is in a unique position to suggest a diagnosis directing the appropriate method of establishing the etiology. Radiologic evaluation is based on the distribution of disease, the presence or absence of distortion of the small bowel folds, the presence or absence of nodularity, and changes in the small bowel caliber. As case experience accumulates, characteristic radiographic patterns are emerging. CT provides important additional information by detecting the presence or absence of solid organ disease or adenopathy in the mesentery or retroperitoneum.

The clinical setting in which the small bowel will be examined includes those patients with diarrhea or malabsorption, or those patients in whom severe rapid

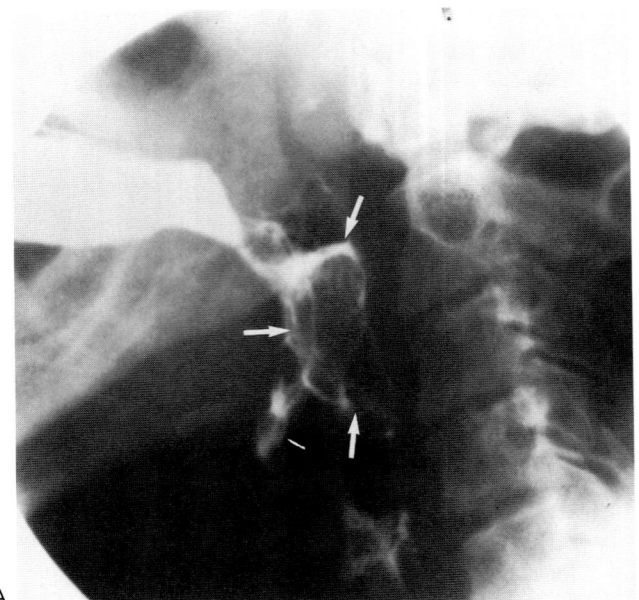

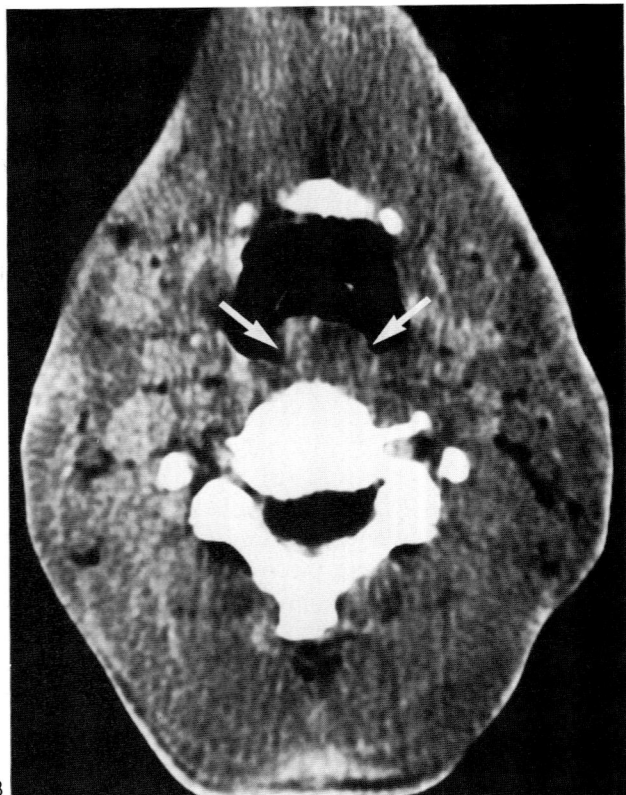

**FIG. 9.** Pharyngeal KS. **A:** Spot film from rapid sequence swallowing study. A large filling defect is seen in the posterior wall of the hypopharynx (*arrows*). **B:** CT reveals lobulated mass (*arrows*). The patient is a 35-year-old i.v. drug user. No skin lesions were present. (Courtesy of Ira Tyler, M.D., Albert Einstein College of Medicine, Bronx, N. Y.).

weight loss, pain, and fever suggests neoplastic involvement. In a prospective evaluation of 22 AIDS patients with diarrhea and/or malabsorption, 10 had infections (cryptosporidia, 3; MAI, 3; campylobacter, 1; candidiasis, 1; salmonella, 1). In two of five patients with malabsorption, no organism was found despite the presence of striking villous atrophy (21).

### Cryptosporidiosis

Cryptosporidial infections may produce a variable pattern of clinical symptoms ranging from moderately severe diarrhea to a choleralike illness that results in uncontrollable dehydration fluid and electrolyte disturbances, and even death. In one clinical series, cryptosporidial infection accounted for nine of 12 patients with GI infection (22). In another report of 80 patients, diarrhea was produced by cryptosporidial infection in 21% (23).

Cryptosporidia is a coccidial protozoan previously known as a cause of bowel disease in domestic animals and poultry. The first reported human case was described in 1976 and seven more cases of self-limiting diarrhea were reported prior to the AIDS epidemic. The diagnosis is usually established by identification of oocysts in the stool. Endoscopic biopsy reveals organisms along the brush border of the intestinal microvilli. The organism is acid-fast and can be stained by a modified Ziehl-Nielson technique (Fig. 21). Treatment has been

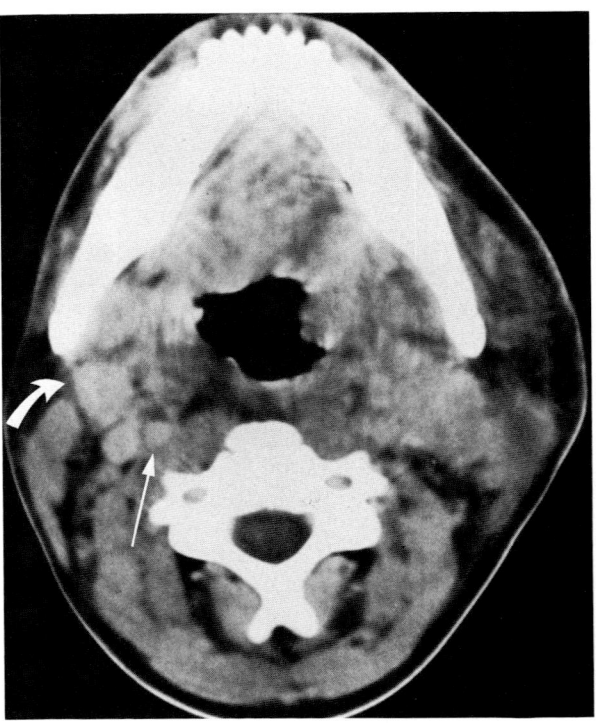

**FIG. 10.** Pharyngeal KS—CT. Pharyngeal space infiltration into the left sternocleidomastoid is demonstrated. *Curved arrow* indicates right submandibular gland. *Straight arrow* indicates right carotid. Compare with loss of this normal anatomy on the left side.

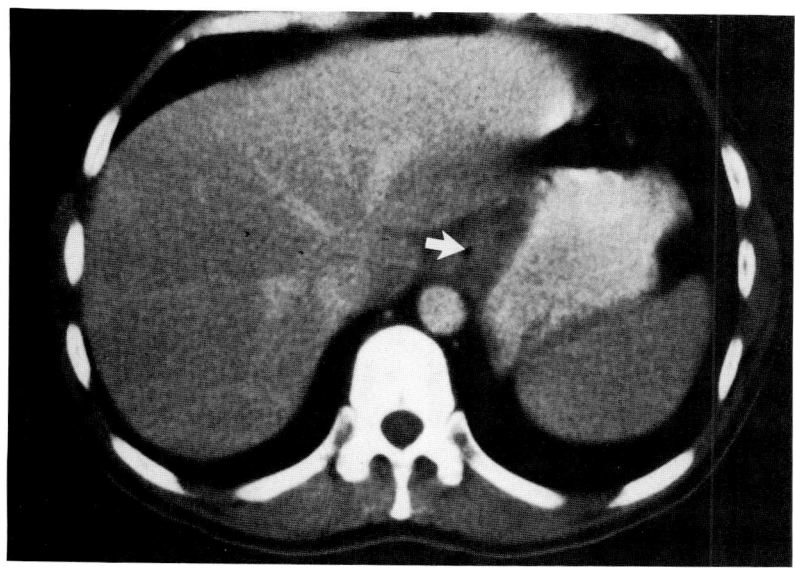

**FIG. 11.** CMV E-G junction—CT scan. The scan was performed to "rule-out" the presence of neoplasm. Marked thickening in the E-G junction is noted. The esophageal lumen is narrowed (*arrow*). The findings are nonspecific, requiring barium radiography or endoscopy for further evaluation. CMV with ulceration was recovered on biopsy.

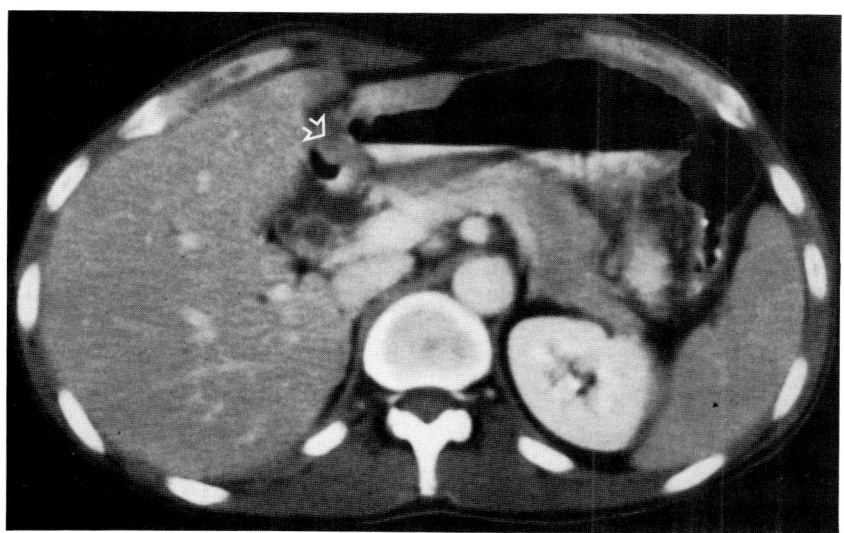

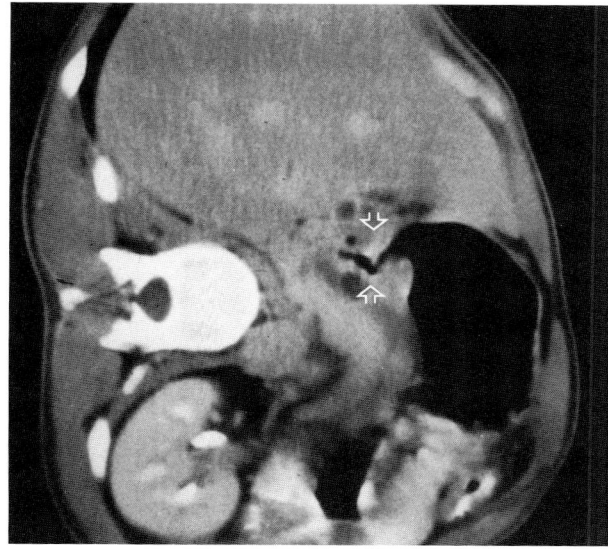

**FIG. 12.** CMV antritis—CT scan—Air contrast. **A:** Routine CT reveals suspicious thickening of the wall of the pyloroantral portion of the stomach (*open arrow*). **B:** Patient scanned in a left side-down decubitus position allowing air to proximally distend distal stomach. Pyloric mural abnormality (*arrow*) is confirmed. **C:** Follow-up barium study revealing submucosal thickening along greater curvature of antrum and in pyloric canal (*arrows*). Endoscopy reveals CMV.

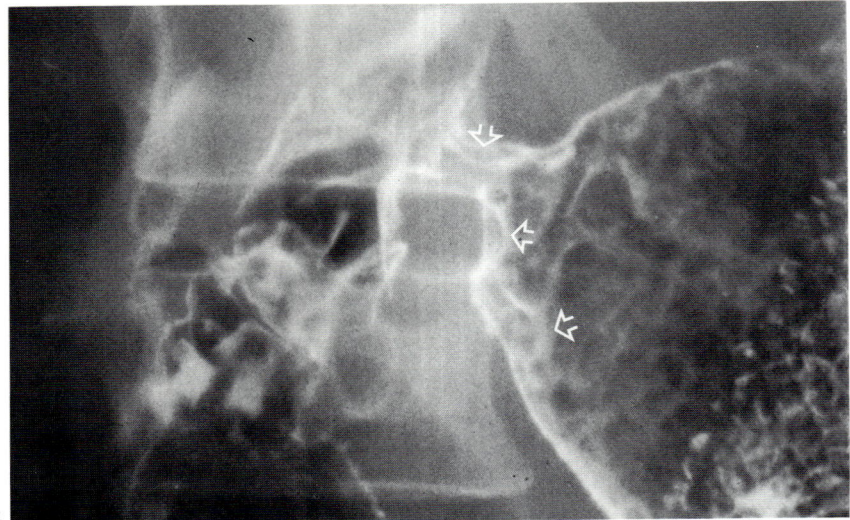

FIG. 12. (Continued)

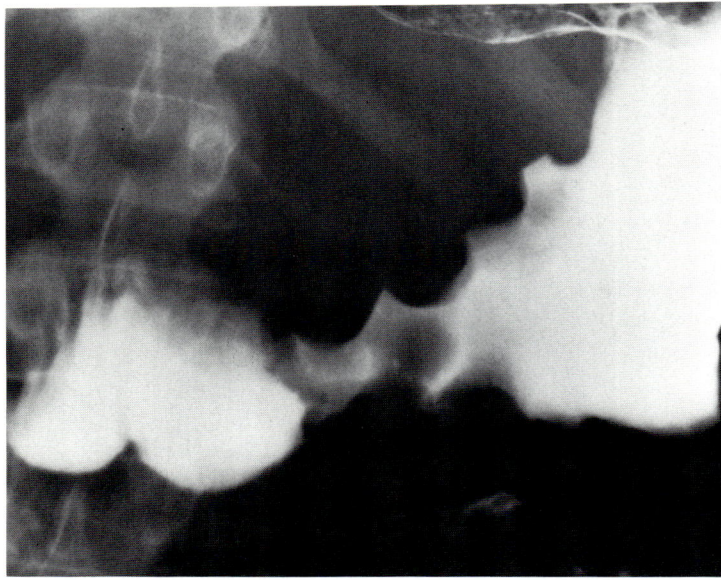

FIG. 13. CMV gastritis. The gastric antrum reveals thumbprinting characteristic of submucosal infiltration. Biopsy revealed CMV inclusion bodies.

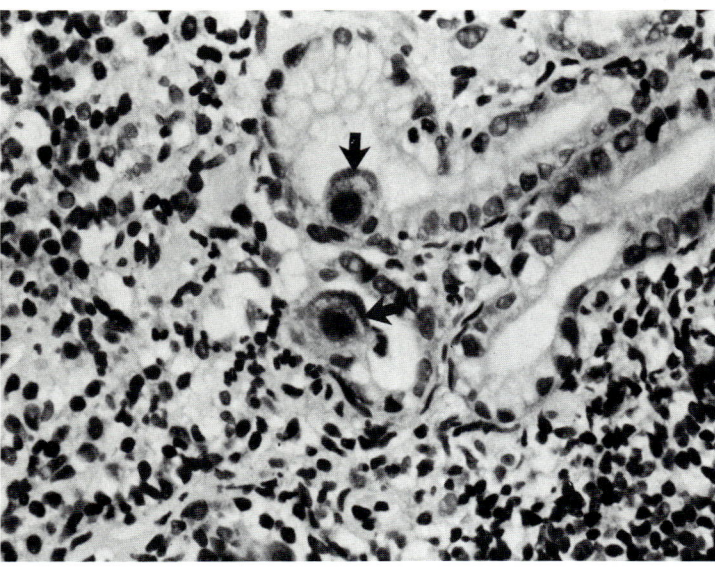

FIG. 14. CMV gastritis—Histologic section. Large nuclear inclusion bodies are easily identified in the bases of the gastric glands (arrows).

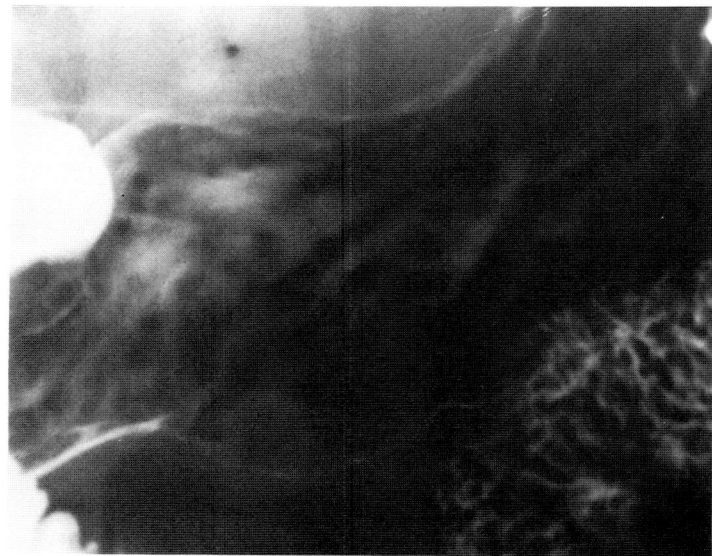

FIG. 15. CMV gastritis. Multiple small nodules are seen in the antrum. Endoscopically these petechial elevations were thought to represent KS. Biopsy revealed CMV.

of limited success, although spiramycin (an antitoxoplasma antibiotic) has provided some control (24). Recently, bovine transfer factor has been used with varying results. The disease usually affects the alimentary canal, but cases of dissemination to the lungs, spleen, and biliary tree are reported (25).

Radiologic features of cryptosporidial enteritis were described by Berk et al. (26). Thirteen of 16 barium studies were abnormal as follows: five patients showed thick folds in the proximal small bowel, four showed fragmentation, three had spasm, and one showed mild dilatation. Most of the involvement was in the proximal intestine with marked thickening and hypersecretion present in the duodenum and jejunum (Fig. 22). In two cases, gastric involvement also was present. Recently we have seen two severe cases in which the intestinal lumen was of normal caliber but there was almost total mucosal atrophy resulting in a "toothpaste" (Fig. 23) appearance. Of note is the high predilection for associated thickening of folds in the duodenum that also may produce findings of marked nodularity or effacement in severe cases (Fig. 24). Differential diagnoses include giardiasis, stronglyoidiosis, Zollinger Ellison syndrome, cystic fibrosis, acquired hypogammaglobulunemia, and Alpha Chain disease. Isospora belli, another coccidial protozoan, may produce identical radiologic features.

### Mycobacterial Infection

Mycobacterial infections of the GI tract are being seen with increasing frequency due in large part to the AIDS

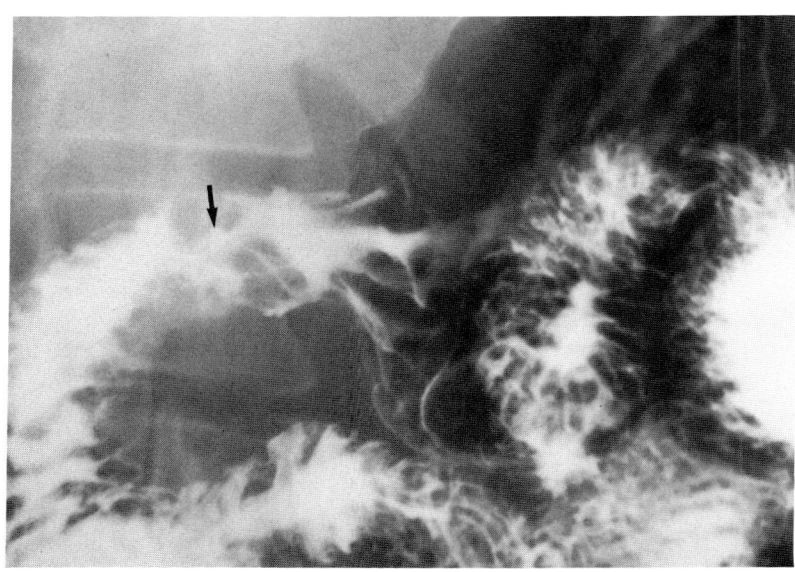

FIG. 16. CMV/cryptosporidial antritis. A small pyloric ulcer is present (arrow); stenosis is seen in the distal antrum. This form of stenotic gastritis is commonly caused by infection with both organisms.

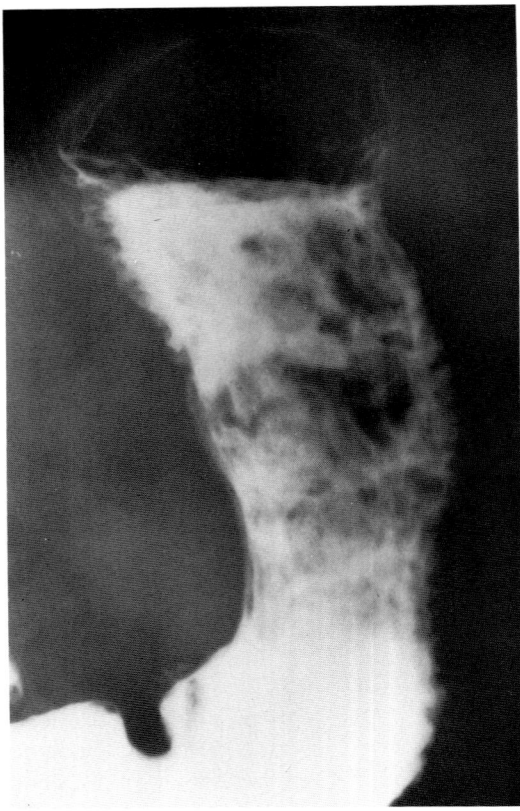

**FIG. 17.** Candida bezoar—Stomach.

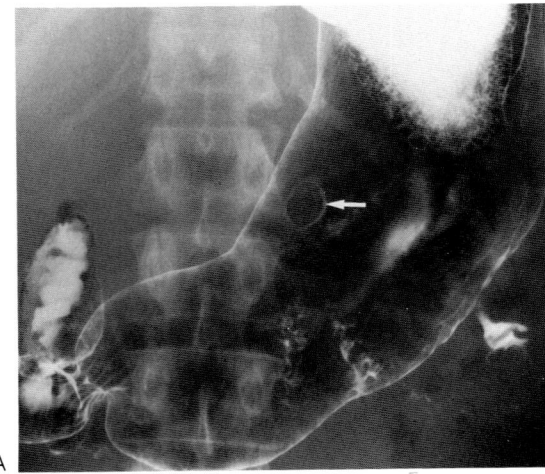

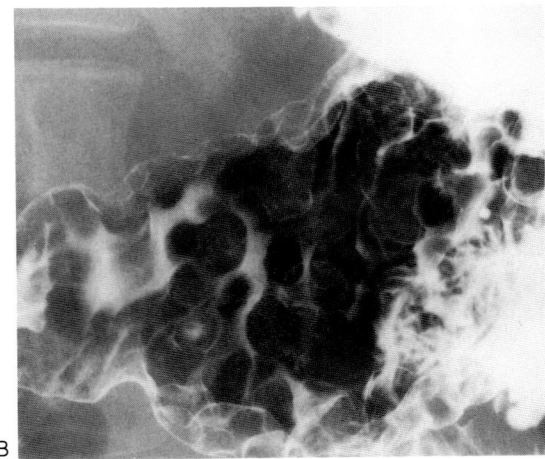

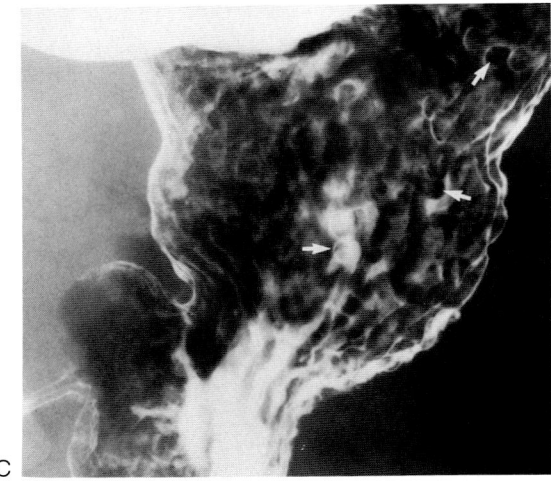

**FIG. 18.** KS—Stomach. **A:** Typical KS lesion (*arrow*) visualized by double-contrast radiography. **B:** Multiple large KS lesions throughout stomach. Despite classic description of "bullseye" lesions, very few KS nodules display central ulceration. **C:** Multiple tiny KS lesions (*arrows*) simulating small gastric polyps.

tention to the presence of MAI in the bowel mucosa simulating Whipple's disease. Vincent and Robbins (31) described the radiographic findings that consisted of epidemic. Both M. tuberculosis and atypical mycobacterial infections may be encountered.

MAI is a slow-growing, nonprotochromogenic, acid-fast bacillus. It is a ubiquitous environmental contaminant rarely producing disease even in patients immunosuppressed for other reasons, and it was rarely implicated in human infections before the AIDS epidemic. This infection has been seen in 20% of AIDS patients followed by the National Institutes of Health (27). The organism is disseminated in the lung, liver, spleen, bone marrow lymph nodes, and GI tract. Histologic examination reveals large "foamy" histiocytes in the lamina propria. Acid-fast staining demonstrates the cells to be filled with numerous bacilli. Granulomas rarely are seen. This lack of granuloma formation is characteristic of AIDS-related MAI infection as opposed to MAI infection in patients with other causes of immunosuppression in whom granulomas do form (Fig. 25) (28).

In the small bowel, MAI infection may produce radiographic findings similar to those of Whipple's disease (Fig. 26). This "pseudo-Whipple" appearance was first described clinically in 1983 in a Haitian woman assumed to have Whipple's disease and associated KS (29). Staining for acid-fast bacillus was not performed on the small bowel mucosa. Roth et al. (30) called at-

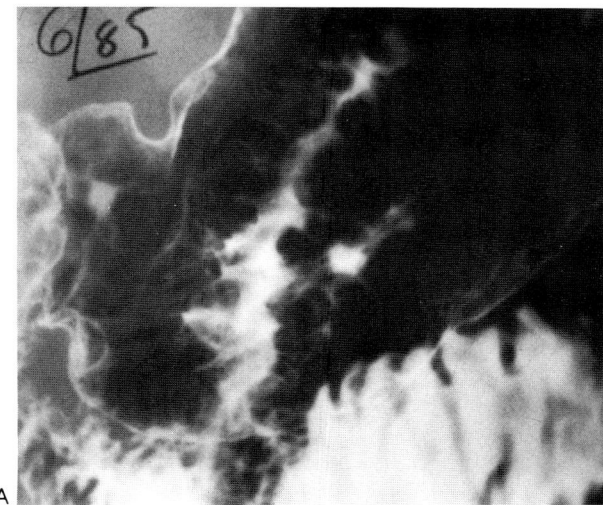 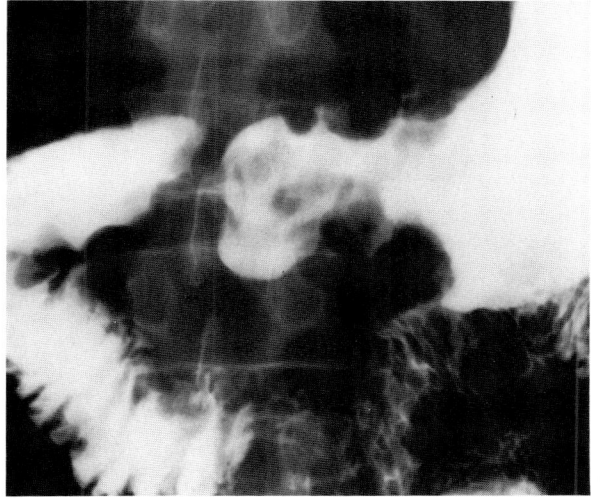

FIG. 19. KS—Progression. **A:** Film from 6/85 reveals discrete nodules in antrum. **B:** Film from 9/85: The nodules have increased in size and number. The antrum is rigid due to the submucosal infiltration by the tumor. Compare this irregular neoplastic nodularity with more symmetric nodularity seen in CMV gastritis (Fig. 11).

mild dilatation of the small bowel with thick undulating folds and fine nodularity. CT scanning reveals mesenteric and retroperitoneal lymphadenopathy, splenomegaly, and ascites (32), and it demonstrates the changes in the small bowel in a small percentage of cases. A more prominent fold pattern is seen without associated thickening of the wall. This is particularly evident in distal ileal loops where marked hypertrophy of the valvulae conniventes can be recognized. This is an unusual appearance for ileal loops and its detection, and the finding supports the diagnosis of MAI infection (Fig. 27). CT often is the first radiographic examination in patients with disseminated MAI infection because this disease may have symptoms suggesting debilitating neoplasm rather than malabsorption or diarrhea. The findings on CT suggest infection rather than neoplasm. This information directs biopsy and proper histochemical analysis to the intestine, bone marrow, or lymph nodes in order to establish the diagnosis. CT appearances of lymphadenopathy in MAI will be discussed in Chapter 5.

## Cytomegalovirus

CMV infection of the small bowel results in a diffuse enteritis or ileo colitis (3,4). It is a severe manifestation of AIDS and it may be preterminal. Intestinal perforation may occur (34), and is attributed to the ischemic necrosis secondary to vasculitis induced by CMV inclusion bodies found in the endothelial cells and the small vessels in the bowel wall (35).

On barium radiography, CMV may produce a diffuse enteritis, but in our experience it more commonly produces findings limited to the distal ileum (Fig. 28). These include narrowing of the terminal ileum with discrete submucosal nodules measuring between 0.25 and 0.75 cm. The colon may be variably involved (Fig. 29). In Teixidor et al.'s (12) series, 7 of 14 patients had CMV enteritis, 3 had barium examinations, and 1 had diffuse jejunal and ileal disease with blunted mucosal folds, narrowing of the lumen, and separation of the loops. A second had deep ulceration of the terminal ileum with fistula formation and a third had a normal barium examination, although distal ileitis was found at autopsy.

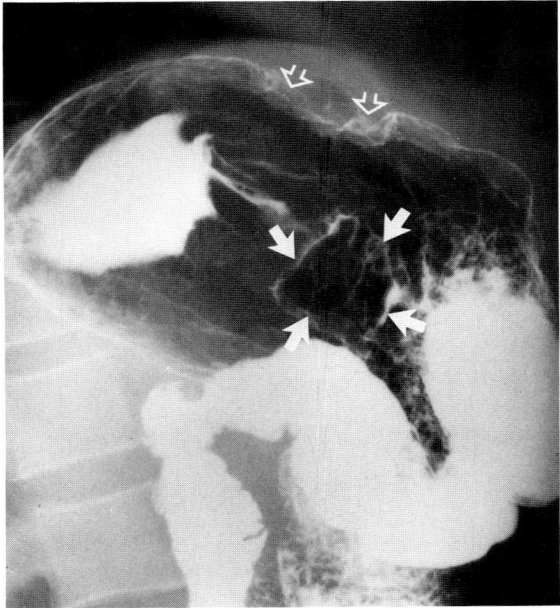

FIG. 20. Gastric lymphoma. A raised submucosal mass is seen along the greater curvature (*open arrows*). The overlapping folds are distorted. A second ulceration is seen "en-face" arising from the pars media (*arrows*).

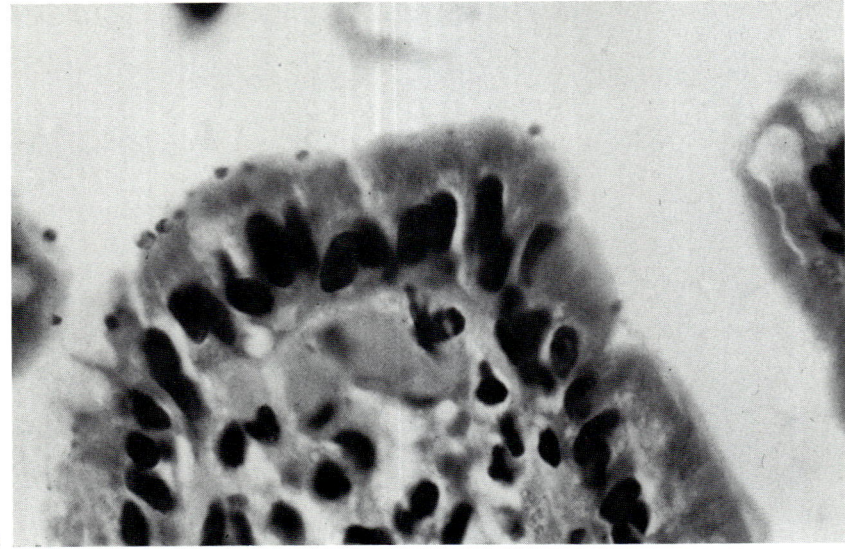

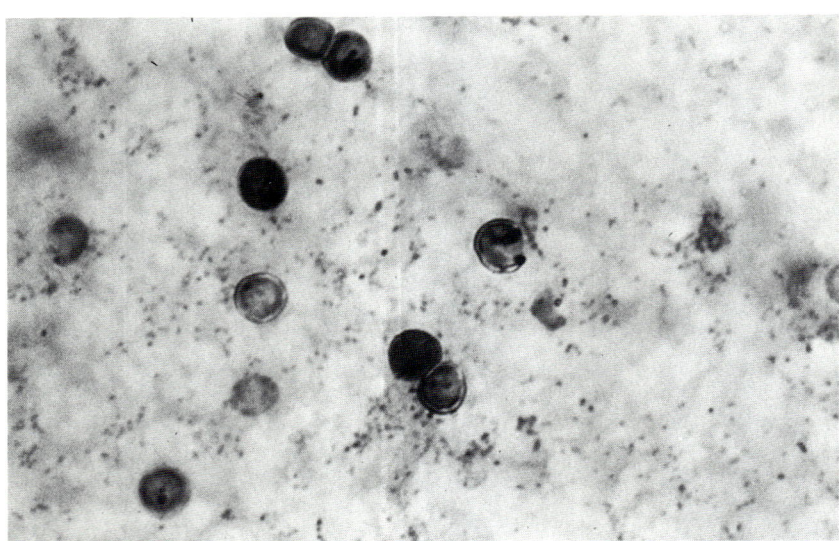

**FIG. 21.** Cryptosporidiosis—Histology and microscopy. **A:** Histologic section of small bowel reveals multiple cryptosporidial oocysts along the brush border of the epithelium. **B:** Stool specimen, acid-fast stain. Multiple cryptosporidial organisms are readily identified.

In the autopsy material 4 patients had involvement of the colon as well.

CT examination in these patients often reveals marked thickening of the wall of the distal ileum with associated colonic disease. The thickening may be so prominent as to produce small bowel obstruction (Fig. 30). Localization of the wall thickening to the terminal ileum, relatively uniform in appearance, lack of mesenteric adenopathy, and associated disease in the colon should lead to a diagnosis of CMV infection of the distal ileum as opposed to lymphoma or other neoplasm.

## NEOPLASMS

KS and lymphoma account for neoplastic complications in the small bowel of AIDS patients. KS lesions present as discrete submucosal nodules (20,36). They generally vary in size from 1 to 2 cm. Preservation of mucosal folds between the lesions distinguishes KS lesions from nodules of lymphoma which are associated with diffuse submucosal infiltration of the bowel wall. When the caliber and fold pattern of the small bowel are distorted, one must consider such complications of KS as intramural hemorrhage or coexistent lymphoma in the differential diagnosis.

The small bowel series is relatively insensitive to KS lesions. Careful fluoroscopy-guided spot filming using graded compression may be necessary to demonstrate the lesions that may be hidden between folds (Fig. 31). Enteroclysis doubtless would improve detection of lesions, but the significance of the finding of KS lesions in the small bowel when demonstrated in the stomach or colon does not warrant putting these ill patients through

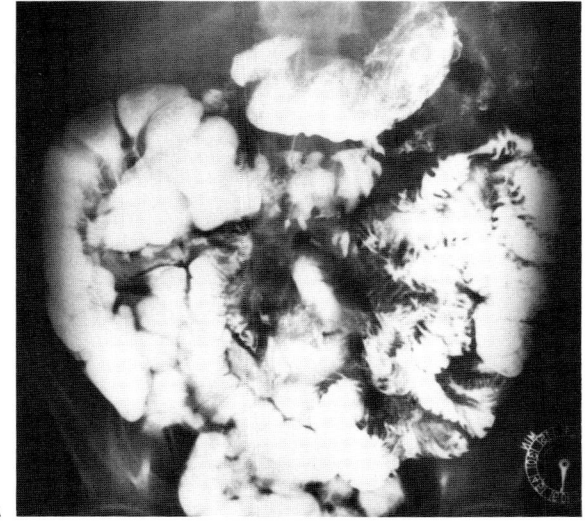
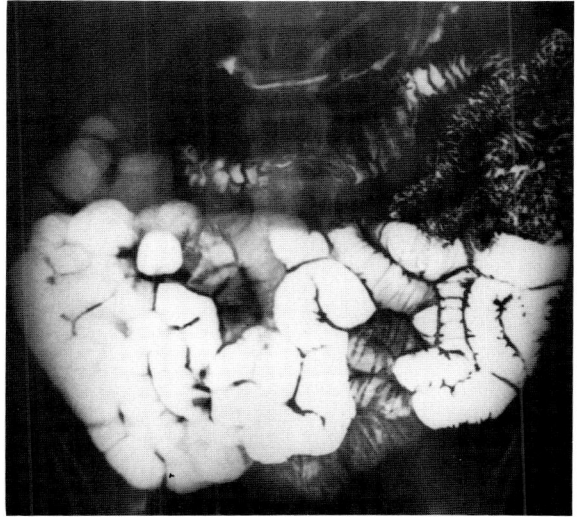
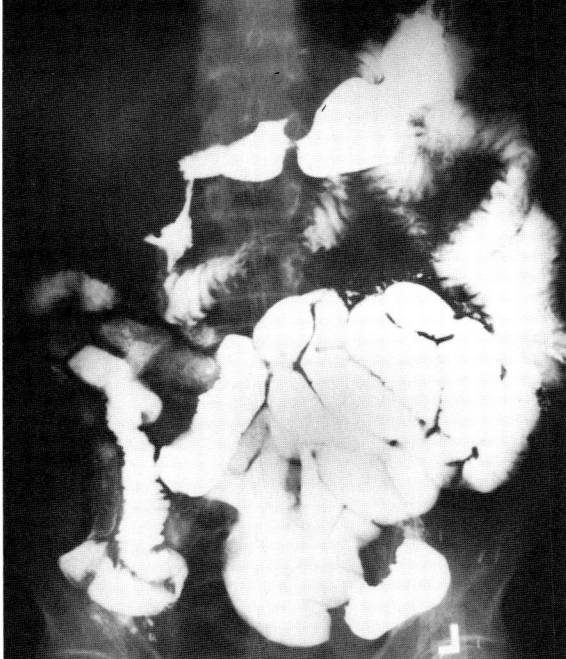

FIG. 22. Cryptosporidiosis typical radiographic patterns. **A:** Dilated bowel loops with hypersecretion are seen. The folds are preserved. **B:** Small bowel series in another patient reveals fragmentation of the barium column and jejunal secretion. The entire bowel is dilated. **C:** Severe cryptosporidial infection with marked dilatation, hypersecretion, and fold preservation. Prominent duodenal disease resulted in stricturing and effacement of the second portion of the duodenum. In these three cases, the pattern is similar to sprue.

this somewhat difficult examination. KS rarely causes complications in the small bowel. Anecdotal cases of KS lesions leading to intussusceptions have been described (Fig. 31C). These lesions rarely bleed unless the patient is on an anticoagulant therapy or has a bleeding diathesis.

Lymphoma may involve the small bowel, producing a variety of radiographic appearances. In our experience focal lesions with discrete, penetrating ulcers or multiple nodules with associated bowel thickening are the most common radiographic appearances in AIDS-related lymphoma. As stated previously, unlike classic GI lymphoma, AIDS-related GI lymphoma is more commonly seen distal to the ligament of Treitz.

CT scanning has a high sensitivity in detection of GI lymphoma (37) and is the imaging modality of choice to exclude this diagnosis in AIDS patients (38). Findings include variably thickened small bowel loops with loss of mucosal features resulting in blunted folds. As opposed to classic small intestinal lymphoma, mesenteric adenopathy is infrequently visualized (Fig. 32). Further detail on the radiographic appearance of mesenteric changes in AIDS-related lymphoma may be found in Chapter 5.

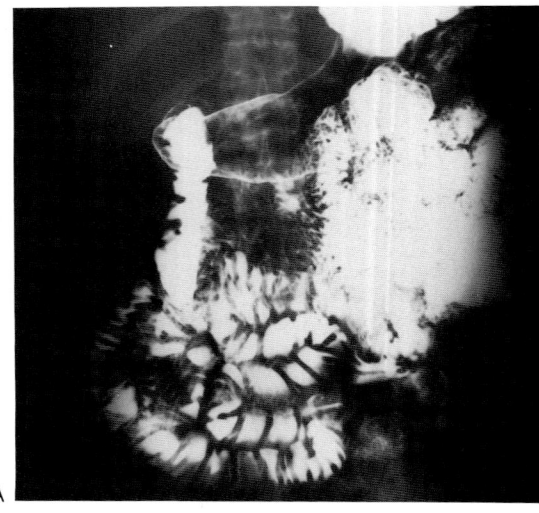 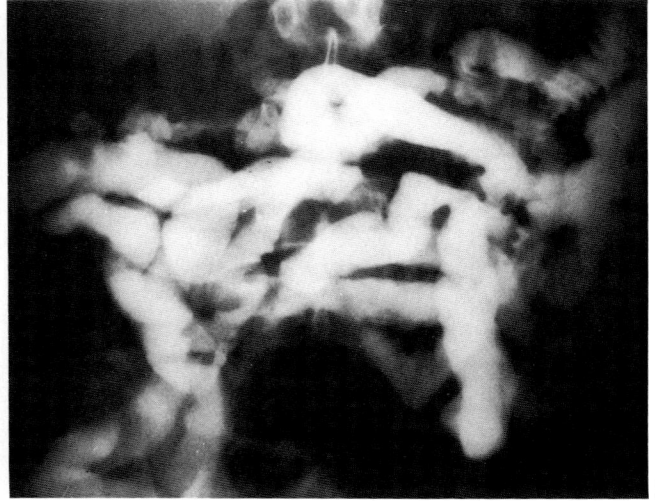

FIG. 23. Cryptosporidiosis—Atypical appearances. **A:** Dilatation of distal small bowel with marked fold thickening. **B:** In another patient, diffuse mucosal sloughing has resulted in a "toothpaste" appearance.

## COLON

### Colitis

Colitis due to a variety of organisms is prevalent in the gay population. Many individuals harbor ameba, gonococcous, shigella, salmonella, or campylobacter. The "gay bowel syndrome" has been described due to a variety of common pathogens (39). These patients also may have a variety of anal infections. Nonspecific periproctitis may be visualized on CT scanning as a hazy increased density in the perianal fat. Moon et al. (40) described the perirectal abnormalities in 23 of 28 (82%) homosexual men with AIDS-related KS and lymphadenopathy syndrome. In 22 of 23, the abnormalities were due to inflammatory disease rather than tumor. Albin et al. (41) reported rectal and perirectal abnormalities visualized by CT in 8 of 30 patients. In this series 6 of 8 had inflammatory disease and 2 had tumor. The CT appearances were identical in both groups.

Several colitides are unique in AIDS patients. Only CMV colitis produces radiographic findings that may be distinguishable from other infectious colitides. Cryptosporidia and MAI infections have been documented in the colon of AIDS patients but they do not produce characteristic x-ray findings. As stated previously, double-contrast studies are essential for demonstrating the radiographic findings in the colon. In Wall et al.'s series (3), 16 of 19 patients had an abnormal barium enema. All segments of the colon were equally involved. In Frager et al.'s series (6) five patients demonstrated colonic disease. In this latter group, all were due to CMV infection.

CMV colitis may run a variable course in AIDS patients (42). The colitis may be mild or there may be fulminant disease with toxic megacolon and multiple sites of gangrenous necrosis of the bowel wall (43). Hemorrhagic colitis may be seen: several cases of CMV producing an endoscopic appearance simulating pseudomembranous colitis have been described (44). CMV must be actively sought in these patients. The predilection of a cecal involvement with multiple deep linear ulcers as seen in renal transplant patients also is seen in the AIDS population (45).

In a review by Hinnant et al. (46), it was shown that CMV is the second most common infection found in

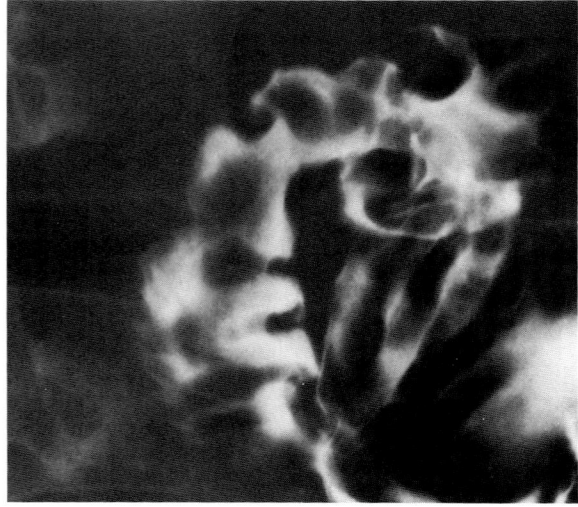

FIG. 24. Cryptosporidiosis—Duodenum. Marked fold thickening simulating nodules is present in the duodenal bulb and sweep in this patient with cryptosporidiosis.

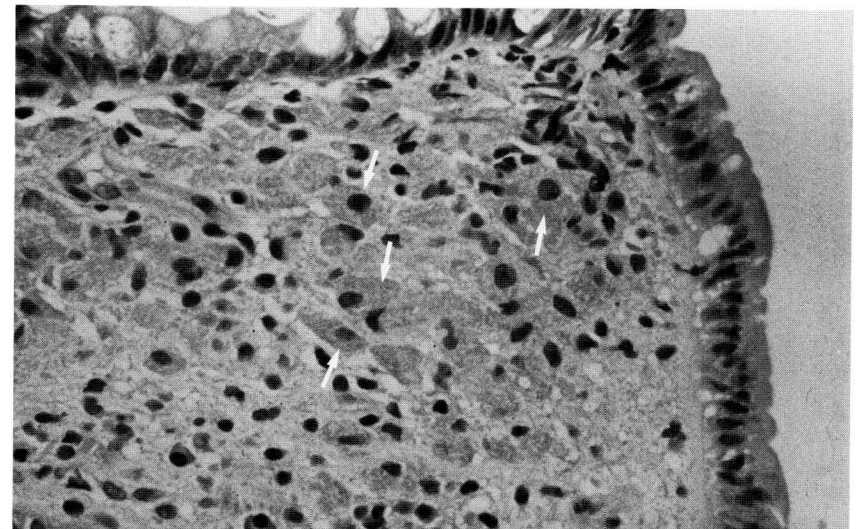
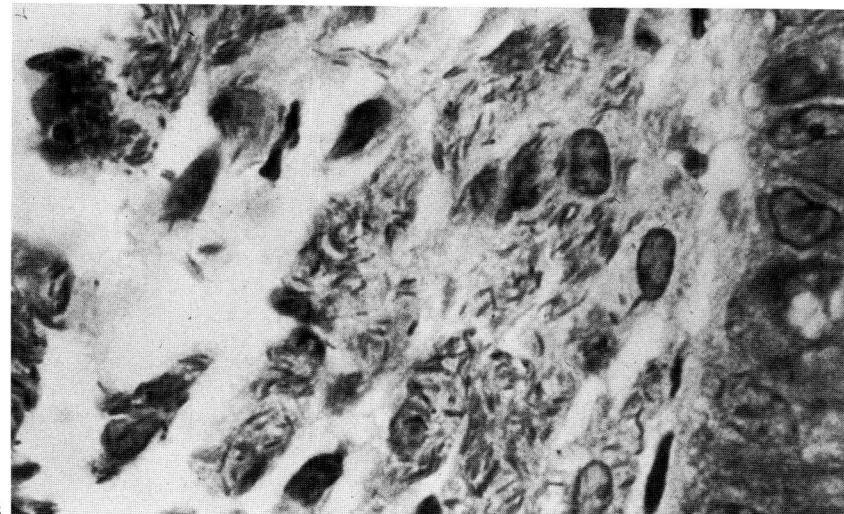

**FIG. 25.** MAI histology. **A:** Rectal biopsy: large "foamy" histiocytes are seen in the colonic lamina propia (arrows). **B:** Same patient, AFB stain. Innumerable acid-fast bacilli choke the histiocytes. The large number of organisms and lack of granuloma formation are characteristic of MAI infection in AIDS.

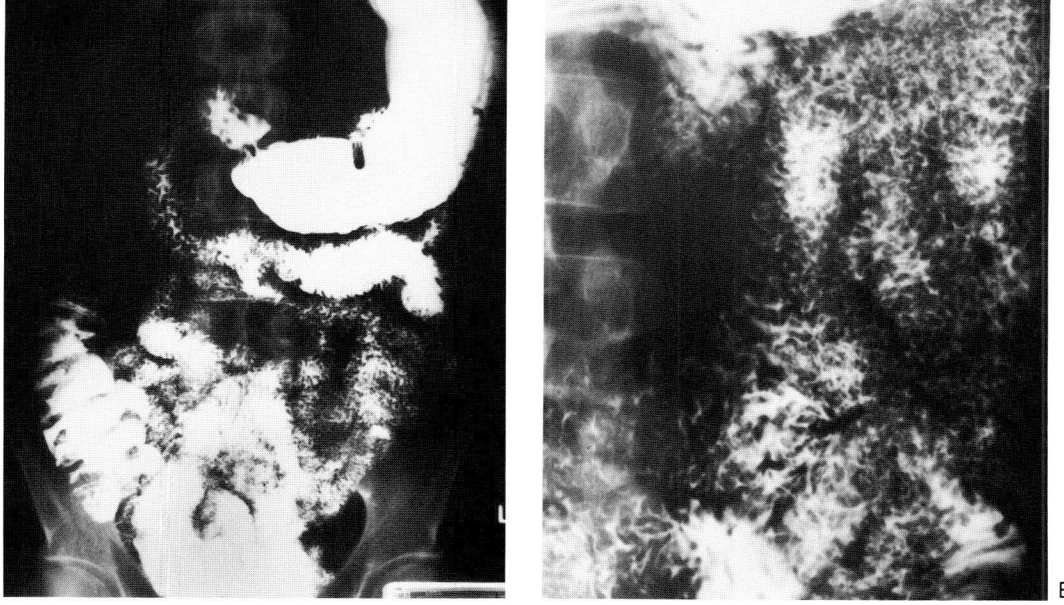

**FIG. 26.** MAI small bowel. **A:** This overhead radiograph reveals a diffuse increase in the folds throughout the jejunum and ileum. KS lesions are present in the duodenal bulb. **B:** Spot film from A. The folds appear "sandy" due to the marked villous hypertrophy. The findings are similar to classic Whipple's disease.

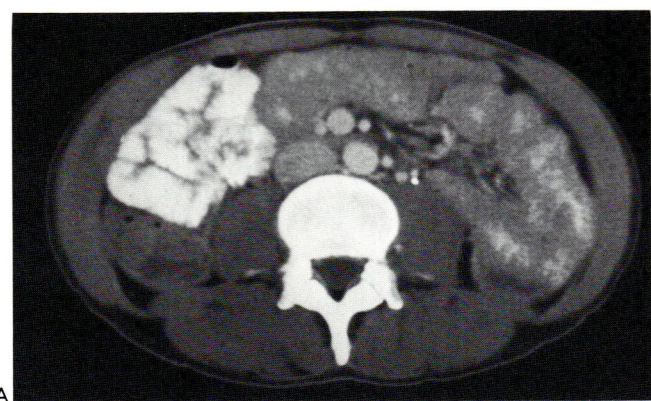
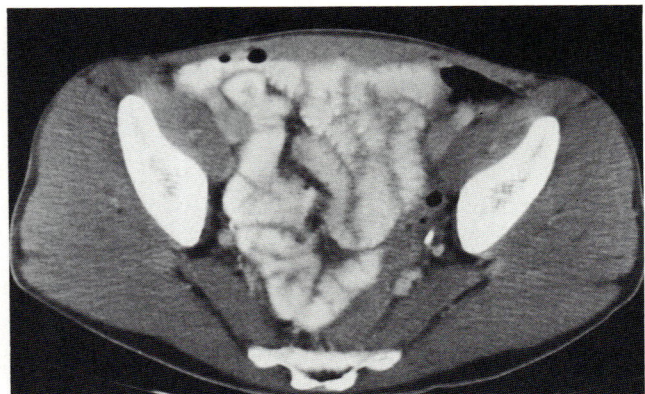
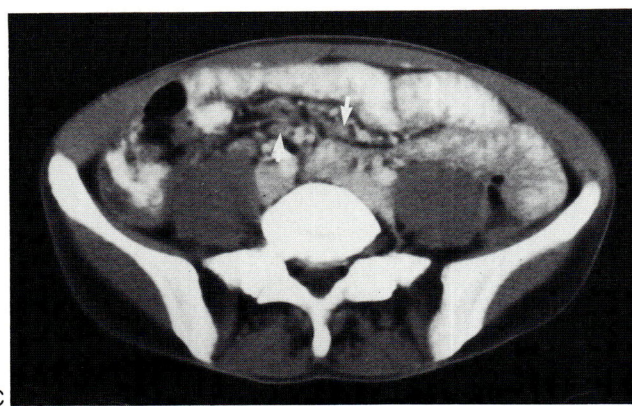

**FIG. 27.** MAI small bowel CT scan. **A:** Mid-abdominal scan reveals secretion in jejunum simulating a thick wall. The folds are prominent in the ileum. **B:** Scan through pelvis reveals the exaggerated fold pattern in ileal loops (pseudo-Whipple appearance). **C:** Scan through pelvic inlet reveals exaggerated small bowel folds. Note the mesenteric lymphadenopathy (*arrows*) seen among the enhanced mesenteric vessels. These scans were performed to rule out lymphoma. The pattern of fold abnormality and mesenteric adenopathy led to the diagnosis of MAI infection confirmed on small bowel biopsy. The small bowel series (see Fig. 25) was performed after this CT.

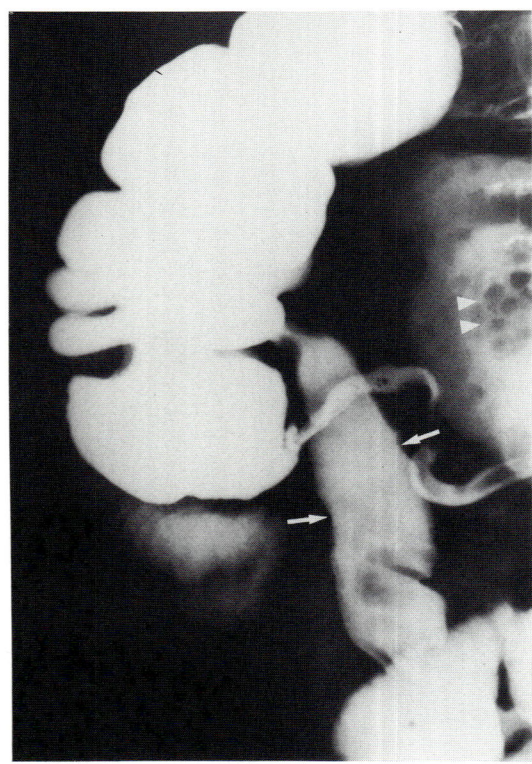

**FIG. 28.** CMV ileitis. The terminal ileal mucosa is absent. Multiple, discrete submucosal elevations are seen (*arrows*). The colon is involved (*arrowheads*) (see Fig. 33B).

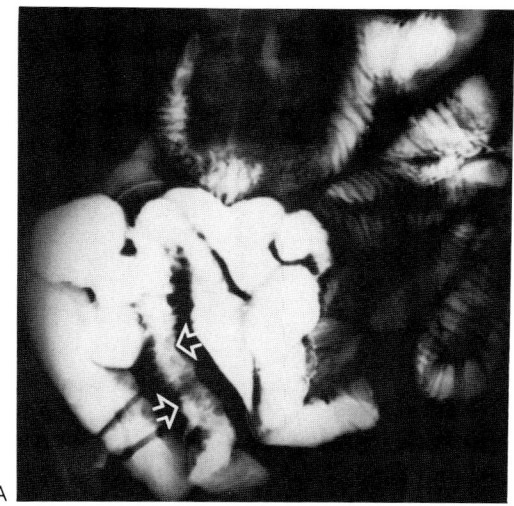
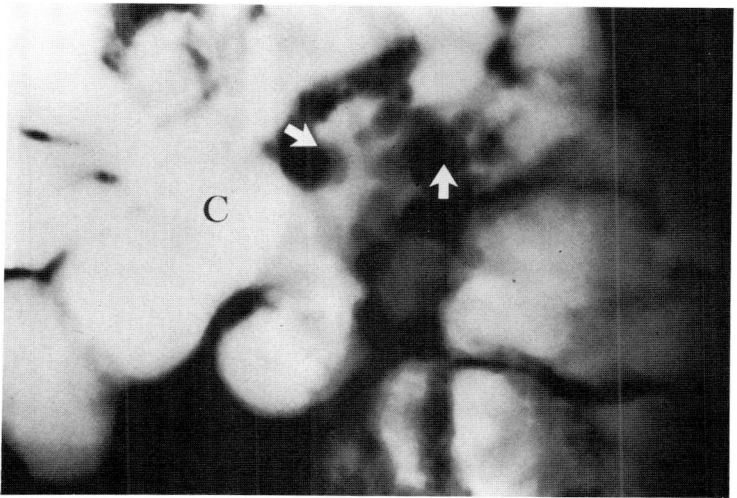

**FIG. 29.** CMV ileitis. **A:** Overhead radiograph reveals marked submucosa infiltration of the distal ileum (*open arrows*). **B:** Spot film reveals submucosal nodularity in terminal ileum (*arrows*). C, cecum.

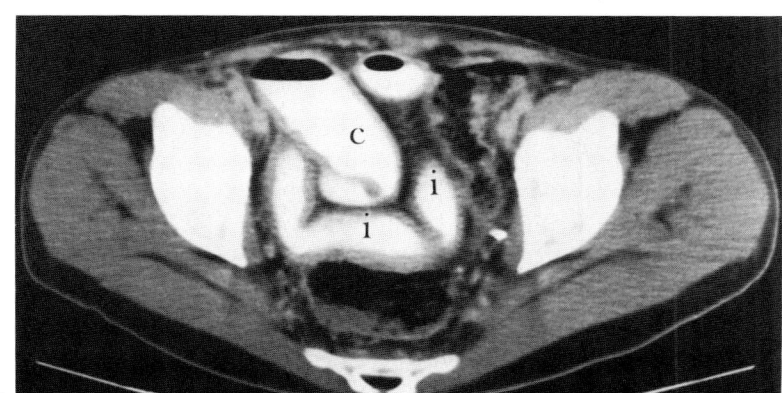
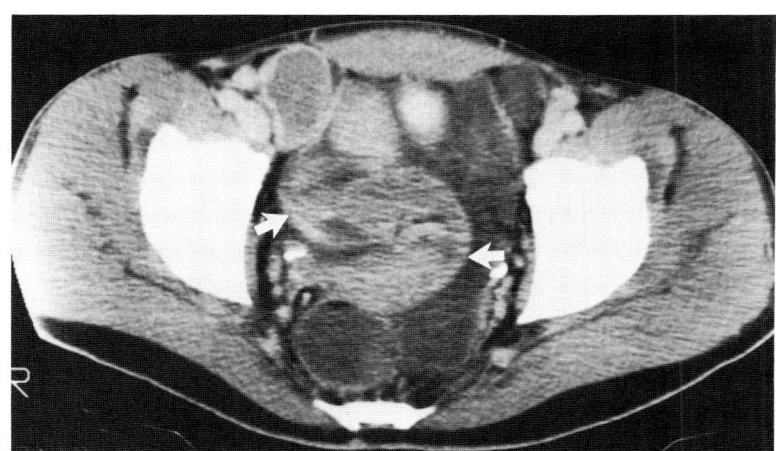

**FIG. 30.** CMV ileitis—CT scan. **A:** Pelvic CT in patients studied to exclude malignancy reveals a continuous segment of intestinal wall thickening in distal ileum (i) and cecum (c). This study led to endoscopic biopsy of the right colon with recovery of CMV inclusions. **B:** CT in another patient (see Fig. 29) with symptoms of small bowel obstruction. Dilated mid-ileal loops are seen in the left pelvis. A contiguous segment of distal ileum (*arrows*) displays a thickened wall with obliteration of the lumen. This patient's distal ileum perforated several days following this scan.

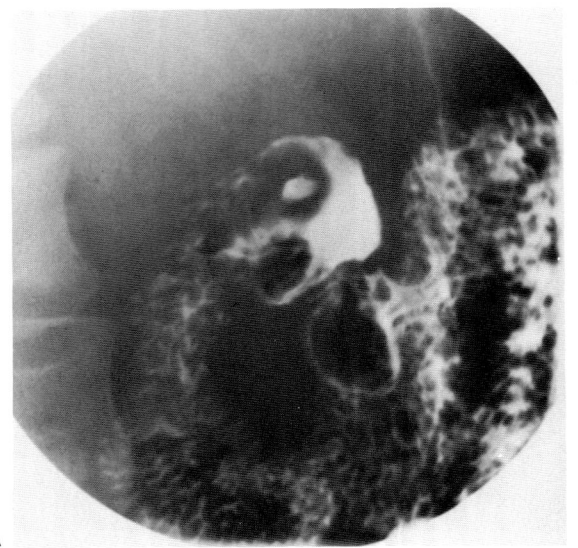
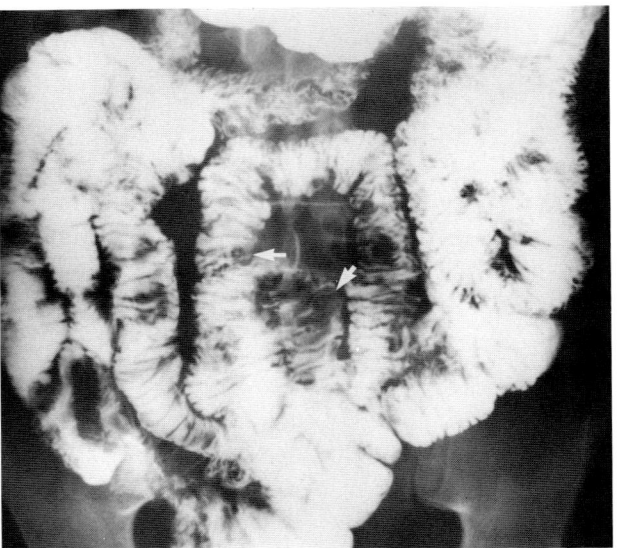
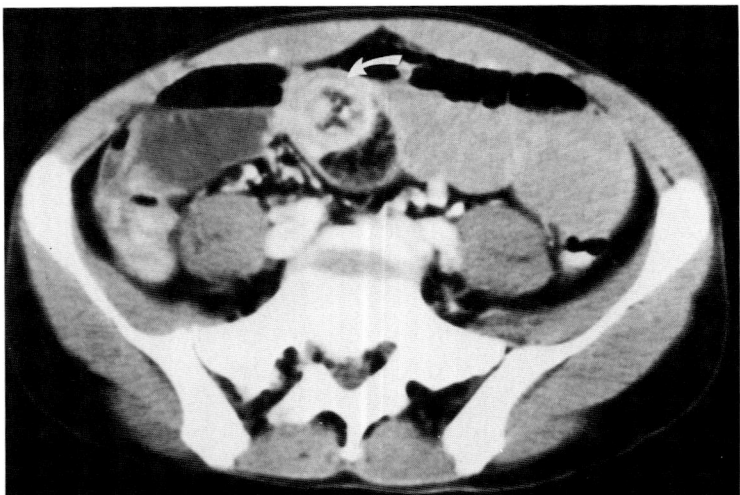

**FIG. 31.** KS—Small bowel. **A:** Focal "bullseye" lesion, duodenal bulb from KS. Ulceration is uncommon in our experience. **B:** Multiple KS nodules throughout small bowel. Occasional umbilications are seen (*arrows*). **C:** Small bowel obstruction resulting from ileo-ileal intussusception led by a Kaposi Sarcoma lesion (curved arrow).

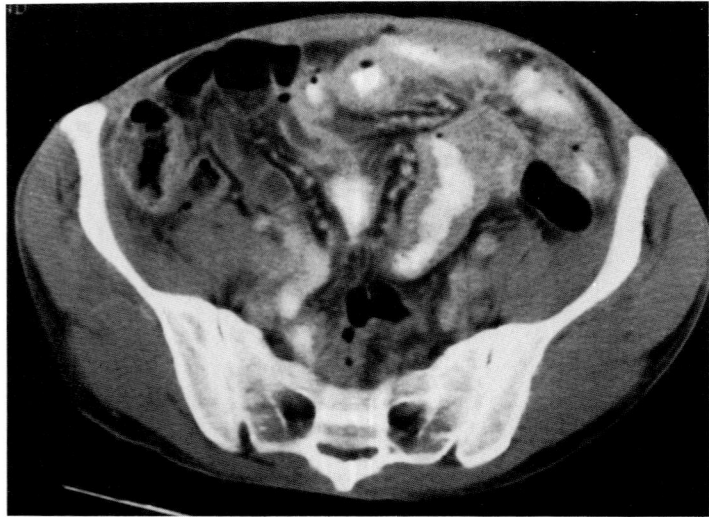
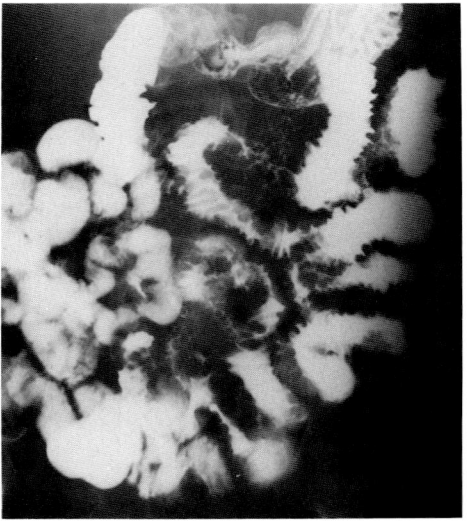

**FIG. 32.** Small bowel lymphoma. **A:** CT shows irregular wall thickening with abnormal luminal contour in the jejunum. Thickened mesenteric leaves are seen but no large node masses are present. **B:** Small bowel series, same patient as A. Note the irregular degree of involvement in multiple loops. Submucosal infiltration (reflected in a "picket-fence" appearance) and multiple-sized submucosal nodules are present. Compare these findings with Fig. 31 in which discrete nodules are recognized against a normal mucosal pattern.

AIDS patients preceded only by PCP. The colon is the most frequent site of CMV 1B infection in AIDS patients. As compared with other immunosuppressed patients, those with AIDS have higher titers to CMV 1B. The colon is more frequently diseased in AIDS patients than is the upper GI tract, which is diseased more frequently in nonAIDS patients. CMV may be more easily cultured from the right colon as opposed to the sigmoid colon (46).

Balthazar et al. (47) described the radiographic findings in 11 patients with CMV colitis. In eight positive cases studied by barium enema, three showed diffuse mucosal granularity involving the entire colon. One patient showed involvement of the left colon. In four cases, cecal spasm with ulceration and terminal ileal fold effacement is present. Since publication of this report, we have noted two cases with classic apthous ulcers (Fig. 33). In Teixidor et al.'s series (12), four of eight patients underwent barium enema. In three, the colonic mucosa showed granularity in superficial or deep ulceration. The fourth patient had a normal barium enema. Frager et al. (48) reported radiologic findings in six cases of CMV colitis. Radiographic changes of mild decrease included a mild reticular granular mucosal pattern and apthous ulcers. Severe disease was characterized by multiple large discrete ulcers and submucosal hemorrhage (Fig. 34).

At our institution, barium enema is used infrequently to diagnose CMV colitis. Many of these patients undergo CT scanning as the primary imaging modality in an attempt to rule out neoplastic disease. CT findings include thickening of the colonic wall (Fig. 35A). A "target sign," due to submucosal edema, usually is present. Visualization of the target sign helps to distinguish inflammatory from neoplastic wall thickening. Most cases show a pancolitis, but right-sided involvement always is present. Sometimes associated thickening of the wall of the distal ileum is noted. Contiguous involvement of ileum and right colon, associated target sign, and variable distal colitis may be considered virtually diagnostic of CMV colitis in an AIDS patient. Obviously, one must interpret films with a history of AIDS because similar findings may be found in Crohn's disease and salmonella infection.

On barium studies, the colonic involvement is generally documented by antegrade opacification during small bowel examination. The abnormal contour of the colon can be sufficiently visualized by this method without performing a retrograde study.

In advanced stages, patients with CMV colitis may present with toxic dilatation of the colon which may progress to perforation. Clinical presentation is severe acute abdominal pain. On plain film one may see a dilated colon with detectable nodularity along the wall (Fig. 36A). CT may reveal a dilated thin-walled colon and serosal enhancement. Intramural gas dissection may be visualized within the wall, indicative of vascular compromise. Peritoneal fluid is seen in association with the dilated colon and CMV organisms may be recovered from it (Fig. 35B). Occasionally patients may present with spontaneous pneumotosis coli (Fig. 36B). These findings result from the vasculitis induced by CMV infection of the colonic submucosa. CMV inclusion bodies may be found in the endothelial cells of the submucosal vessels and may lead to ischemic necrosis of the bowel wall (Fig. 36C, D).

We recently have seen two cases of isolated cecal ulceration as a manifestation of CMV colitis (49,50). This

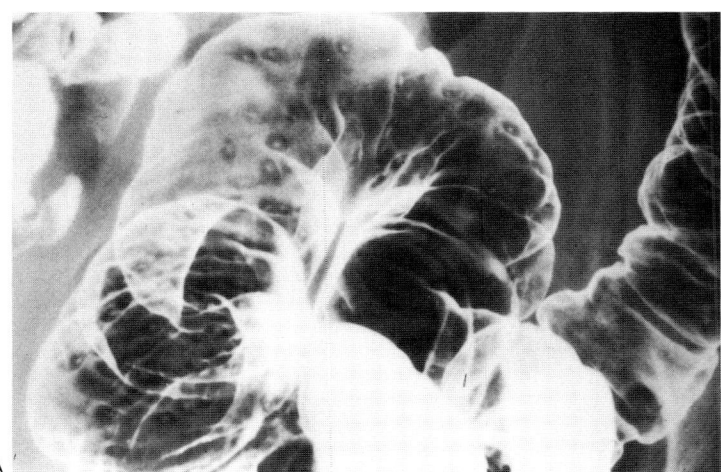
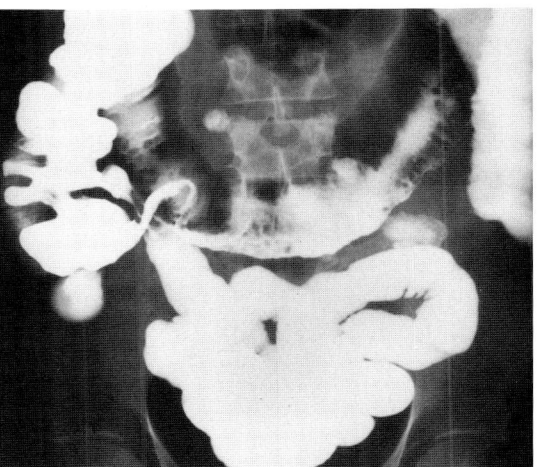

FIG. 33. CMV colitis. A: Multiple apthous ulcers. B: Follow-through examination from small bowel series in a different patient. Multiple raised lesions are seen in the transverse colon (same patient as Fig. 28).

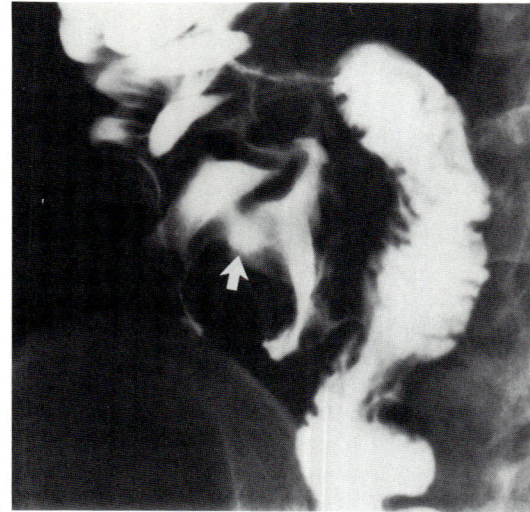
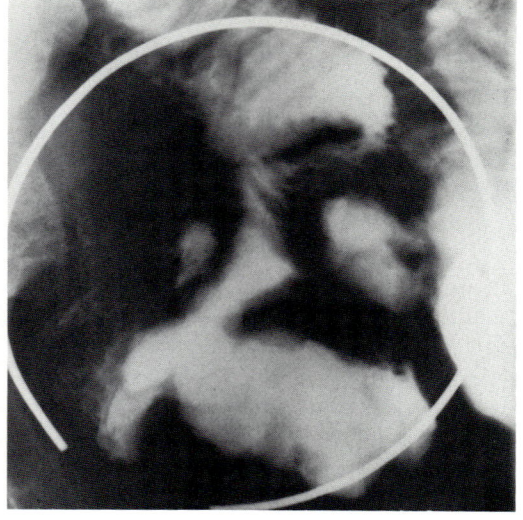

**FIG. 34.** CMV colitis—Cecal ulcer. **A:** Spot film from small bowel series reveals marked spasm in cecum with large ulceration (*arrow*). The terminal ileum and remaining colon are spared. **B:** Compression spot in another patient. Barium in the cecum has been compressed revealing a deep ulcer. Graded compression must be used in these cases due to the intense spasm in the ileocecal region.

finding has been described in renal transplant patients with CMV colitis but to our knowledge has not been described previously in AIDS patients. In one case the ulcer in the cecum was the only finding of CMV colitis. In the other patient, distal ileal involvement was associated.

Other organisms, such as cryptosporidia, MAI, and histoplasmosis, may produce colitis in AIDS patients. Insufficient radiographic case material has been accumulated to allow definition of characteristic radiologic features (Fig. 37).

### Neoplasms

KS and lymphoma are the two major neoplasms found in the colon of AIDS patients. KS presents with either isolated submucosal plaques or focal areas of submucosal infiltration. This submucosal infiltration may be reflected as a localized cluster of undulating filling defects that narrows the colonic lumen, or as a granular focal plaquelike lesion along various segments of the bowel (Fig. 38). Both institutions have seen patients who have presented with acute appendicitis caused by KS lesions occluding the appendiceal orifice leading to per-

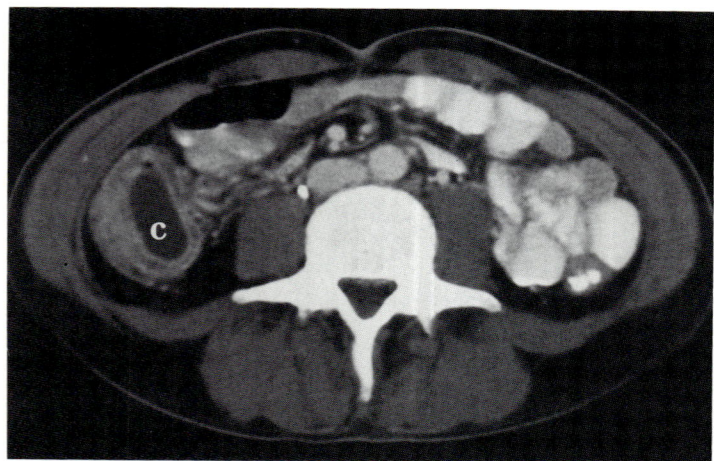
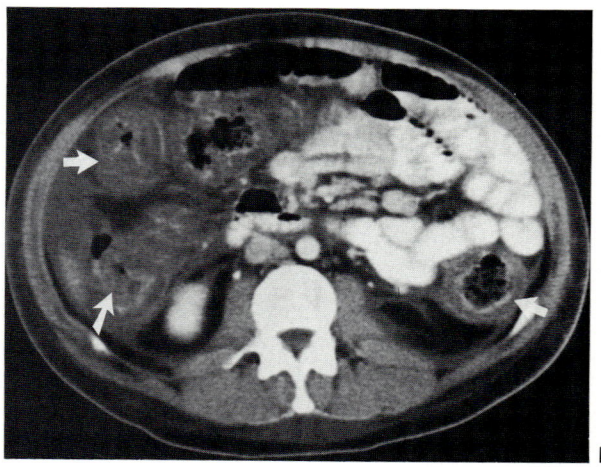

**FIG. 35.** CMV colitis CT. **A:** Marked thickening of the wall of the ascending colon (c) is seen. A target sign is present. **B:** CT in another patient with fever reveals a marked colon wall thickening. The serosa appears hyperemic (*arrows*). Marked submucosal edema is evident with the attenuation values of the clonic wall approaching water density ascites. Ascites, due to CMV peritonitis, is seen.

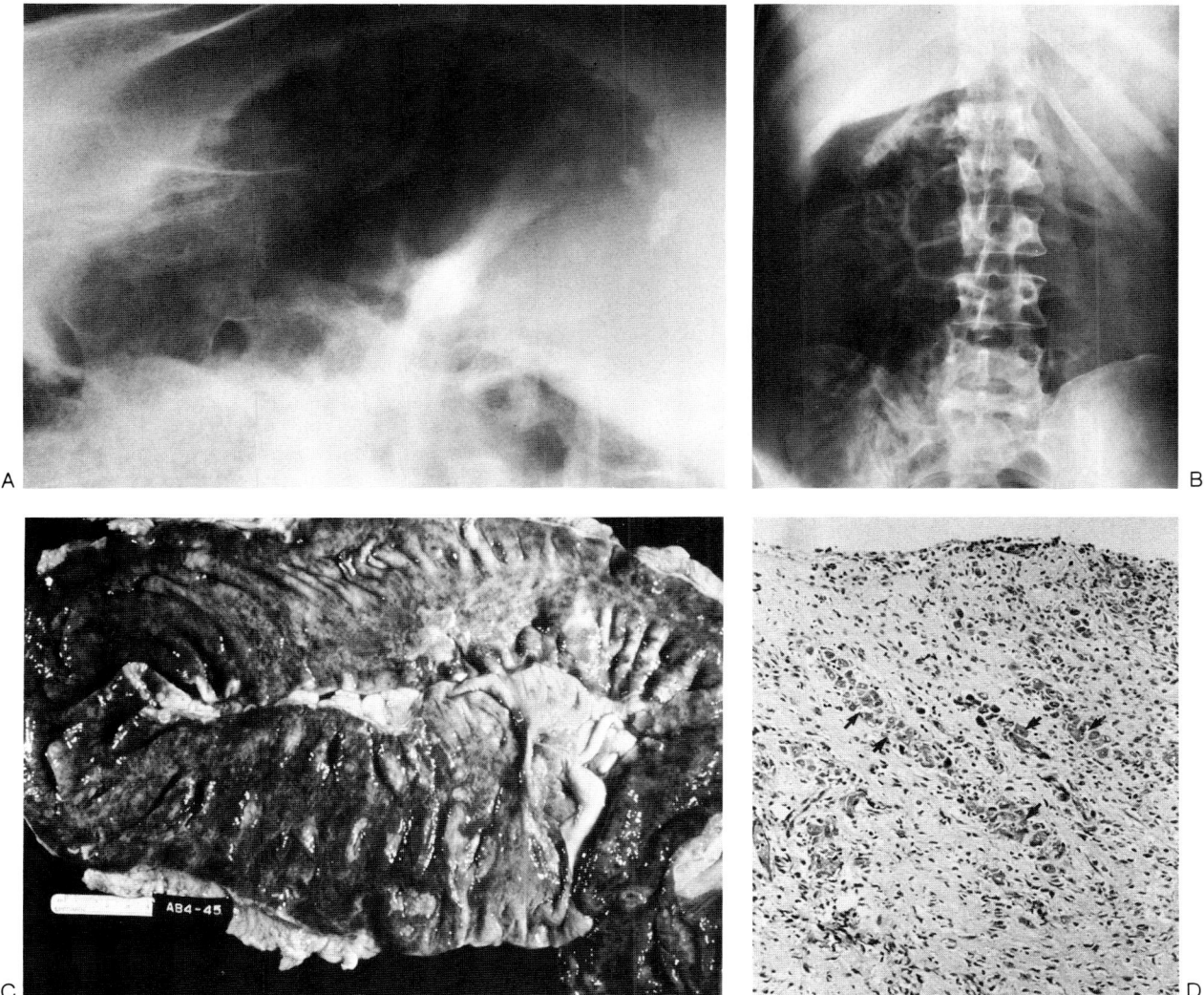

FIG. 36. CMV colitis. **A:** Plain film, left side-down decubitus, reveals dilated, ahaustral right colon with a nodular wall. **B:** Plain film in another patient. Pneumatosis coli due to breakdown of colonic mucosa is present. This patient died within 24 hours of this film. **C:** Autopsy specimen in another patient with CMV colitis revealing areas of mucosal ulcerations and diffuse hemmorrhage. **D:** Histologic section reveals loss of colonic mucosa. The endothelial cells are enlarged and contain inclusion bodies (*arrows*). This "vasculitis" results in the hemorrhagic, ischemic necrosis seen in terminal CMV colitis.

foration and abscess. In neither case was a preoperative diagnosis made.

Colonic lymphoma is more common in the AIDS population than in nonAIDS patients with bowel lymphoma. In our own population of patients with AIDS-related lymphoma we have seen four cases of colonic lymphoma, a higher percentage of colonic involvement than seen in classical lymphoma. The appearances are variable. Polypoid lesions simulating adenocarcinoma and bulky masses leading to intussusception have been seen. There is a high predilection of rectal involvement in AIDS-related lymphoma; these have been seen in both the N.Y.U. and California case experiences. Bulky infiltrating masses surrounding the rectum, infiltrating the pelvic floor are seen (Fig. 39). We have seen two patients who presented with discrete perianal masses. Both were presumed to have perirectal abscesses, and CT was performed to evaluate the extent of the disease. Burkitt's lymphoma was found in the perianal biopsy (Fig. 40) of both patients. Thus, any perianal mass in an AIDS patient that does not respond clinically to abscess treatment should be biopsied to rule out lymphoma. As in our cases of small bowel lymphoma, there often is a striking lack of nodal disease in these patients.

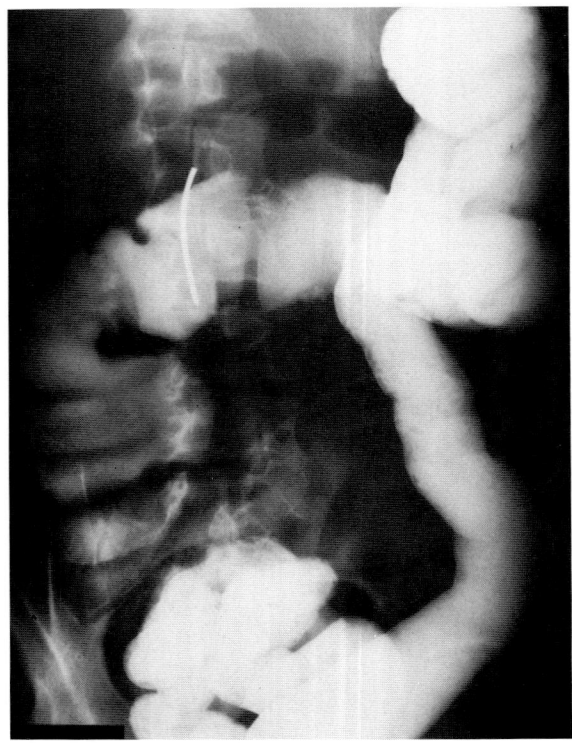

**FIG. 37.** Cryptosporidial colitis. Diffuse "vesicular" filling defects are seen as well as a focal nodular mass at the hepatic flexure (same patient as Fig. 22A).

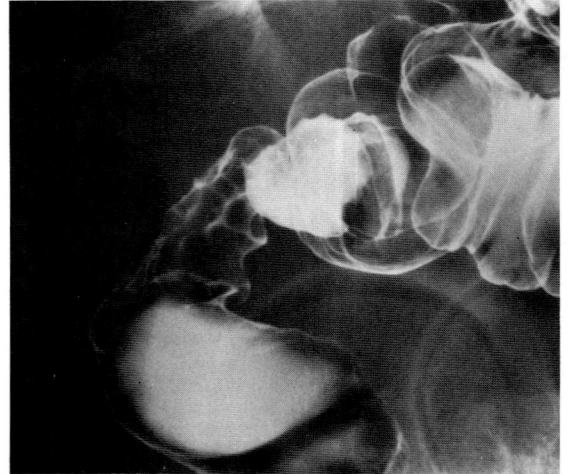

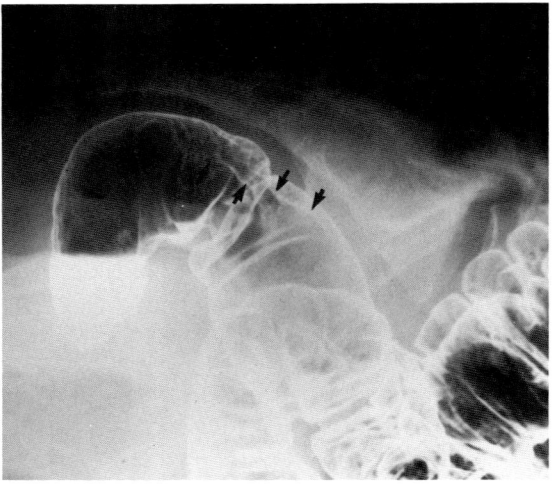

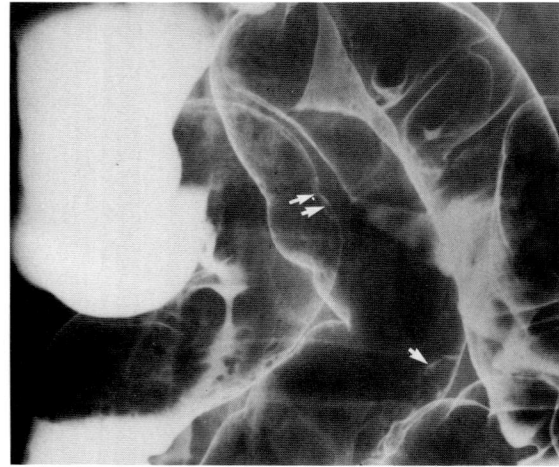

**FIG. 38.** KS—Colon. **A:** Confluent submucosal masses narrow rectal lumen. The features (simulating varices) are characteristic of a submucosal colonic process. **B:** Mild granularity and wavy lines (arrows) indicate that submucosal infiltration is present. **C:** Multiple tiny plaquelike elevations due to KS in sigmoid (arrows).

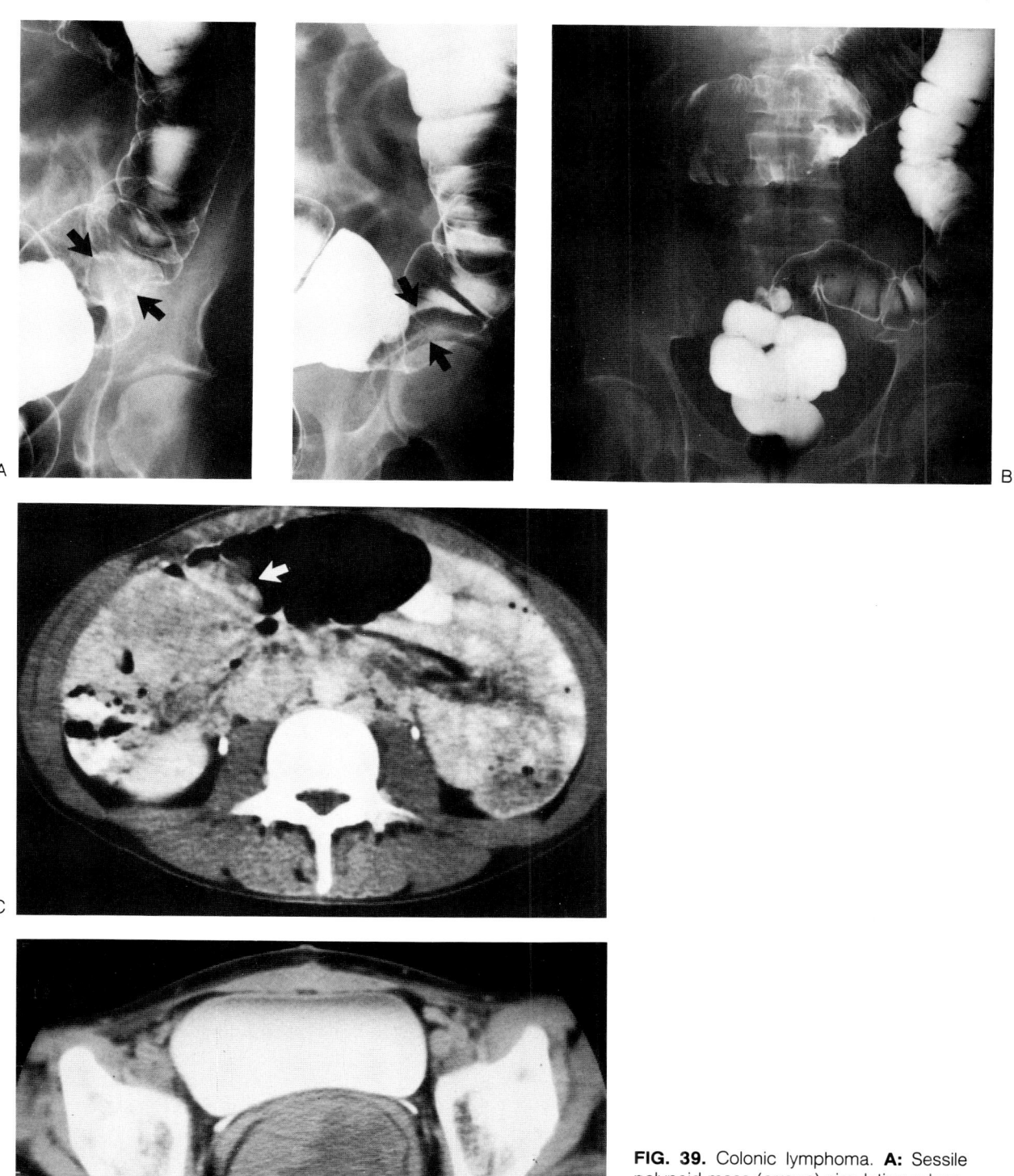

**FIG. 39.** Colonic lymphoma. **A:** Sessile polypoid mass (*arrows*) simulating adenocarcinoma seen in sigmoid colon of a 39-year-old patient with AIDS-related lymphoma. **B:** Intussuscepting cecal Burkitt's lymphoma into the transverse colon. **C:** CT in same patient reveals lobulated mass leading intussusception (*arrow*) into the air-filled transverse colon. **D:** Bulky pelvic mass from rectal/perirectal AIDS-related B-cell lymphoma.

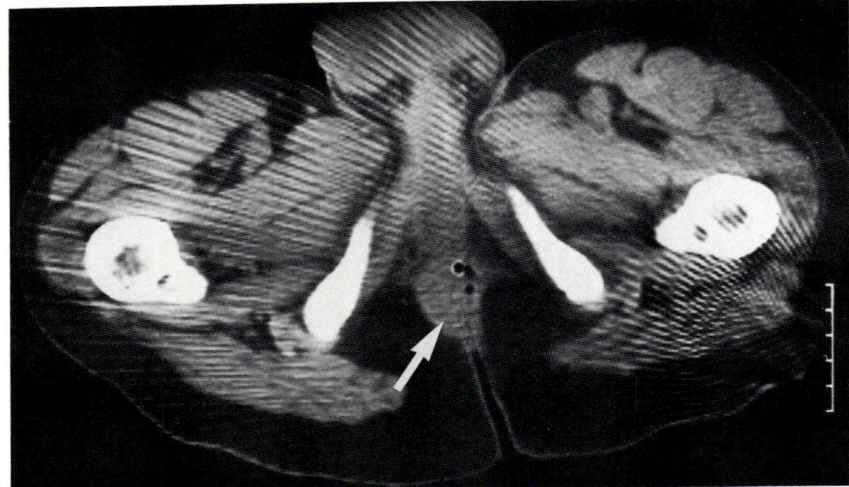

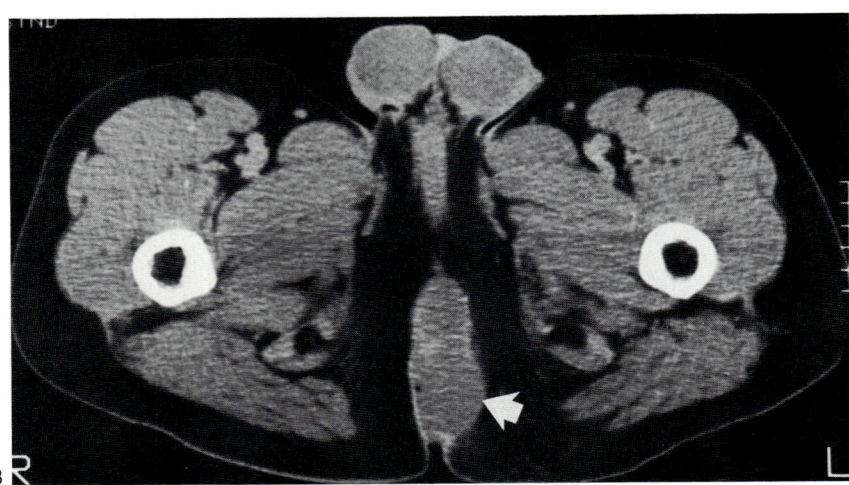

**FIG. 40.** Burkitt's lymphoma—Anal canal. **A, B:** CT scan in two patients thought to have crypt abscess. Homogeneous masses (*arrows*) are seen in both. Biopsy revealed Burkitt's lymphoma.

## BILIARY DISEASE

Recent attention has been directed at involvement of the biliary tract in AIDS patients. Most reported cases described acalculous cholecystitis secondary to CMV or cryptosporidial infection (51,52).

A recent report documented the radiographic findings in nine AIDS patients with right upper quadrant pain, jaundice, or abnormal liver function tests. Eight of the nine imaging studies disclosed intrahepatic or extrahepatic bile duct changes identical to those seen in sclerosing cholangitis. Isolated papillary stenosis in ductal dilatation was present in one patient. Eight patients had some stricturing of the distal common bile duct (Fig. 41). Cholangitis caused by CMV or cryptosporidium is the proposed pathogenic mechanism (53). In Teixidor et al.'s series (12), one patient was shown to have CMV infection of the biliary tree. The finding in this case was that of a stenosing papillitis. We have seen two patients at N.Y.U. with AIDS-related biliary tree disease. Both were studied by CT to evaluate abnormal liver function tests. In both cases dilated intra- and extrahepatic ducts were seen without evidence of a pancreatic mass. In one patient there was diffuse dilatation of the entire intra- and extrahepatic duct system. ERCP revealed a dilated common bile duct with multiple vesicular filling defects seen within it. Cryptosporidial organisms were found in the common duct (Fig. 42). In the second patient, CT revealed findings suggestive of sclerosing cholangitis. Segmental intrahepatic bile duct dilatation was seen. In this patient it was interesting to note the enhancement of the wall of the common hepatic duct, common bile duct, and gall bladder. Furthermore, a small amount of pericholecystic fluid was seen. On ERCP, segmental intrahepatic bile duct dilatation is seen associated with marked irregularity of the common hepatic duct and common bile duct. Similar to the previous case, intraductal vesicular protuberances were noted. This patient was found to have both CMV and cryptosporidial organisms in the common duct (Fig. 43). CMV and reo-

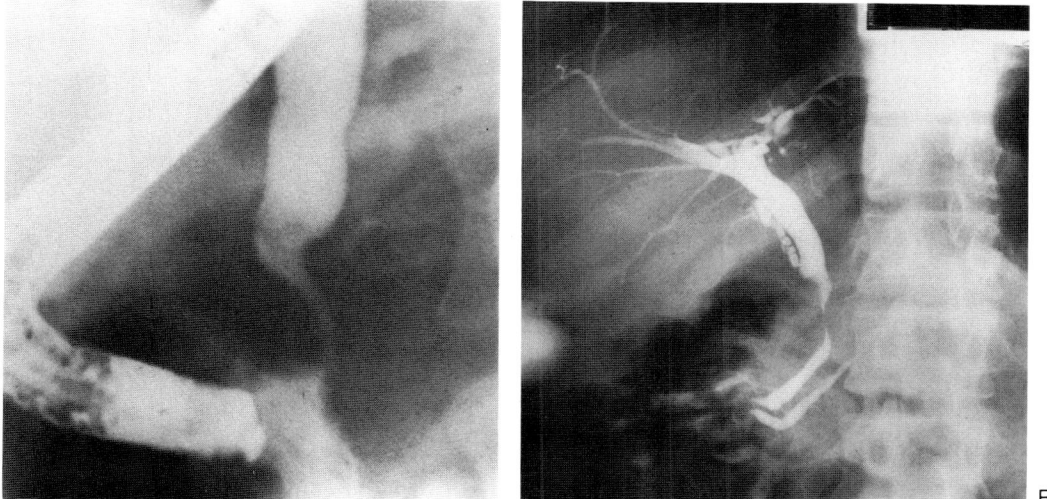

**FIG. 41.** AIDS cholangitis. **A:** Stenosing papillitis, CMV infection. **B:** Stricture mid-common duct, CMV cholangitis.

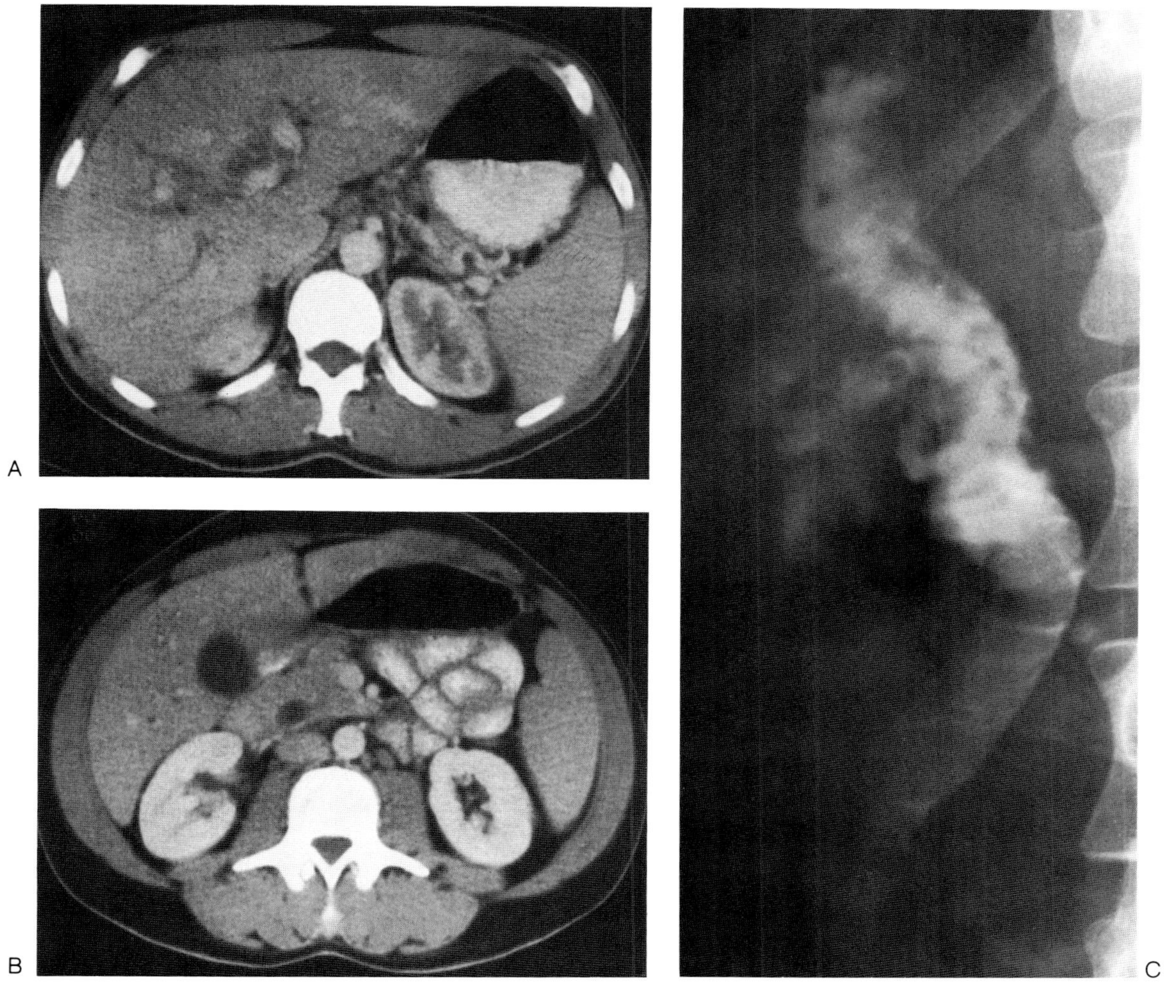

**FIG. 42.** AIDS cholangitis. **A:** CT in patient with abnormal liver function tests reveals dilated intrahepatic ducts. **B:** Scan through pancreatic head reveals dilated common bile duct. No masses are present. **C:** ERCP revealing dilated common bile duct with multiple filling defects along wall. Cryptosporidial infection was documented.

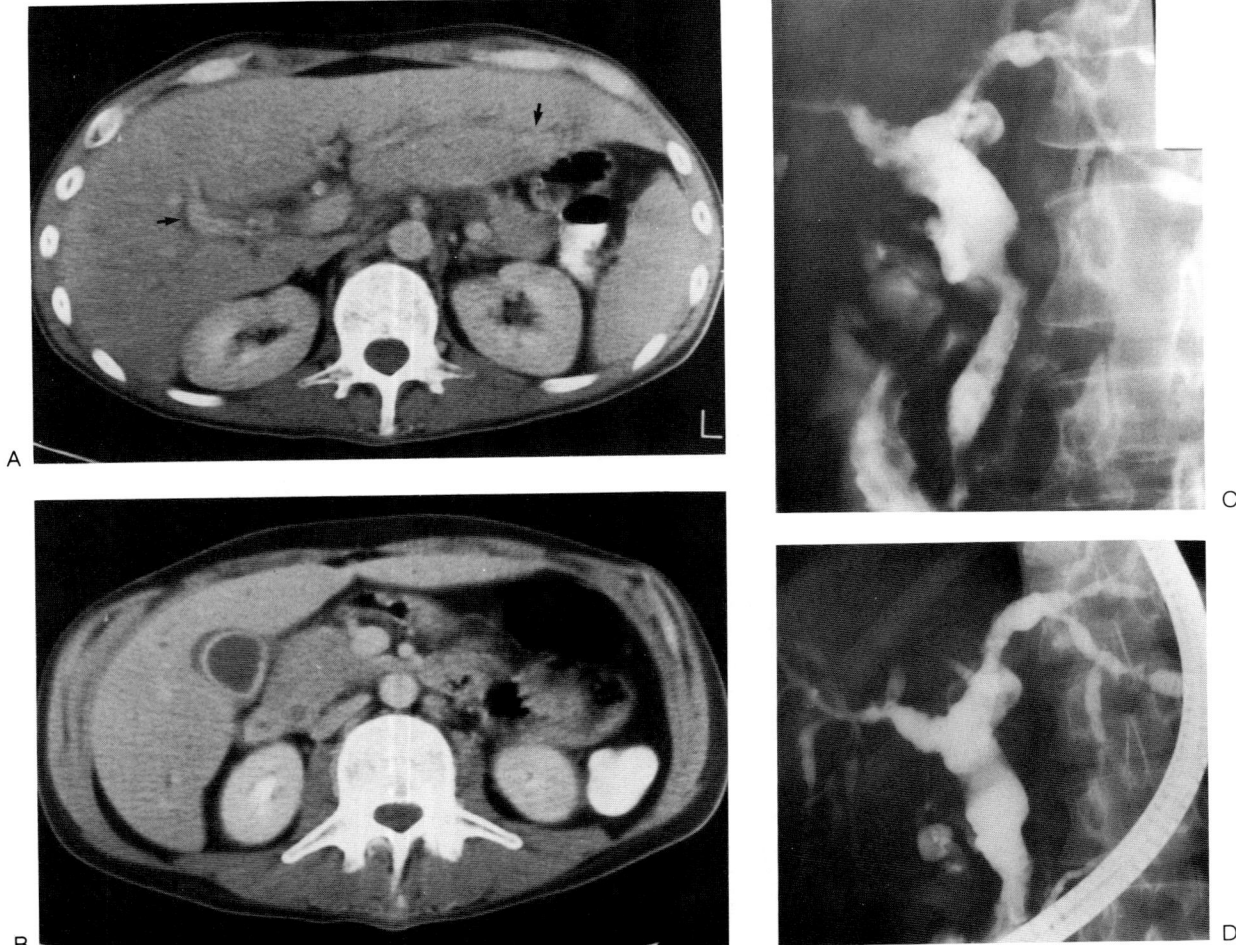

FIG. 43. AIDS cholangitis. **A:** CT scan revealing peripheral duct dilatation in the liver (*arrows*). **B:** The common duct is slightly dilated and pericholecystic fluid is seen. **C:** ERCP: There is a stricture in the distal common duct. Multiple vesicular filling defects are seen along the course of the common bile duct. **D:** Intrahepatic ducts reveal varying strictures and dilatation reminiscent of the classic pattern of sclerosing cholangitis. This patient had combined CMV and cryptosporidial infection.

virus III have a tropism for bile duct epithelium in the neonate (54). Reflux of the organisms through the ampulla of Vater presumably when there is superinfection in the duodenum or small bowel may be responsible for this disorder.

In any AIDS patient with abnormal liver function tests, imaging generally will be performed to evaluate the presence of hepatomegaly or space-occupying lesions within the liver. Careful attention should be paid to the bile ducts. If segmental dilatation of any portion of the biliary tree is seen, direct cholangiography may be useful to document the presence of AIDS-related cholangitis. Ultrasonic visualization of gallbladder wall thickening or bile duct dilatation has been shown to be significant for AIDS-related cholangitis (55).

## REFERENCES

1. Centers for Disease Control (1987): Revision of the CDC surveillance care definition for acquired immunodeficiency syndrome. *M.M.W.R.*, 62–70.
2. Fauci, A. S. (1985): Acquired immune deficiency syndrome: An update. *An. Intern. Med.*, 102:800–813.
3. Wall, S. D., Ominsky, S., Altman, D. F., et al. (1986): Multifocal abnormalities of the gastrointestinal tract in AIDS. *A.J.R.*, 146:1–7.
4. Laufer, I. (1979): *Double Contrast Gastrointestinal Radiology with Endoscopic Correlation.* W. B. Saunders Co., Philadelphia.
5. Alpern, M. B., Lawson, T. L., Foley, W. D., et al. (1986): Focal hepatic masses and fatty infiltration detected by enhanced dynamic CT. *Radiology,* 158:51–55.
6. Frager, D. H., Frager, J. D., Brandt, L. J., et al. (1986): Gastrointestinal complications of AIDS. Radiologic Features. *Radiology,* 158:597–605.
7. Klein, R. S., Harris, C. A., and Small, C. B. (1984): Oral candi-

diasis in high risk patients as initial manifestation of acquired immune deficiency syndrome. *N. Engl. J. Med.,* 311:354–358.
8. Roberts, L., Gibbons, R., Gibbons, G., et al. (1987): Adult esophageal candidiasis: A radiographic spectrum. *Radiographics,* 7:289–307.
9. Goldberg, H. I., and Dodds, W. J. (1968): Cobblestone esophagus due to monilial infection. *A.J.R.,* 104:608–612.
10. Levine, M. S., Macones, A. J., and Laufer, I. Candida esophagitis: Accuracy of radiographic diagnosis. *Radiology.*
11. Balthazar, E. J., Megibow, A. J., and Hulnick, D. H. (1985): Cytomegalovirus esophagitis and gastrites in acquired immune deficiency syndrome. *A.J.R.,* 144:1201–1204.
11a. Balthazar, E. J., Megibow, A. J., Hulnick, D., Chok, C., Beranbaum, E. (1987): Cytomegalovirus esophagitis in AIDS: Radiographic features in 16 patients. *A.J.R.,* 149:919–925.
12. Teixidor, H. S., Honig, C. L., Norsoph, E., Albert, S., Mouradian, J. A., and Whalen, J. P. (1987): Cytomegalovirus infection of the alimentary canal: Radiologic findings with pathologic correlation. *Radiology,* 163:317–325.
13. St. Onge, G., Bezahler, G. H. (1982): Giant esophageal ulcer associated with cytomegalovirus. *Gastroenterology,* 83:127–130.
14. Farman, J., Tavitian, L. E., Rosenthal, G. E., et al. (1986): Focal esophageal candidiasis in acquired immunodeficiency syndrome (AIDS). *Gastroint. Radiol.,* 11:213–218.
15. Levine, M. S., Laufer, I., Kressel, H. Y., and Friedman, H. (1981): Herpes esophagitis. *A.J.R.,* 863–866.
16. Emery, C. D., Wall, S. D., Federle, M. P., and Sooy, C. D. (1986): Pharyngeal Kaposi Sarcoma in patients with AIDS. *A.J.R.,* 147:919–922.
17. Elta, G., Turnage, R., Eckhauser, F. E., Agha, F., and Ross, F. (1986): A submucosal antral mass caused by cytomegalovirus infection in a patient with acquired immunodeficiency syndrome. *Am. J. Gastroenterol.,* 81:714–717.
18. Soulen, M. C., Fishman, E. K., Scatarige, J. C., et al. (1986): Cryptosporidiosis of the gastric antrum: Detection using CT. *Radiology,* 159:705–706.
19. Brody, J. M., Miller, D. K., Zeman, R. K., et al. (1986): Gastric tuberculosis: A manifestation of AIDS. *Radiology,* 159:347–348.
20. Rose, H. S., Balthazar, E. J., Megibow, A. J., et al. (1982): Alimentary tract involvement in Kaposi sarcoma. Radiographic and endoscopic findings in 25 homosexual men. *A.J.R.,* 139:661–666.
21. Dworkin, B., Wormser, G. P., Rosenthal, W. S., et al. (1985): Gastrointestinal manifestations of acquired immune deficiency syndrome: A review of 22 cases. *Am. J. Gastroenterol.,* 80:774–778.
22. Barone, J. E., Gingold, B. S., Nealon, T. F., and Arvanitis, M. L. (1986): Abdominal pain in patients with acquired immune deficiency syndrome. *Ann. Surg.,* 204:619–623.
23. Gelb, A., and Miller, S. (1986): AIDS and gastroenterology. *Am. J. Gastroenterol.,* 81:619–622.
24. Cooper, A., Wodak, A., Marriot, D. J. E., et al. (1984): Cryptosporodiosis in AIDS. *Pathology,* 16:455–457.
25. Gross, T. L., Wheat, J., Bartlett, M., and O'Connor, K. W. (1986): AIDS and multisystem involvement with cryptosporidium. *Am. J. Gastroenterol.,* 81:456–458.
26. Berk, R. N., Wall, S. D., McCardle, C. B., et al. (1984): Cryptosporidiosis of the stomach and small intestine in patients with acquired immune deficiency syndrome. *A.J.R.,* 143:549–554.
27. Greene, J. R., Sidhu, S., Lewin, S., et al. (1982): Mycobacterium Avium-Intracellulare: A case of disseminated life-threatening infection in homosexual drug abusers. *Ann. Intern. Med.,* 97:539–546.
28. Sohn, C. C., Schroff, R. W., Kliewer, K. E., Lebel, D. M., et al. (1983): Disseminated Mycobacterium Avium-Intracellulare infection in homosexual men with acquired cell-mediated immunodeficiency: A histologic and pathologic study of two cases. *Am. J. Clin. Pathol.,* 79:247–252.
29. Autran, B., Gorin, I., and Leibowitch, M. (1983): Acquired immune deficiency syndrome in a Haitian woman with cardiac Kaposi sarcoma and Whipple's disease. *Lancet,* 1:767–768.
30. Roth, R., Owen, R. L., and Keven, D. F. (1983): Acquired immune deficiency syndrome with Mycobacterium Avium-Intracellulare lesions resembling those of Whipple's disease. *N. Engl. J. Med.,* 309:1324–1235.
31. Vincent, M. E., and Robbins, A. R. (1985): Mycobacterium Avium-Intracellulare complex enteritis: Pseudo-Whipple's disease in acquired immune deficiency. *A.J.R.,* 144:921–922.
32. Nyberg, D. A., Federle, M. P., Jeffrey, R. B., et al. (1985): Abdominal CT findings in disseminated Mycobacterium Avium-Intracellulare. *A.J.R.,* 145:297–299.
33. Knapp, A. B., Horst, D. A., Eliopoulos, G., et al. (1983): Widespread cytomegalovirus gastroenterocolitis in a patient with acquired immune deficiency syndrome. *Gastroenterology,* 85:1399–1402.
34. Frank, D., and Raicht, R. F. (1984): Intestinal perforation with CMV in patients with acquired immune deficiency syndrome. *Am. J. Gastroenterol.,* 79:201–205.
35. Goodman, M. D., and Poster, D. D. (1973): Cytomegalovirus vasculitis with fatal colonic hemorrhage. *Arch. Pathol.,* 96:281–284.
36. Hill, C. A., Harle, T. S., and Mansell, P. W. A. (1983): The prodrome. Kaposi sarcoma and infection associated with acquired immune deficiency syndrome. Radiologic findings in 39 patients. *Radiology,* 149:393–399.
37. Megibow, A. J., Balthazar, E. J., Bosniak, M. A., Naidich, D. P. (1983): Computed tomography of gastrointestinal lymphoma. *Am. J. Roentgenol.,* 141:541–548.
38. Nyberg, D. A., Jeffrey, R. B., Federle, M. P., et al. (1986): AIDS-related lymphomas: Evaluation by abdominal CT. *Radiology,* 159:59–63.
39. Sider, L., Mintzer, R. A., and Mendelson, E. B. (1982): Radiologic findings of infections proctitis in gay men. *A.J.R.,* 139:667–672.
40. Moon, K. L., Federle, M. P., Abrams, D. I., et al. (1984): Kaposi's sarcoma and lymphadenopathy syndrome: Limitations of abdominal CT in acquired immunodeficiency syndrome. *Radiology,* 150:479–485.
41. Albin, J., Lewis, E., Eftekhari, F., and Shirkhoda, A. (1987): Computed tomography of rectal and perirectal disease in AIDS patients. *Gastroint. Radiol.,* 12:67–71.
42. Levinson, W., and Bennetts, R. W. (1985): Cytomegalovirus in acquired immune deficiency syndrome: A chronic disease with varying manifestations. *Am. J. Gastroenterol.,* 80:445–447.
43. Meiselman, M. S., Cello, J. P., and Margareten, W. (1985): Cytomegalovirus colitis in acquired immune deficiency syndrome. *Gastroenterology,* 88:171–175.
44. Gertler, S. C., Pressman, J., Price, P., et al. (1983): Gastrointestinal CMV infection in a patient with acquired immune deficiency syndrome. *Gastroenterology,* 85:1399–1402.
45. Foucar, E., Mukai, K., Foucan, K., et al. (1981): Colon ulceration in lethal cytomegalovirus infection. *Am. J. Clin. Pathol.,* 76:788–801.
46. Hinnant, R., Rotterdam, H. Z., Bell, E. T., and Tapper, M. L. (1986): Cytomegalovirus infection of the alimentary tract: A clinicopathological correlation. *Am. J. Gastroenterol.,* 81:944–950.
47. Balthazar, E. J., Megibow, A. J., Fazzini, E., et al. (1985): Cytomegalovirus colitis: Radiographic findings in 11 patients. *Radiology,* 155:585–589.
48. Frager, D. H., Frager, J. D., Wolfe, E. L., et al. (1986): Cytomegalovirus colitis in acquired immune deficiency syndrome: Radiologic spectrum. *Gastroint. Radiol.,* 11:241–246.
49. Sutherland, D. E. R., Chan, F. Y., Foucar, E., et al. (1979): The bleeding cecal ulcer in transplant patients. *Surgery,* 86:386–398.
50. Wolf, B. M., and Cherry, J. D. (1973): Hemorrhage from cecal ulcers of cytomegalovirus infection. *Ann. Surg.,* 177:490–494.
51. Kavin, H., Jonas, R. B., Choudhury, L., et al. (1986): Acalculous cholecystitis and cytomegalovirus infection in acquired immune deficiency syndrome. *Ann. Intern. Med.,* 104:53–54.
52. Blumberg, R. S., Kelsy, P., Perrone, T., et al. (1984): Cytomegalovirus and cryptosporidia associated acalculous cholecystitis. *Am. J. Med.,* 76:118–123.
53. Dolmatch, B. L., Laing, F. C., Federle, M. P., et al. (1987): AIDS-related cholangitis: Radiographic findings in nine patients. *Radiology,* 163:313–317.
54. Margulis, S. J., Honig, C. L., Soave, R., et al. (1986): Biliary tract obstruction in the acquired immune deficiency syndrome. *Ann. Intern. Med.,* 105:207–210.
55. Romano, A. J., van Sonnenberg, E., Casola, G., et al. (1988): Gallbladder and bile duct abnormalities in AIDS: Sonographic findings in eight patients. *A.J.R.,* 15:123–129.

CHAPTER 5

# Malignant Neoplasms: Kaposi's Sarcoma, Lymphoma, and Other Diseases with Similar Radiographic Features

Michael P. Federle, David A. Nyberg, Donald H. Hulnick, and R. Brooke Jeffrey, Jr.

Patients with acquired immune deficiency syndrome (AIDS) and AIDS-related disorders are predisposed to develop certain neoplasms, especially Kaposi's sarcoma (KS) and lymphoma (1–8). A previously rare disease, KS has notoriety as one of the primary manifestations of AIDS, seen in 27% of all reported cases (9). Malignant lymphoma, the second most common neoplasm associated with AIDS, occurs approximately one tenth as often as KS (10). However, present figures may underestimate the future incidence of lymphoma, based on the estimated 1 million individuals who already have been infected with the AIDS virus and who are at risk for developing AIDS-related disorders (11) and an apparent longer "lead time" for development of lymphoma. We have seen a recent dramatic increase in AIDS-related lymphomas while the incidence of KS has decreased. Other neoplasms also have been reported in patients with AIDS, e.g., squamous cell carcinoma of the oral pharynx (12) and cloacogenic carcinoma of the rectum (13).

The relationship between human immunodeficiency virus (HIV) infection, KS, and lymphoma is under extensive investigation (1–11, 14–18). HIV infection is associated with multiple clinical syndromes resulting from severe cellular immunodeficiency; the formation of secondary cancers is recognized as a distinct, classifiable clinical entity. Some neoplasms, including KS and lymphoma, are probably induced by tumor-specific viruses (8). Cytomegalovirus (MV) has been implicated as a possible cause of KS (15,16) and Epstein-Barr virus is known to induce Burkitt's lymphoma (17,18). A wide geographic difference in the incidence of KS and Burkitt's lymphoma, with a strikingly high incidence in equatorial Africa, supports the contention of an infectious etiology for these neoplasms (19). Interaction between viruses may explain the association of KS and lymphomas in both AIDS and nonAIDS patients. Of nonAIDS patients with KS, 37% developed second neoplasms, and 58% of these are lymphomas or leukemia (20).

Evidence suggests that both lymphomas and KS originate from the lymphoreticular system (21). Prior to the current AIDS epidemic, lymphoreticular neoplasms were also a well-known complication in patients immunosuppressed from other causes, particularly organ donor recipients (22–24). Among recipients of renal transplants, for example, 4.9% developed KS and 26% of new tumors are non-Hodgkin's lymphoma (NHL). The incidence of KS in renal allograft recipients is believed to be between 150 and 200 times the expected incidence for the interval between transplantation and the development of KS (about 16 months). The form of the disease may vary from indolent cutaneous involvement to aggressive infiltrative and lymphadenopathic.

The clinical manifestations of both KS and AIDS-related lymphomas (ARLs) are highly variable and difficult to distinguish from other concurrent illness. Fever, weight loss, headache, diarrhea, and malaise are common complaints in many patients with AIDS, whether or not they have KS or lymphoma. Excluding mucocutaneous lesions, the usual sites of ARL and KS also are similar. Attempting to distinguish these neoplasms may be particularly difficult when they coexist, which is not infrequent.

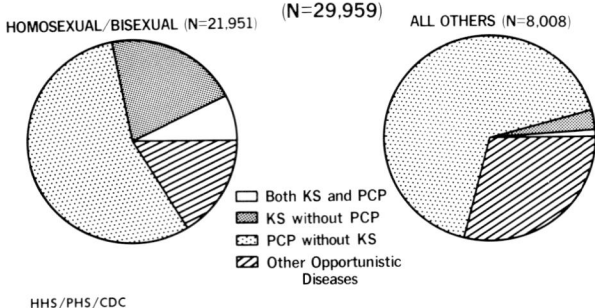

**FIG. 1.** Graphs of data from the CDC. Note the increased incidence of KS in homosexual/bisexual men compared with other risk groups (1981 to Feb. 2, 1987).

ARL and KS demonstrate wide radiographic spectra that often overlap. Typical radiographic findings of each condition have been described that may suggest the specific diagnosis. In this chapter we discuss the pathologic and radiologic findings in AIDS-related malignancies with emphasis on KS and ARL. Opportunistic infections may produce similar radiographic findings (see Chapter 4). The role of CT scanning will be emphasized because it plays a central role in the evaluation of AIDS patients with suspected neoplasms.

## KAPOSI'S SARCOMA

Despite extensive clinical and pathological studies since its initial description in 1872, the origin and clinical significance of KS remain poorly understood. The clinical course and aggressiveness of KS may vary markedly, depending on the patient population and country of origin (19). In its classic form, KS was described as an

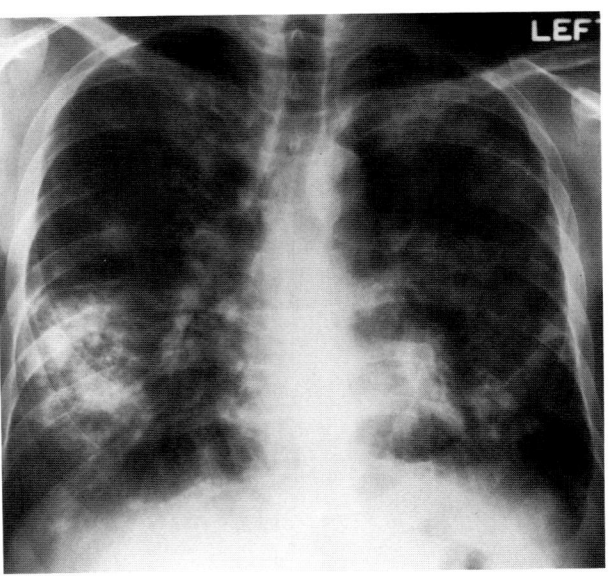

**FIG. 2.** Diffuse, poorly defined nodular infiltrates of KS. Small left pleural effusion.

indolent cutaneous neoplasm, most often found on the lower extremities of elderly eastern European and East Mediterranean subjects. In equatorial Africa, where KS has long been endemic, at least four clinical subtypes are recognized (25–28): 1) the nodular form, 2) the aggressive form, 3) the generalized form, and 4) the lymphadenopathic form (see Chapter 1).

The clinical course of KS in patients with AIDS also is variable (10,29). Most patients have disseminated and progressive disease that closely resembles the generalized form of African KS or the lymphadenopathic form. For unknown reasons, the incidence of KS is much

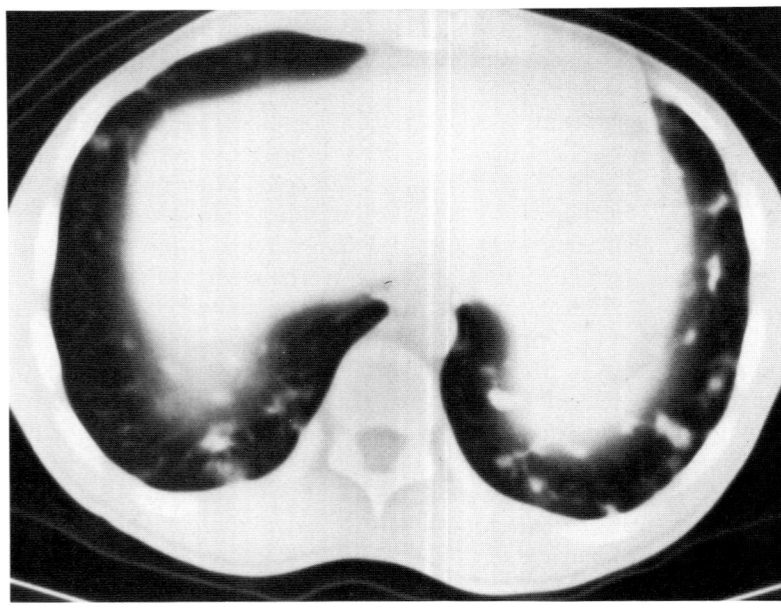

**FIG. 3.** CT scan of lung bases in another patient demonstrates multiple irregular nodular densities.

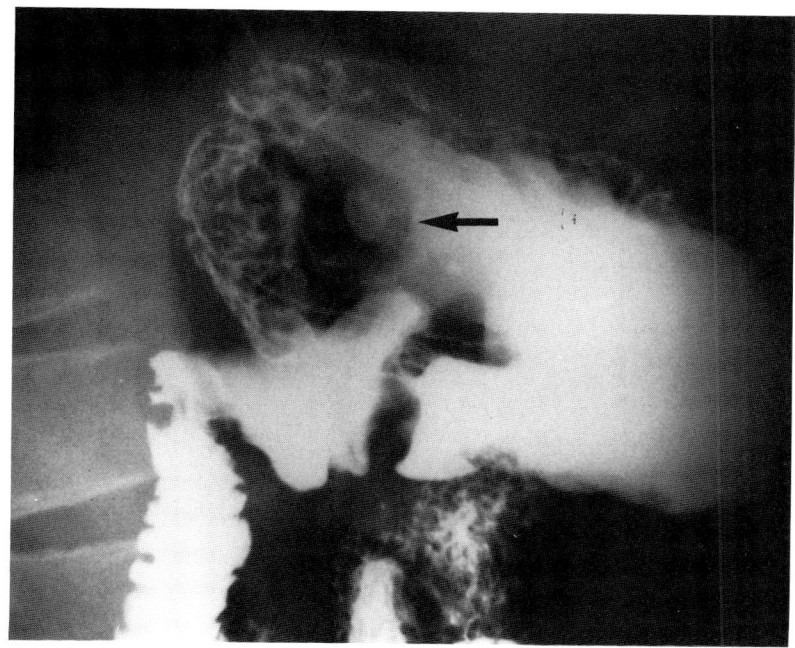

**FIG. 4.** KS involvement of the stomach, seen as a large, well-defined target lesion (*arrow*) with central umbilication.

higher among homosexual men than in other AIDS patients. Approximately 93% of all male cases of KS in the United States have been diagnosed in homosexuals and bisexuals. Almost 50% of all homosexual men with AIDS present with or eventually will develop KS during the course of their illness. By comparison, only 4% of all heterosexual i.v. drug abusers with AIDS and about 12% of Haitian AIDS patients develop epidemic KS (30) (Fig. 1). Very few women or pediatric AIDS patients have developed KS. These epidemiologic observations raise interesting speculation as to the cause of KS in this population. Among the homosexual men with epidemic KS, the incidence of multiple sexually transmitted diseases is extremely high. Among the various pathogens, CMV has attracted attention as a potential cause of KS, and for many years has been felt to be associated with the African form of KS. Antibodies to CMV have been found in 94% of gay men at a venereal disease clinic (versus 54% of heterosexual controls) and CMV has been isolated from blood, semen, gut, and brain lesions in AIDS patients. CMV deoxyribonucleic acid (DNA) sequences have been identified in biopsy specimens and tissue cultures from KS patients (31,32).

Approximately 95% of AIDS patients with KS have visible cutaneous or oral lesions (33). The development of KS lesions is an ominous sign, invariably followed by death within months to three years. However, KS itself appears to be less responsible for this grim prognosis than the severe concurrent infections that usually dominate the clinical course of patients with AIDS (10). KS lesions may not explain the systemic symptoms, since even disseminated KS is usually asymptomatic.

Multiple cutaneous lesions and visceral lesions usually are present at autopsy, representing multicentric involvement, rather than metastases from a primary focus (36–39). In one autopsy series, 29 of 56 (52%) patients with AIDS had KS and all but one had disseminated disease. Common sites of involvement in that study included the skin (93%), lymph nodes (72%), lung (52%), gastrointestinal (GI) tract (48%), liver (34%), and spleen (34%) (37).

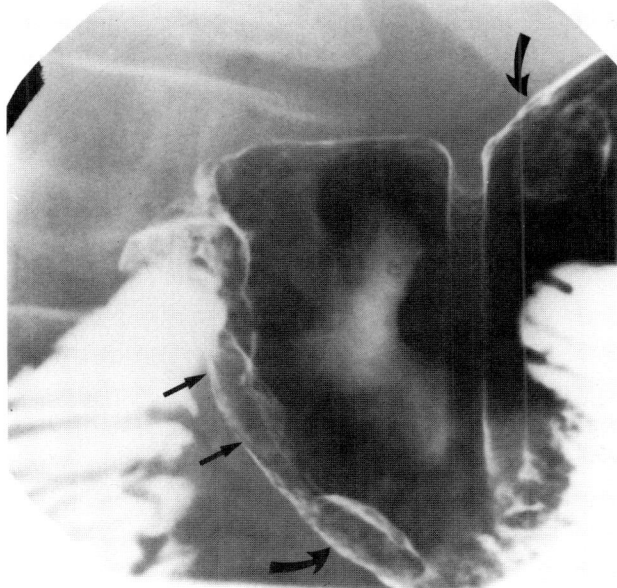

**FIG. 5.** Gastric KS. Nodularity (*straight arrows*) and submucosal nodules (*curved arrows*) of the gastric antrum on double contrast examination.

Brain involvement with KS is relatively rare (38–40). Due to the paucity of cases reported, it is impossible to state whether a characteristic appearance exists on computed tomography (CT). A homogeneously enhancing pattern that should be distinguished from primary brain lymphoma has been reported (38). Magnetic resonance imaging (MRI) appears to be more sensitive than CT for detecting cerebral KS, although the diagnostic specific-

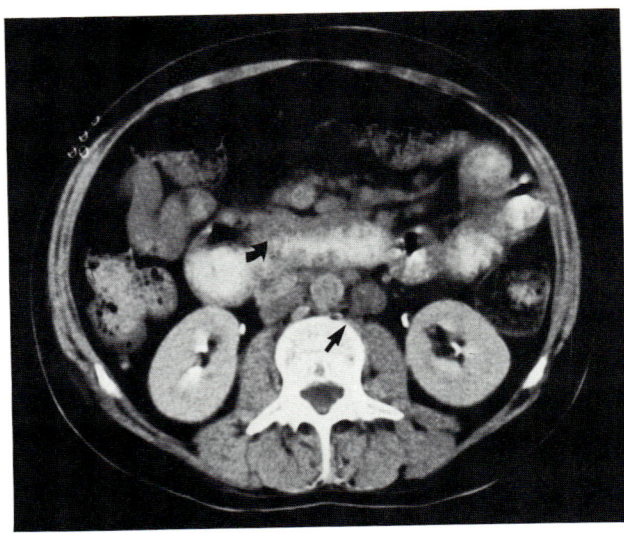

**FIG. 7.** Lymphadenopathy in KS. CT demonstrates enlarged retroperitoneal nodes (*arrow*) as well as marked thickening of the transverse duodenum (*curved arrow*).

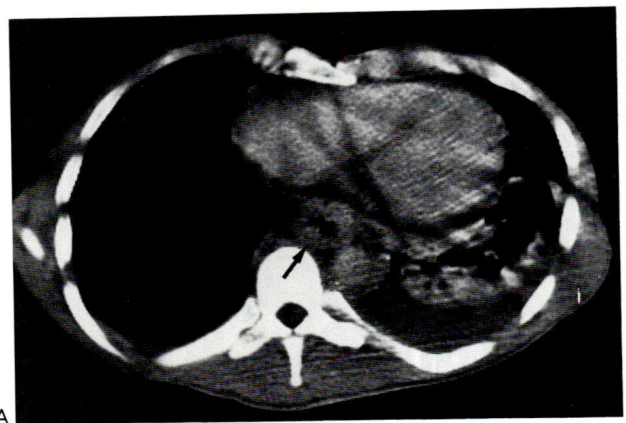

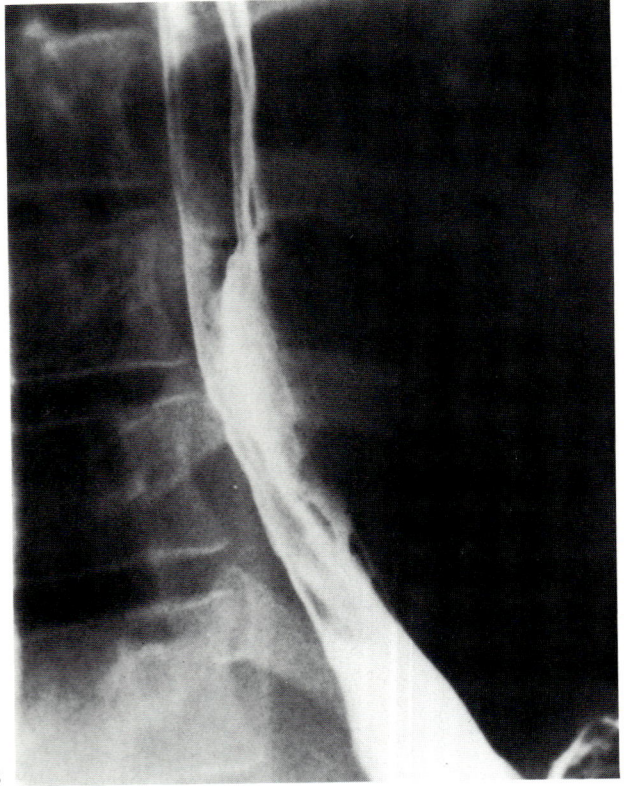

**FIG. 6.** KS of the esophagus. **A:** CT scans of the lung base demonstrates marked esophageal wall thickening (*arrow*). **B:** Subsequent esophagram confirms narrowing and nodularity of the distal esophagus.

ity probably is not improved (40).

KS is a much less common cause of pulmonary disease than opportunistic infections. In a large clinical series of 441 AIDS patients with lung disease, KS was diagnosed in only 8% (41). However, this figure undoubtedly underestimates the true incidence of pulmonary KS because of the difficulty in premortem diagnosis. Bronchoscopy appears to be ineffective for diagnosis of pulmonary KS and an open-lung biopsy often is required. Pulmonary involvement is present in about 50% of autopsy AIDS patients who have KS (37). The radiographic appearance of pulmonary KS is not specific, but typical patterns have been recognized (42,43). A pattern of poorly defined diffuse nodular densities on conventional radiographs (Fig. 2) or CT (Fig. 3) is suggestive of KS. A diffuse course pattern is more common, but may simulate opportunistic infections, including Pneumocystis carinii pneumonia. A high percentage of patients with pulmonary KS have pleural effusion (Fig. 2). Usually the chest abnormalities appear late in the course of the disease, although there have been a few reports of pulmonary KS that predate the mucocutaneous manifestations (see Chapter 3, Table 2).

The GI tract is a common site of involvement for AIDS-related KS (2,44–46). Involvement of the oropharynx and nasopharynx occurred in 51% of AIDS patients in one study (47). While clinical examination may permit accurate detection of such lesions, the evaluation of a bulky tumor may require barium pharyngography or esophagography. When KS extends to the deeper tissues of the neck or produces cervical lymphadenopathy, either CT or MR may be necessary to evaluate the extent of involvement.

KS lesions involving the gut usually are submucosal in location and have a characteristic violaceous appearance at endoscopy. The lesions may involve any portion of the gut. Barium studies reveal one or more submucosal nodules with or without central umbilication, a finding highly suggestive of KS (Fig. 4) (48–52). More subtle nodularity, thickened folds, polypoid lesions, and plaque formation are less specific (Fig. 5). Using double-contrast studies, Wall et al. (52) detected one or more of these findings in 12 of 44 (27%) AIDS patients. CT is also useful for detecting KS of the GI tract by demonstrating bowel wall thickening (Figs. 6–8).

With the exception of mucocutaneous lesions, lymph nodes are the most common site of KS in AIDS (35). Pathologically, KS usually involves multiple lymph node groups, including abdominal nodes. Paraaortic and mesenteric lymph nodes are demonstrated in most patients with KS, although these are usually normal in size or mildly enlarged. Lymphadenopathy detected by CT is nonspecific and may represent a variety of disorders, including reactive hyperplasia in patients with persistent generalized lymphadenopathy (Figs. 9,10) (51,53). Marked contrast enhancement of KS-infiltrated nodes is a distinctive, though uncommon, feature (Fig. 11).

Visceral organs are commonly involved with KS at autopsy (37). However, since KS tends to produce microscopic infiltration along the vascular tracts, imaging studies of the liver and spleen during life usually are normal. Mild splenomegaly is a nonspecific finding, commonly seen in patients who have the lymphadenopathy syndrome or concurrent infection (51,53). Occasionally, focal liver or splenic lesions are demonstrated on CT or ultrasound (Fig. 12).

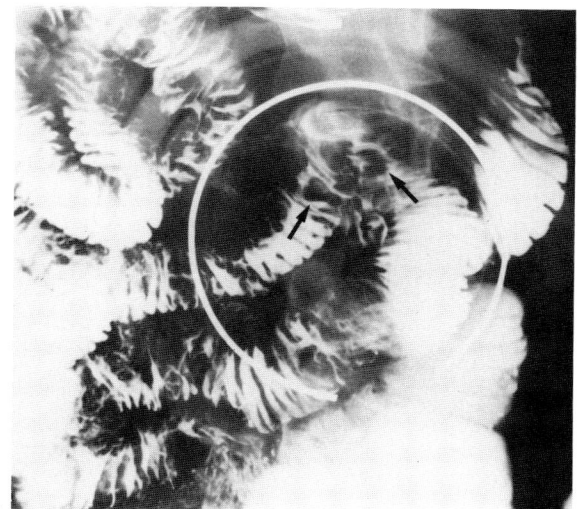
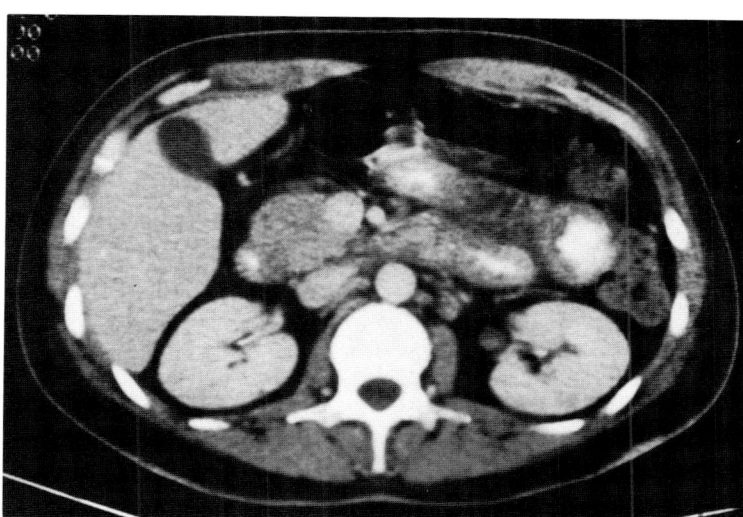
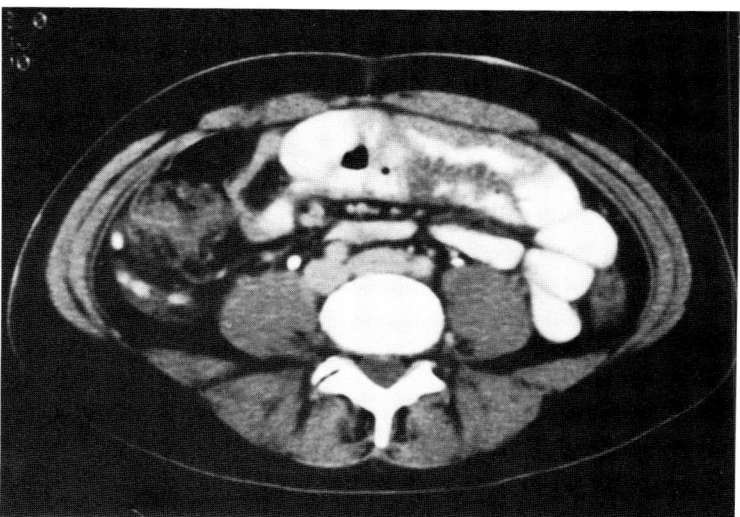

**FIG. 8.** A 29-year-old male with cutaneous KS and sudden onset of severe cramping abdominal pains and falling hematocrit. Patient on coumadin therapy for recurrent pulmonary emboli. **A:** Barium small bowel study demonstrates nodular submucosal masses in proximal jejunum (*arrows*) along with more diffuse irregular fold thickening due to hemorrhage. **B, C:** Diffuse mural thickening of the proximal jejunum. KS lesions are very vascular and prone to hemorrhage with trauma or anticoagulation.

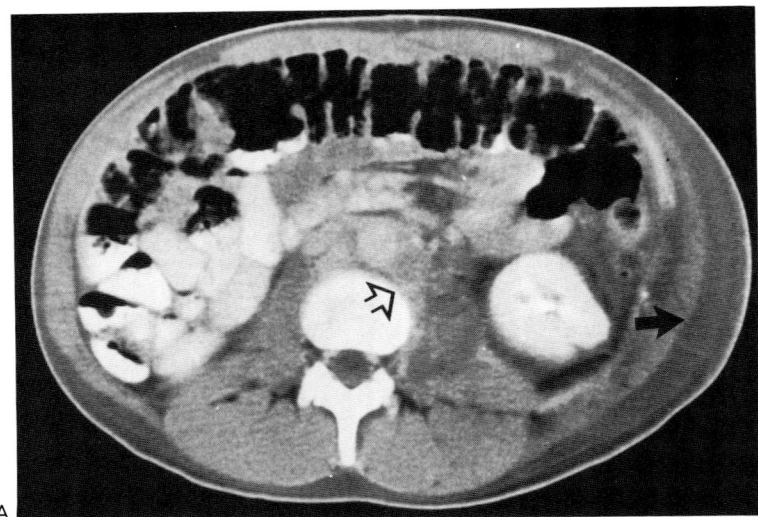
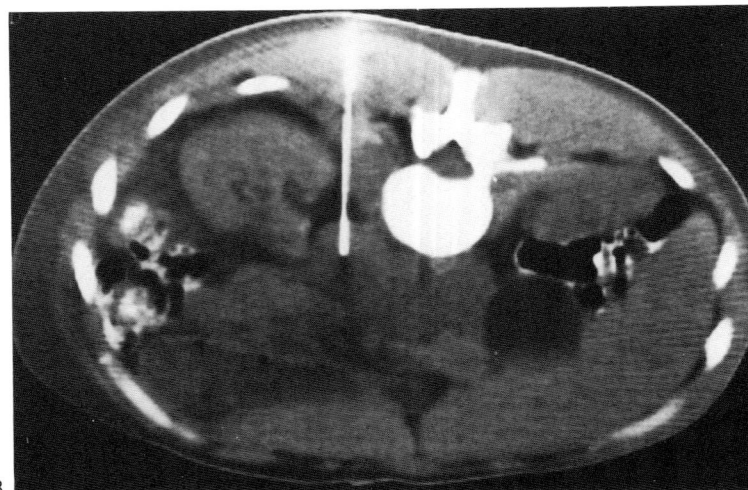

**FIG. 9.** Widespread abdominal involvement in KS. **A:** Paraaortic nodal disease (*open arrow*) and diffuse infiltration of psoas muscle and left abdominal wall (*straight arrow*). **B:** Percutaneous thin-needle biopsy of psoas mass confirmed KS invasion.

## LYMPHOMA

Primary brain lymphoma, small noncleaved lymphoma (either Burkitt or nonBurkitt type), and immunoblastic sarcoma diagnosed in patients with laboratory evidence of HIV infection are recognized indicator diseases establishing diagnosis of AIDS (1–5). T-cell phenotypes, lymphocytic, lymphoblastic, small-cleaved, and plasmacytoid lymphocytic lymphomas are not considered indicator diseases. The ARLs are aggressive neoplasms but have distinct clinical features compared with lymphomas in the general populations. Extranodal lymphoma may occur at any site; it commonly involves the bowel, visceral organs, and bone marrow. In a multiinstitutional review of 90 patients with ARL, Ziegler et al. (5) found extranodal involvement in all but two cases. Similar findings have been reported by others (6,7), including our own review of 29 patients with abdominal ARL (54).

Clinical symptoms in ARL often are different from those in nonAIDS lymphoma patients, and it may be difficult to distinguish from other AIDS-related disorders. Altered mentation is a common symptom of central nervous system (CNS) lymphoma, but similar symptoms may be experienced by other AIDS patients without lymphoma (55,56) (see Chapter 2).

Patients with abdominal lymphoma commonly present with nonspecific systemic symptoms, including weight loss, fever, and night sweats. Peripheral lymphadenopathy may be absent, as in 14 of 29 (49%) of patients in our study (54). The onset of lymphoma may precede other manifestations of AIDS. KS or an opportunistic infection developed after the onset of lymphoma in 17 of 90 (19%) of homosexual men studied by

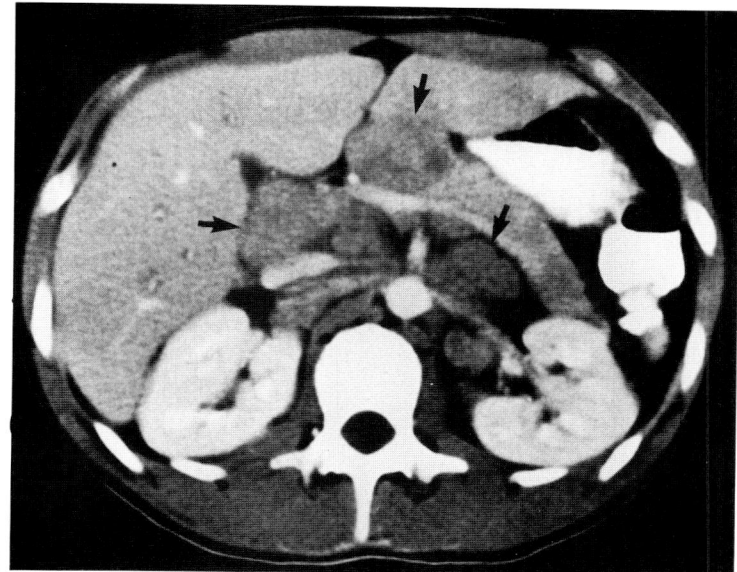
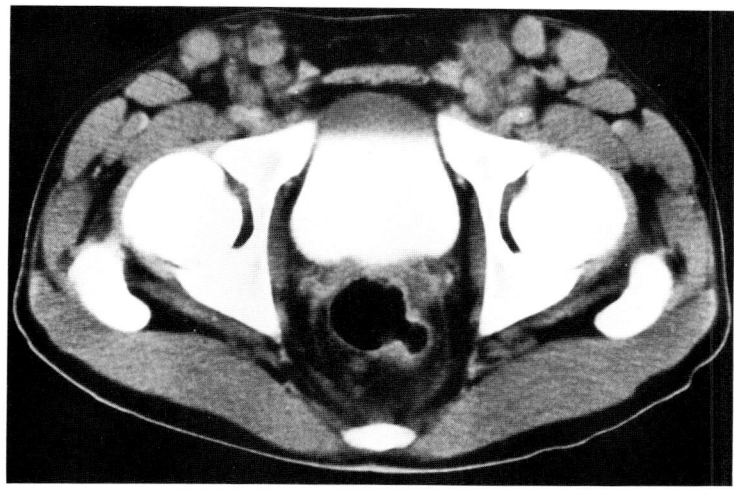

**FIG. 10.** Lymphadenopathic form of KS. **A:** Bulky peripancreatic, periportal, and retroperitoneal adenopathy (*arrows*). **B:** Extensive inguinal adenopathy proven to be KS by fine-needle aspiration biopsy.

Ziegler et al. (5) and in seven of 29 (24%) patients with abdominal ARL (54).

Persistent generalized lymphadenopathy (PGL) associated with or indicative of ARC appears to predispose to ARL, as well as to other AIDS-related disorders (57). PGL was present for months to 3 years before the diagnosis of lymphoma was made in 33 of 90 (33%) patients with NHL (5), and in 7 of 29 (24%) patients with abdominal lymphoma (54). Biopsy of these lymph nodes prior to the development of lymphoma typically demonstrates marked follicular hyperplasia (6,57).

The mortality for ARL is significantly higher than lymphomas of similar histology and clinical staging in the generalized population (5). The outcome appears to depend more on the presence of concurrent infection or illness than on the histologic subtype or extent of disease. In the study by Ziegler et al. (5), death occurred in 15 of 21 (71%) patients who had preexisting AIDS, 19 of 23 (58%) who presented with PGL, and four of 12 (33%) who had no prodromal symptoms. Similar results were noted in 29 patients with abdominal lymphoma, in whom the mortality was greater among those who developed Pneumocystis pneumonia (83%) or PGL (53%) than in the remaining group (13%) (54).

Pathologic findings of ARL depend on the specific histologic subtype. An increased incidence of Burkittlike lymphomas was initially reported among homosexual men (3). However, subsequent studies have demonstrated a frequent association of small noncleaved lymphoma, immunoblastic sarcoma, or primary brain lymphoma (4–7) (Fig. 13). In any HIV-seropositive patient, the onset of any of these forms of lymphoma is diagnostic of AIDS. Primary CNS lymphoma is considered supportive evidence of AIDS even in the absence of labora-

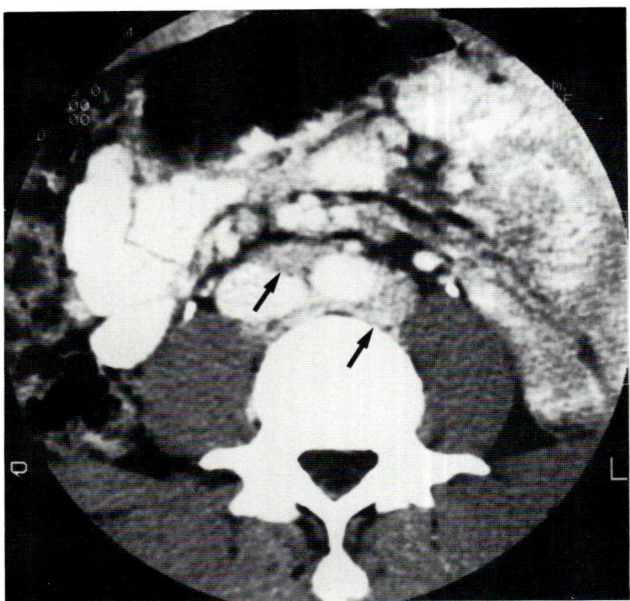

**FIG. 11.** KS in retroperiteonal nodes (*arrows*). Note the striking contrast enhancement of nodes compared with muscle. This is an uncommon finding but is suggestive of KS due to the vascular nature of the tumor.

tory evidence of HIV infection. Recently, Hodgkin's disease, especially with a high-grade mixed cellularity subtype, also has been implicated with AIDS, although less frequently than NHL (8,54,59). Review of our own experience in San Francisco suggests that the incidence of Hodgkin's disease is not increased in AIDS patients, although the clinical and radiographic manifestations are atypical. The most recent Centers for Disease Control (CDC) case surveillance criteria does not yet include Hodgkin's disease as an indicator disease of AIDS (58).

Primary CNS lymphoma is a relatively common autopsy finding in patients with AIDS (5,60–62) as it is in other immunosuppressed patients (63). Of 90 patients with NHL reported by Ziegler et al. (5), 21 patients (23%) had primary brain lymphoma. However, brain lymphoma in AIDS is less frequently reported in clinical and radiographic studies, probably because of the difficulty in establishing the premortem diagnosis. Typical CT findings include areas of homogeneous enhancement, often periventricular in location (38,39,61,62). Ring enhancement may occur. The lesions may be solitary or multiple.

Spinal involvement also may occur in patients with ARL. Paraspinal involvement was reported in 5 of 90 patients (6%) with NHL (5). One patient in our series developed leg weakness due to epidural lymphoma (54) (Fig. 14).

ARL may occur in the neck from involvement of cervical lymph nodes or as a primary neoplasm. In AIDS patients, Burkitt's lymphoma may be in the oral cavity, as in most African patients. In contrast, the American form of Burkitt's lymphoma usually presents with an abdominal mass.

Patients with ARL seldom have thoracic involvement. Ziegler et al. (5) reported lung involvement in 8 of 90 (9%) patients with NHL; we have encountered even fewer cases (Fig. 15). The manifestations of Hodgkin's disease in AIDS may be atypical (e.g., absence of mediastinal lymphadenopathy in patients with bibasilar infiltrates). Pleural effusion has been reported (64).

Mediastinal and hilar lymphadenopathy is unusual in uncomplicated AIDS. Although it does occur in ARL,

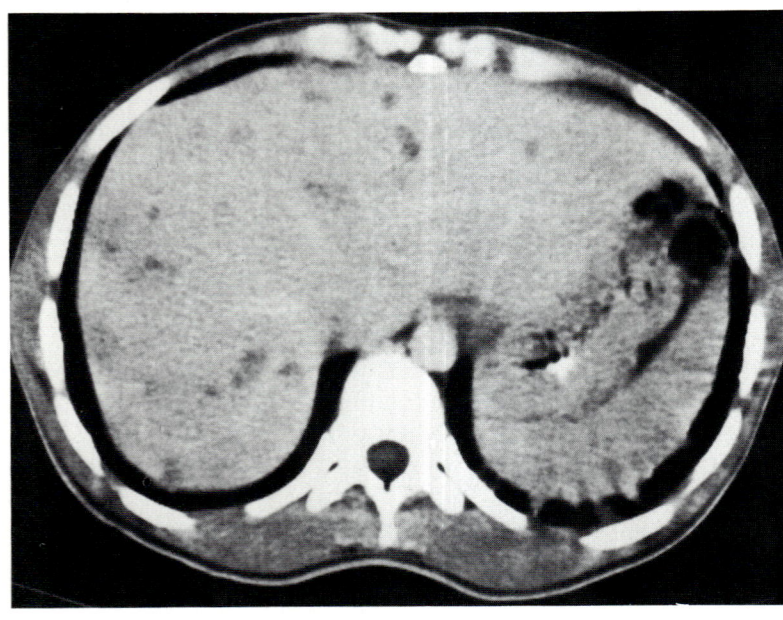

**FIG. 12.** KS lesions throughout the liver on an abdominal CT scan. Although one-third of AIDS patients have liver and/or spleen involvement by KS at autopsy, this is uncommonly evident during life either clinically or radiographically.

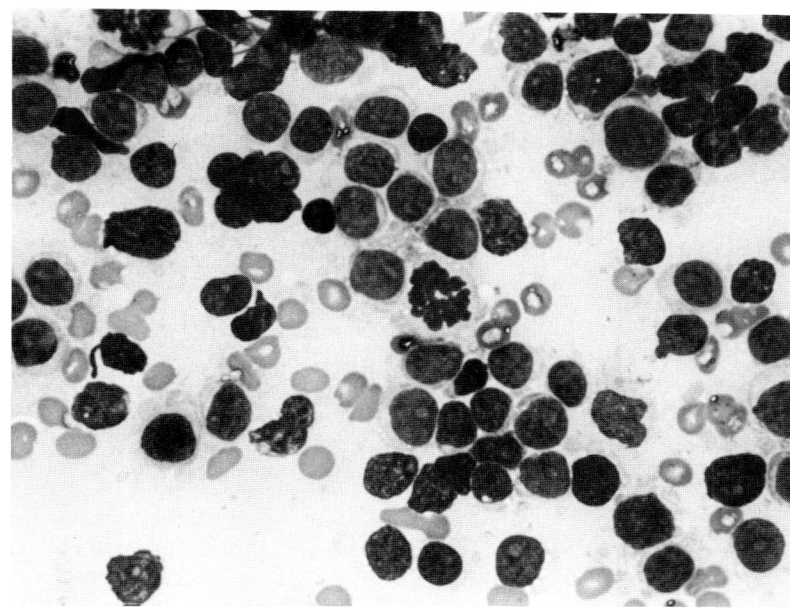

FIG. 13. NHL. Photomicrograph of diffuse large cell NHL showing a monomorphic population of malignant cells. (May-Grunwall-Giemsa stain, ×280).

more often it is the result of an indolent infection such as tuberculosis or fungus disease (64,65). In ARL, we have observed absence of mediastinal lymphadenopathy despite the presence of abdominal lymphadenopathy. Other unusual patterns have been previously noted in ARL, such as bone marrow without splenic involvement in AIDS patients with Hodgkin's disease (59).

ARL commonly involves multiple abdominal sites, including lymph nodes, solid visceral organs, and bowel (5,8,54). Because of this, we consider CT the imaging method of choice for examining the abdomen in AIDS patients. In a study of 29 patients with ARL, CT demonstrated involvement in multiple abdominal sites, including paraaortic lymph nodes (52%), mesenteric lymph nodes (24%), pelvis (24%), liver (21%), spleen (21%), bowel (17%), and kidneys (7%) (54). Frequency of involvement in these areas was greater for NHL than for Hodgkin's disease.

Abdominal lymph nodes are commonly involved with ARL, including the paraaortic and mesenteric lymph groups (Figs. 16–21). CT and ultrasound are useful for evaluating this lymphadenopathy. Identification of bulky abdominal nodes is important in AIDS, since it suggests the presence of a serious complication. In our experience the most common causes of bulky abdominal lymphadenopathy (greater than 1.5 cm) are lym-

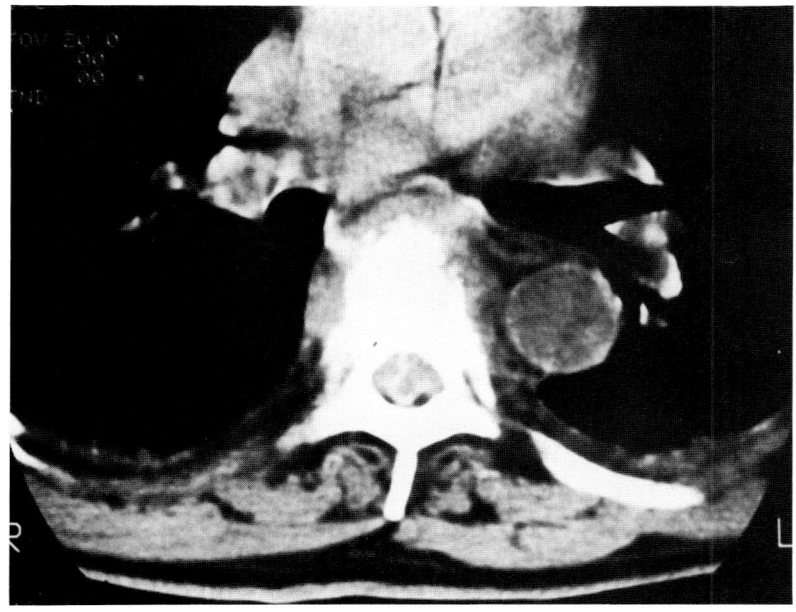

FIG. 14. Spinal involvement with AIDS-related NHL, vertebral destruction of T6-9 along with paravertebral soft tissue mass. Metrizamide-enhanced thecal sac is compressed by epidural tumor.

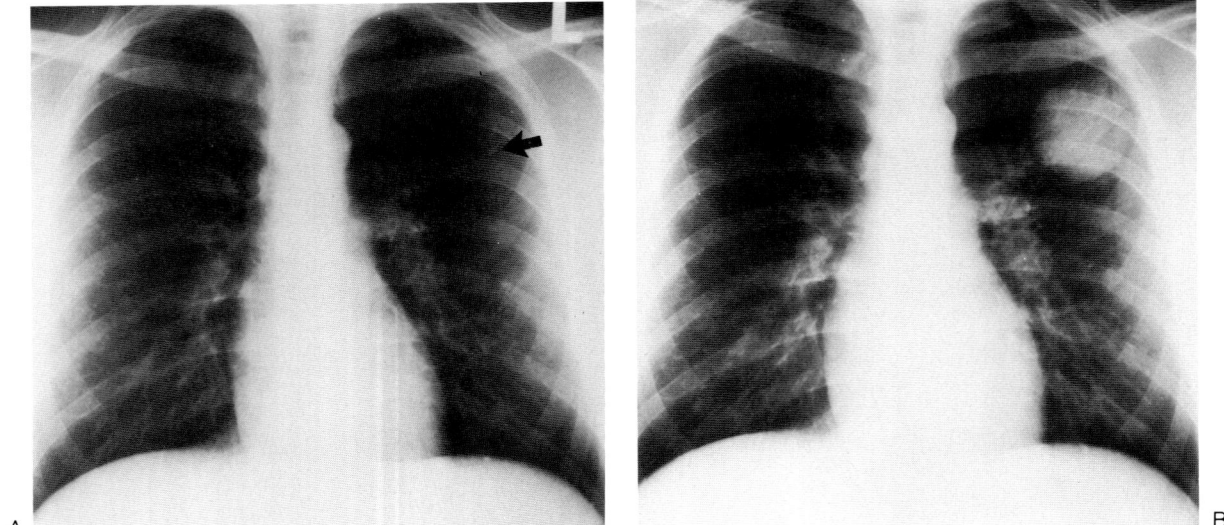

**FIG. 15.** Unusual manifestation of thoracic ARL. **A:** Initial chest radiograph unremarkable except for small nodular density (arrow). **B:** Six months later. Large pulmonary neoplasm without apparent mediastinal or hilar adenopathy. Biopsy proved immunoblastic sarcoma.

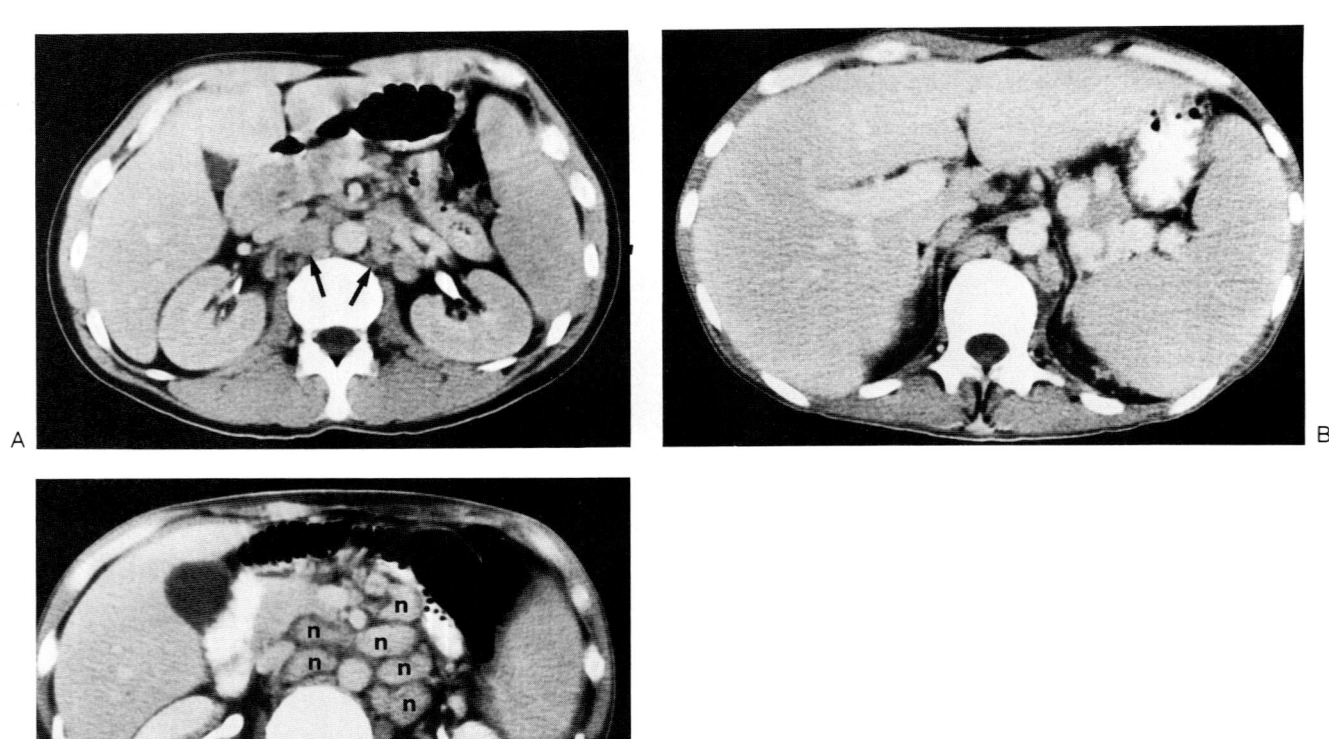

**FIG. 16.** Three patients with adenopathy from ARL. **A:** Multiple discretely enlarged retroperitoneal nodes (arrows). **B:** Retrocrural adenopathy. **C:** Extensive retroperitoneal and mesenteric adenopathy (n).

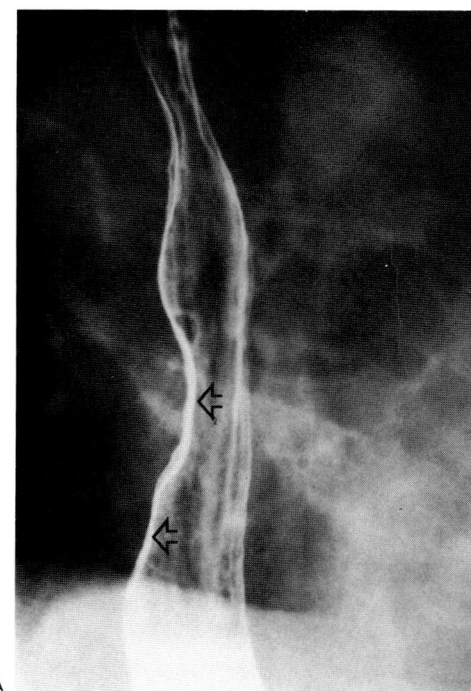
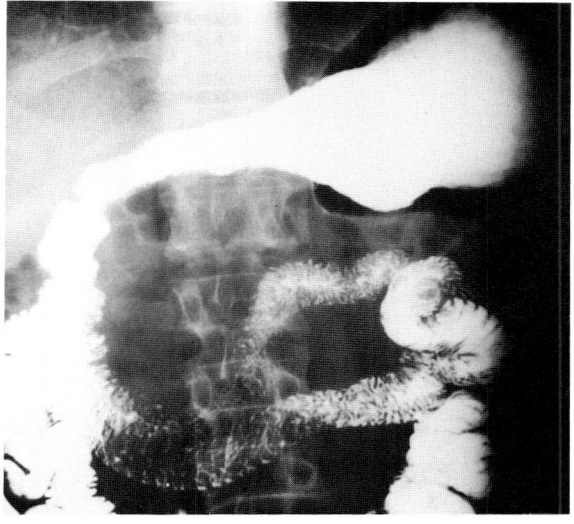

**FIG. 17.** Upper GI series obtained because of dysphagia, satiety, and weight loss. **A:** Air-contrast view of esophagus demonstrates extrinsic indentations by mediastinal nodes (*arrows*). **B:** Mass effect lifts stomach, depresses duodenojejunal flexure, and displaces small bowel loops. CT confirmed extensive adenopathy from NHL.

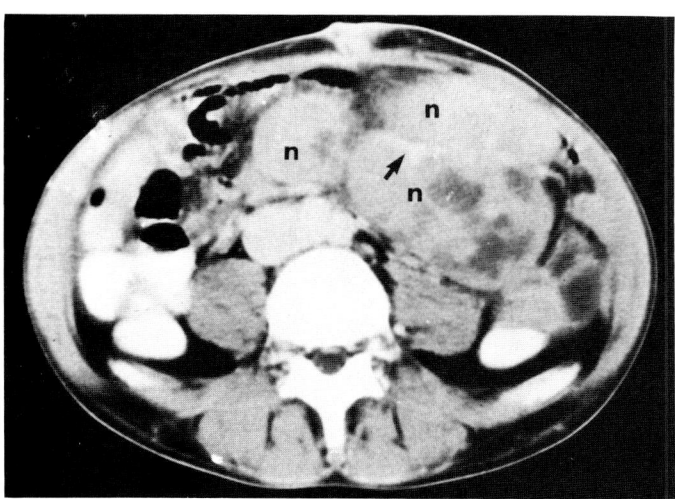

**FIG. 18.** Large mesenteric nodal mass (n) surrounding mesenteric vessel (*arrow*) in a patient with Hodgkin's disease. This patient was HIV antibody-positive following multiple transfusions for sickle cell anemia. Mesenteric adenopathy is an uncommon finding (<5%) in nonAIDS patients with Hodgkin's disease.

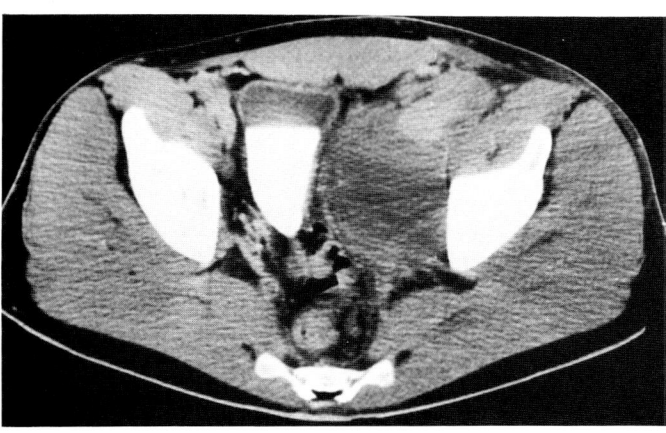

**FIG. 19.** Pelvic mass representing Hodgkin's disease. Little paraaortic adenopathy was noted at other levels, an unusual distribution of adenopathy in Hodgkin's disease.

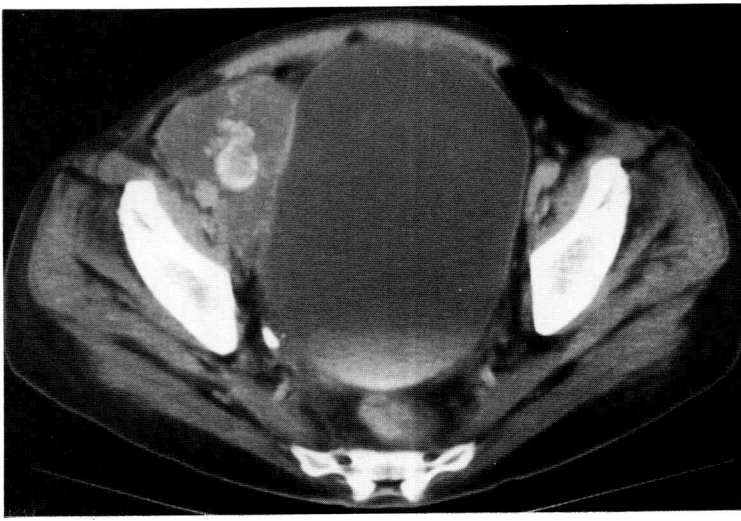

**FIG. 20.** NHL. Partially calcified right pelvic nodal mass is an unusual manifestation of untreated Burkitt's lymphoma.

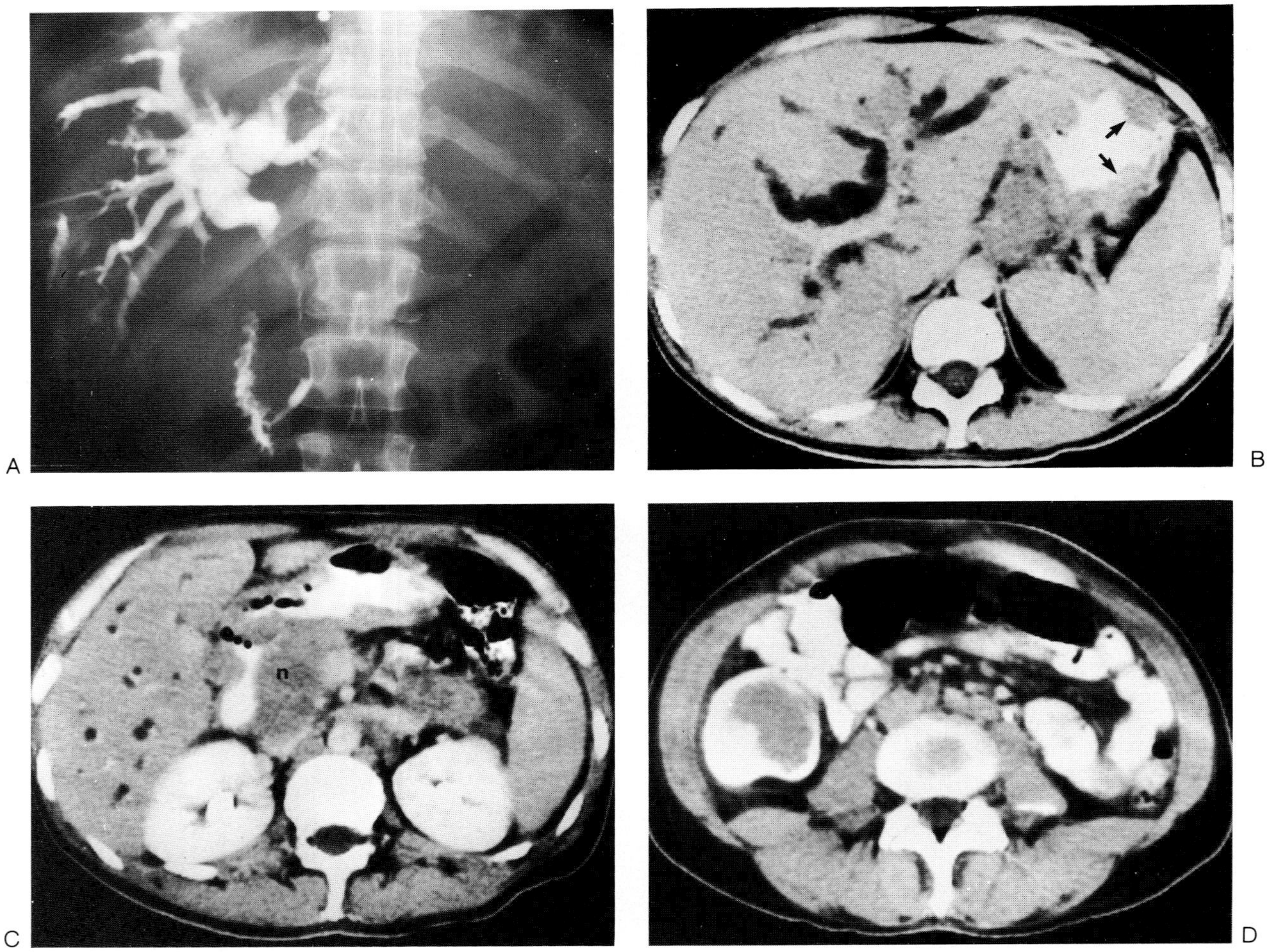

**FIG. 21.** NHL. **A:** Cholangiogram shows long obstructed portion of extrahepatic bile duct. **B:** CT demonstrates dilated bile ducts and adenopathy as well as a thick gastric wall (*arrows*). **C:** Adenopathy (n) causes mass effect in pancreatic head and obstructs the common bile duct. **D:** Cecal mass. All visceral and nodal masses proved to be Burkitt's lymphoma.

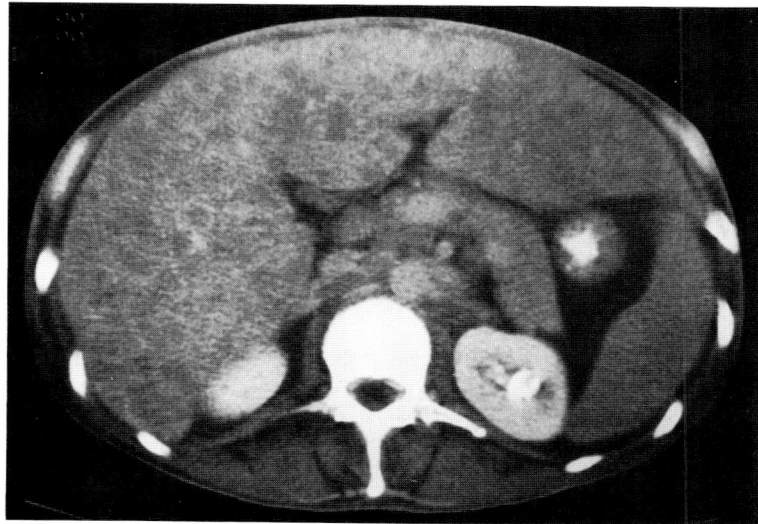

FIG. 22. Diffuse hepatic tumor and adenopathy from Burkitt-type lymphoma.

phoma and infection (particularly by Mycobacterial avium-intracellulare; MAI). KS less frequently causes bulky abdominal lymphadenopathy. We have observed that multiple low-density, unenhanced areas within enlarged lymph nodes suggest the presence of MAI (66), while coexisting hepatic, splenic, or other visceral lesions favor lymphoma (54). Nodes between 1 and 1.5 cm are seen more commonly in patients with PGL.

Since radiographic and CT findings alone are rarely diagnostic, biopsy of enlarged lymph nodes often is necessary to establish the diagnosis. Peripheral lymph nodes, when enlarged, are in more convenient sites of biopsies. Chapter 1 outlines the clinical situations in which peripheral lymph node biopsies are undertaken. Abdominal nodes often are the predominant or only site of involvement; in this situation, CT or ultrasound-guided fine-needle aspiration biopsy (FNAB) and/or core-needle biopsy may be performed. An experienced cytopathologist usually can distinguish between the major diagnostic possibilities in AIDS patients (67). In other cases, complete excision of a node may be necessary to evaluate the nodal architecture, which some oncologists believe is important for determining the appropriate treatment of the variety of lymphomas encountered in these patients.

Visceral organs are common sites of involvement for ARL, reflecting the high frequency of extranodal disease compared with lymphoma in the general population. In a study of 29 patients with abdominal ARL, CT demonstrated liver involvement in 6% of patients with NHL (Figs. 22–27) and 10% of patients with Hodgkin's disease (54). Similarly, in a series of AIDS patients with NHL (excluding primary brain lymphoma) 12% had liver involvement (5). Splenic (26%) and renal (11%)

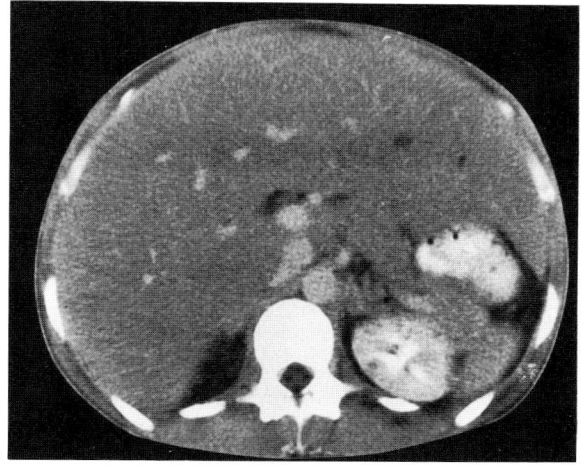 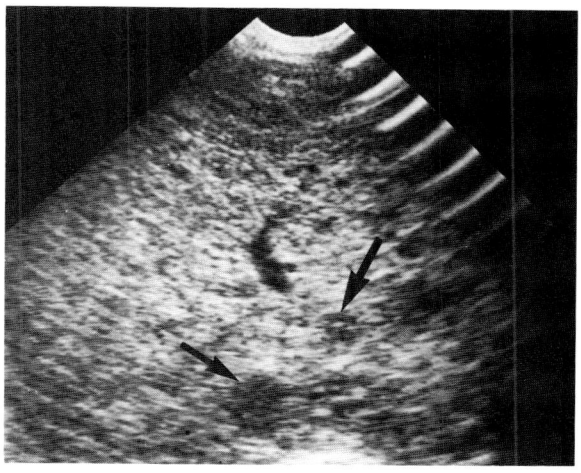

FIG. 23. NHL. **A:** CT. Diffuse hepatomegaly with only a few hypodense focal lesions noted in the liver and kidney. **B:** Hepatic sonogram. Diffuse distortion of echopattern and numerous focal lesions (*arrows*).

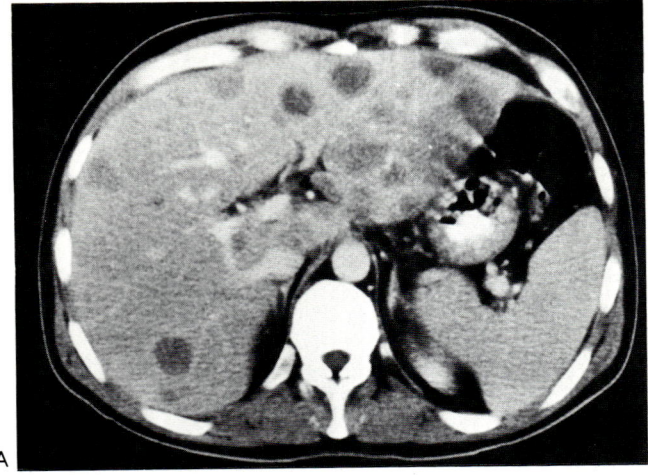
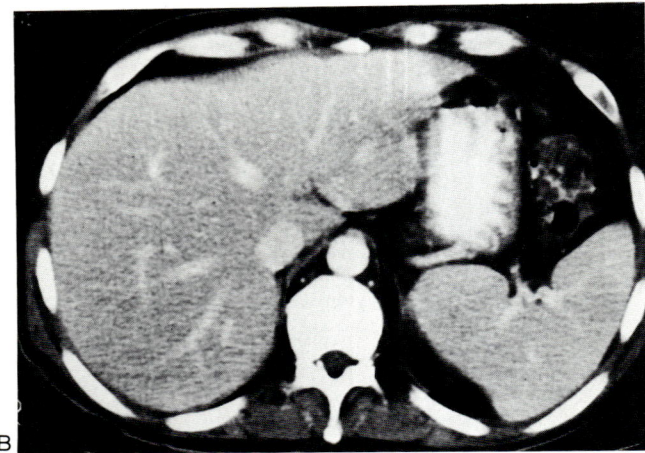

**FIG. 24.** NHL. **A:** Multiple well-defined hypodense hepatic lesions due to undifferentiated NHL. No retroperitoneal or peripheral adenopathy. **B:** Six months later, after chemotherapy, the liver appears normal. This rare patient remains clinically free of tumor 2 years after his initial diagnosis of ARL.

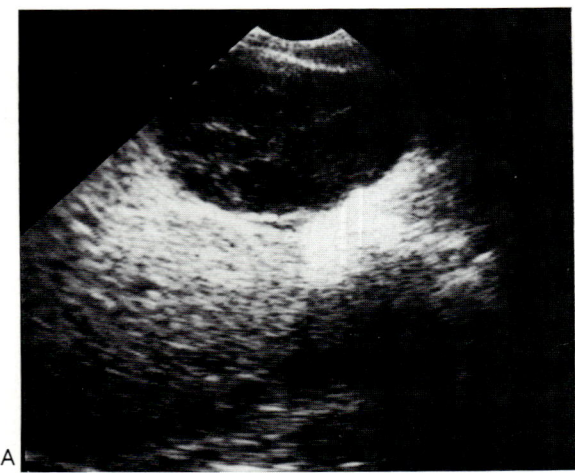
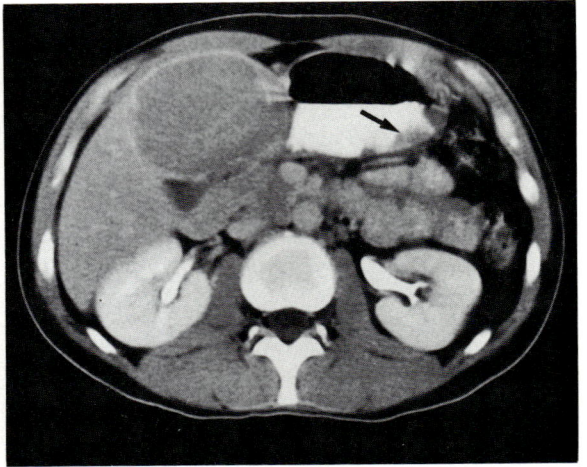

**FIG. 25.** Unusual appearance of hepatic lymphoma (NHL). **A:** Hepatic sonogram demonstrates a solitary large hypoechoic mass with acoustic enhancement and internal septations that suggested the presence of a complex fluid collection. **B:** CT demonstrates a solid-appearing mass (38 H) with a capsule. Also note focal thickening of the gastric wall (arrow). Biopsy of each lesion showed undifferentiated NHL.

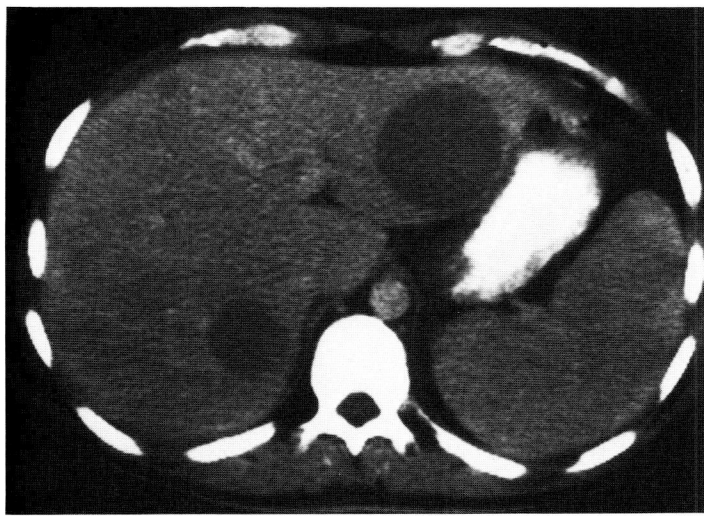

**FIG. 26.** Burkitt's lymphoma. Multiple hepatic lesions simulate cysts on CT.

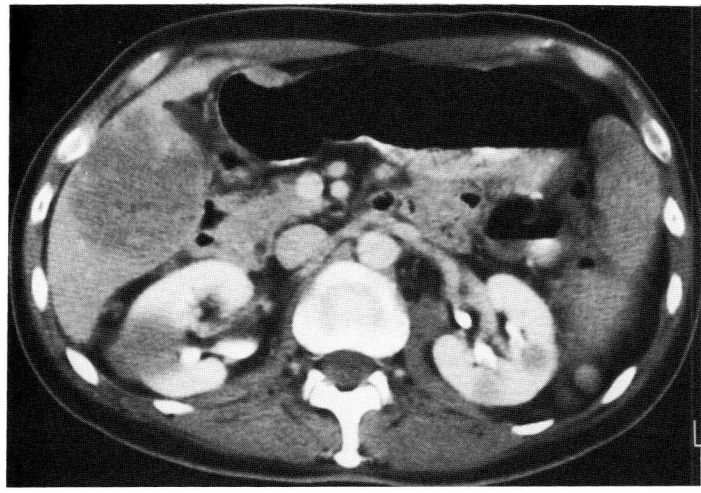

**FIG. 27.** NHL. Hepatic and bilateral renal involvement.

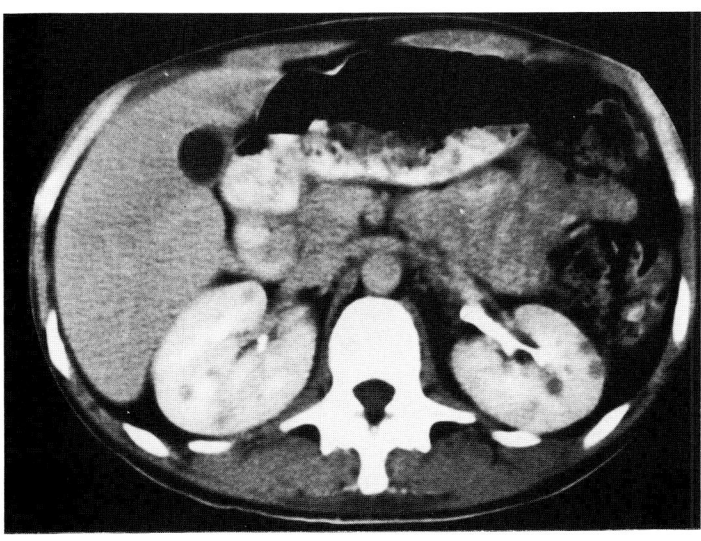

**FIG. 28.** Undifferentiated NHL. Bilateral renal involvement was the only radiographic finding.

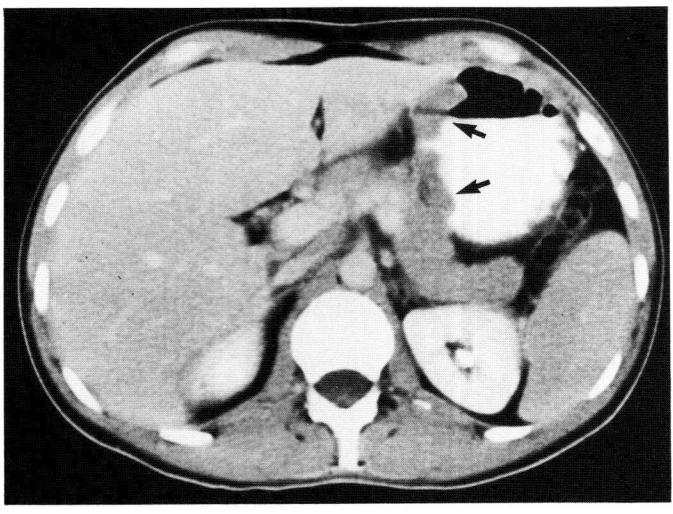

FIG. 29. Extranodal site of involvement in AIDS-related NHL. Focal gastric mass along lesser curve (arrows).

involvement also are frequently demonstrated (Figs. 27,28) (5). Demonstration of focal hepatic, splenic, or renal lesions in patients with AIDS or considered at risk for AIDS should suggest disseminated lymphoma, although other neoplastic and infectious etiologies are possible.

The alimentary tract is a common site of involvement for ARL (Figs. 21,25,29–31). Of 19 patients with AIDS-related NHL, 5 (26%) demonstrated bowel involvement on CT (54). A high frequency of bowel involvement in patients with AIDS and NHL (excluding primary brain lymphoma) also has been reported by Ziegler et al. (5) (22%) and by Ioachim et al. (8) (33%). Although any portion of the GI tract may be involved, oral, rectal, and distal ileal sites are most common (Figs. 30 and 31).

The clinical presentation of patients with bowel lymphoma also may be atypical. One patient in our series presented with hematochezia due to rectal lymphoma; another had a perforation of the distal ileum that simulated a periappendiceal abscess (Fig. 31). An abdominal or pelvic mass is frequently palpable. One patient with Hodgkin's disease presented with a huge mesenteric mass; this is more commonly seen in Burkitt's lymphoma or NHL (Fig. 18). Because of this spectrum of findings, abdominal CT complements barium studies in detecting involvement of the bowel and other abdominal sites.

## DIFFERENTIAL DIAGNOSIS

Patients fulfilling the CDC criteria for a diagnosis of AIDS constitute only a small part of a larger group of

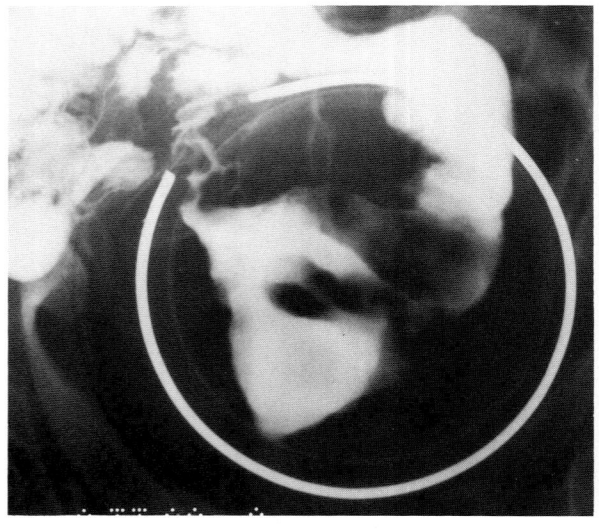
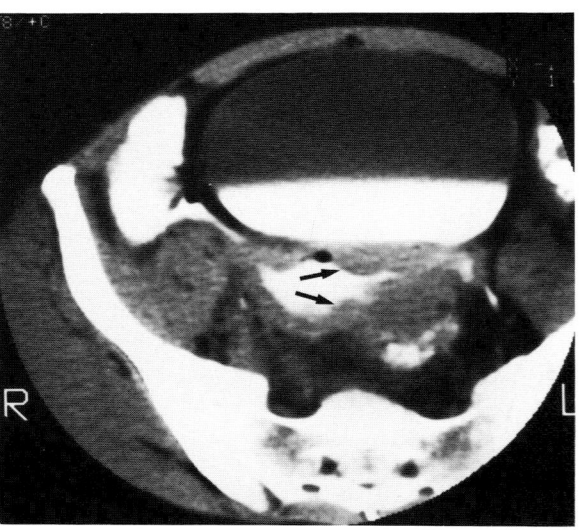

FIG. 30. NHL (large cell, uncleaved). A: Barium small bowel series shows distortion, nodularity, and aneurysmal dilitation of the ileum. B: CT shows distorted lumen and mural soft tissue mass (arrows).

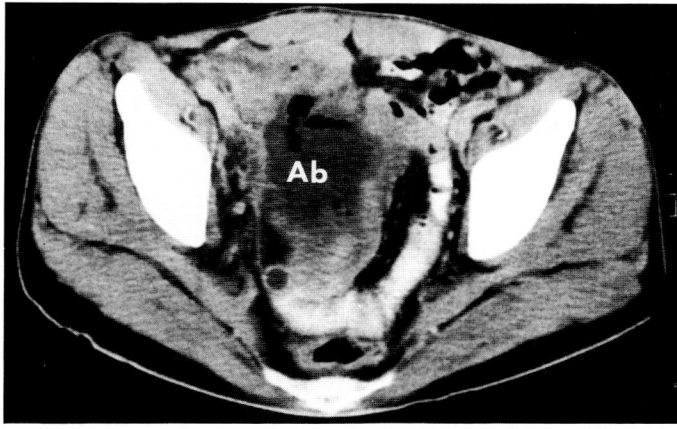

FIG. 31. Pelvic abscess (Ab) clinically and radiographically felt to be periappendiceal. Surgery found perforated ilieal NHL.

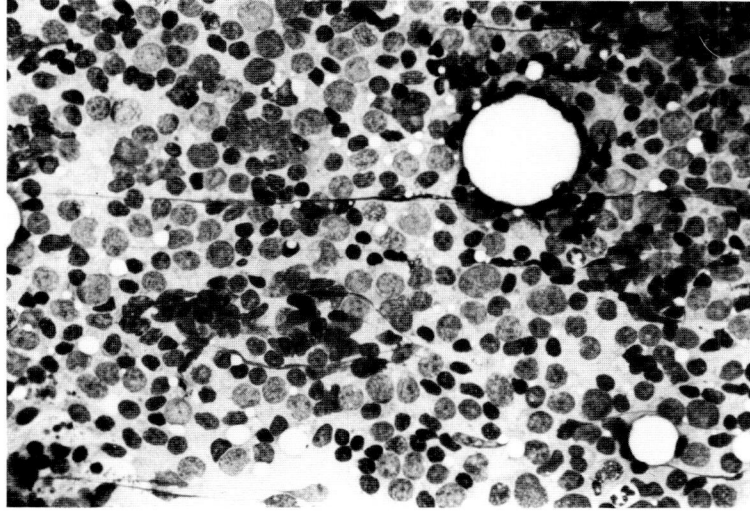

FIG. 32. Benign reactive hyperplasia. Photomicrograph of a FNAB sampled hyperplastic node with a pleomophic population of various lymphoid elements. (May-Grunwald-Giemsa stain, ×60).

patients with HIV infection that includes patients with signs of acute viral infection and asymptomatic carriers with PGL. In addition, PGL may be present and often is referred to as the lymphadenopathy syndrome. The diagnostic criteria for PGL are chronic lymphadenopathy of at least three months' duration involving two or more extrainguinal sites. There is no concurrent illness or drug use that may cause lymphadenopathy, and lymph node biopsies demonstrate reactive hyperplasia without evidence of tumor (Fig. 32) (see Appendix A).

Initial reports of abdominal CT in patients with PGL have emphasized a characteristic triad of: 1) mild lymphadenopathy (clusters of lymph nodes ranging from 5 mm to 1 cm) involving the retroperitoneal, mesenteric, or pelvic lymph nodes chains, (Fig. 33); 2) splenomegaly; 3) abnormal soft-tissue infiltration of the rectal wall or perirectal fat (53). The perirectal disease commonly seen in these patients (often asymptomatic) presumably is the result of chronic proctitis from repeated venereal infections (Figs. 34,35). It should be

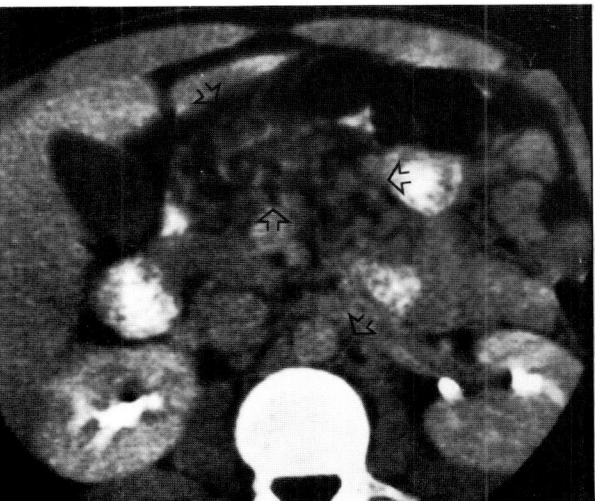

FIG. 33. Clusters of small (<1 cm) nodes in the retroperitoneum and mesentery (arrows) are a nonspecific finding, frequently found in patients with ARC. Biopsy usually reveals benign reactive hyperplasia.

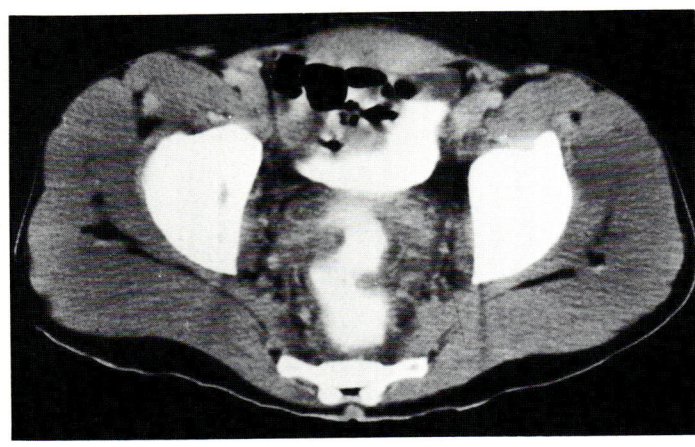

**FIG. 34.** Perirectal inflammation in ARC. Diffuse soft-tissue infiltration of perirectal space.

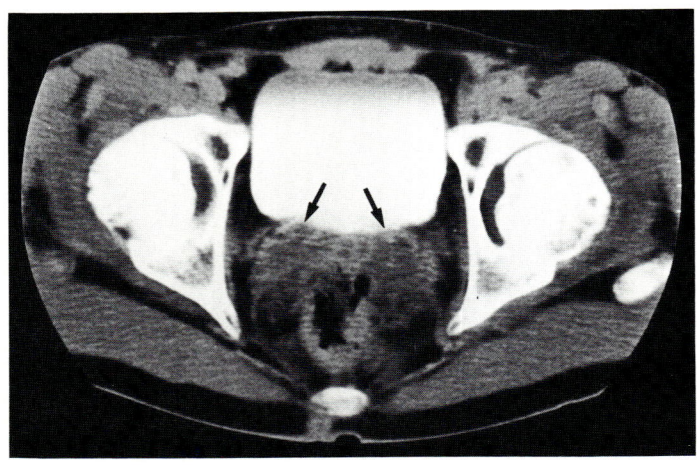

**FIG. 35.** Diffuse inflammation and swelling of the seminal vesicles (*arrows*) frequently accompanies perirectal infiltration in ARC.

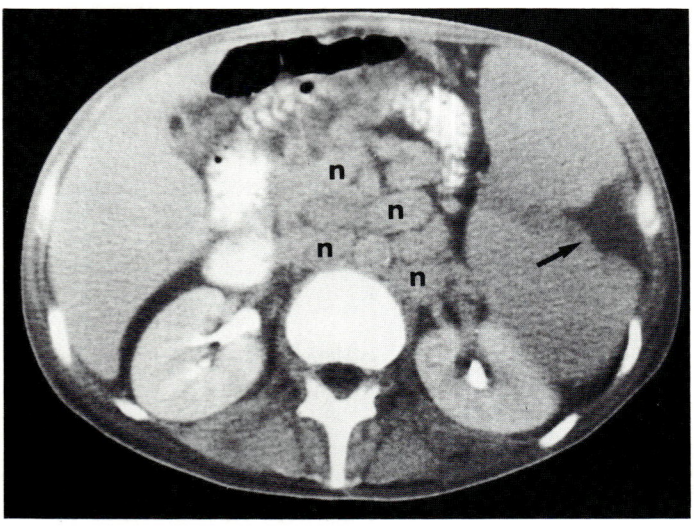

**FIG. 36.** Mesenteric and retroperitoneal lymphadenopathy (*n*) indistinguishable from lymphoma or KS on CT. Biopsy characteristic of MAI. Incidental splenic infarct (*arrow*).

emphasized that abdominal nodal enlargement greater than 1.5 cm, however, is unusual in the lymphadenopathy syndrome and should prompt CT-guided biopsy to exclude neoplastic or infectious nodal disease.

## CT of Abdominal Opportunistic Infections in AIDS

The clinical and radiographic features of enteric infections are discussed in detail in Chapter 4. CT is rarely a primary method of diagnosis, except in cases of MAI, where mesenteric retroperitoneal adenopathy is the striking radiographic feature. In general, the CT findings of AIDS-related opportunistic GI infections are nonspecific and include focal bowel wall thickening, adjacent mesenteric edema or adenopathy, and thickened small bowel folds.

In immunocompetent individuals, MAI is rarely a pathogen. However, it is an increasingly important source of morbidity in patients with AIDS and is often seen in its disseminated form as a preterminal event. Cultures are necessary to distinguish MAI precisely from Mycobacterium tuberculosis (MTB), although MAI has proven, in our experience, to be significantly more common than MTB.

Abdominal CT may be the first imaging study to suggest the diagnosis of MAI, which frequently results in bulky mesenteric and retroperitoneal nodal masses that may have characteristic areas of low density. Unless present, the lymphadenopathy caused by MAI cannot be reliably distinguished from KS or ARL (Fig. 36). In a series at San Francisco General Hospital of 17 patients with biopsy-proven MAI, 14 (82%) had bulky mesenteric or retroperitonal nodes measuring greater than 1 to 1.5 cm in size on CT (66). Focal hepatic and splenic low-density lesions occasionally may be detected by CT (Fig. 37); however, diffuse microscopic involvement of the liver by MAI may not be detectable by CT and can only be confirmed by needle biopsy. In patients with persistently abnormal liver function tests and clinical suspicion of MAI, a core liver biopsy may be required to establish the diagnosis.

The low-density areas within MAI nodes are quite characteristic of this disorder (Fig. 38) but are not generally seen in AIDS-related KS or ARL. CT-guided FNAB of nodes in visceral lesions is a highly reliable technique for diagnosing MAI; microscopy characteristically demonstrates foamy histiocytes laden with acid-fast bacilli (Fig. 39) (67). Thus, in addition to routine viral culture, acid-fast stains should be performed on all FNAB specimens in AIDS. At present, combination chemotherapy is used in treatment (see Chapter 1).

Perirectal inflammatory disorders on CT are common in both ARC and AIDS patients. These are generally secondary to chronic proctitis from repeated venereal infections with syphillis, gonococci, CMV, herpes simplex virus, or lymphogranuloma venereum. On the basis of CT alone, it may be difficult to distinguish proctitis from rectal KS, lymphoma, or cloacogenic carcinoma. The CT demonstration of soft-tissue infiltration of the perirectal space and mild thickening of the perirectal fascia may be seen in relatively asymptomatic individuals with AIDS. However, in patients with symptomatic perirectal inflammatory disease, CT may be of value in distinguishing perirectal cellulitis from a true abscess and in localizing complex abscesses to either the supralevator or infralevator perirectal compartments (68).

## OTHER MALIGNANCIES

Recent reviews suggest that several malignancies other than KS and NHL may be associated with AIDS, including chronic lymphocytic leukemia, adenosquamous carcinoma of the lung, hepatocellular carcinoma, and carcinoma of the oropharynx. Homosexual men

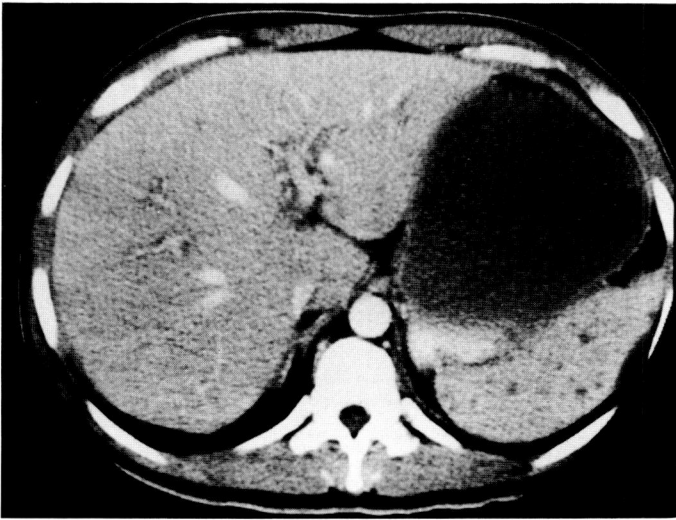

**FIG. 37.** Focal splenic lesions; biopsy-proven MAI.

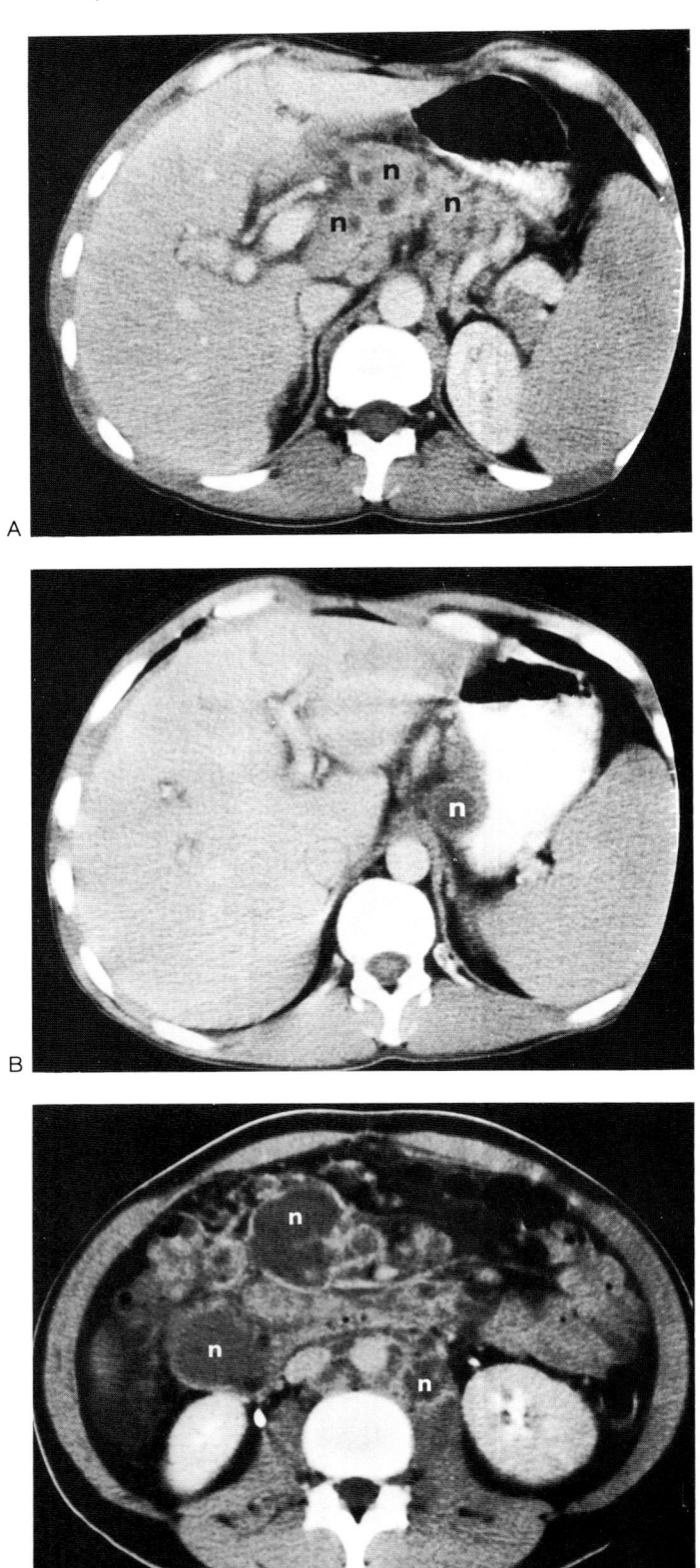

**FIG. 38. A, B, C, D:** Four patients with low-density, necrotic-appearing lymph nodes (n) due to MAI. All had clinical evidence of disseminated MAI and splenomegaly.

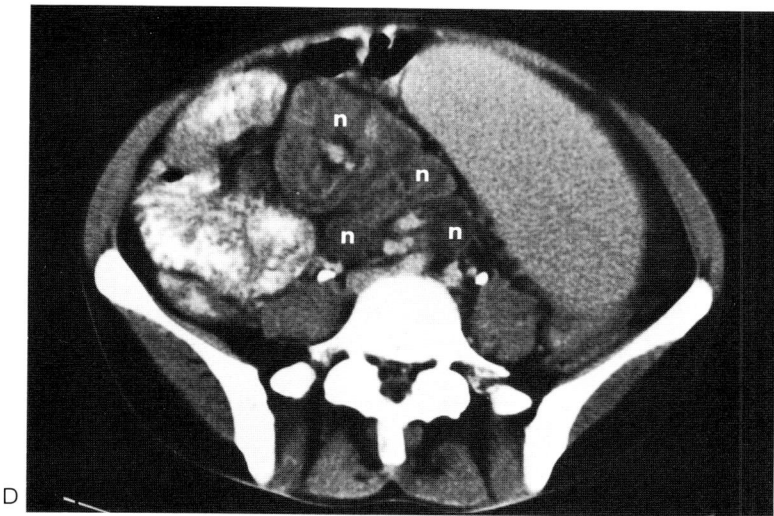

FIG. 38. (Continued)

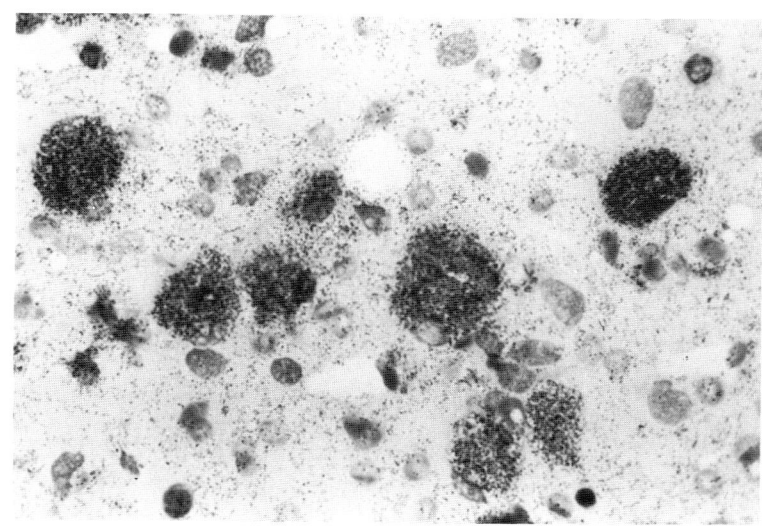

FIG. 39. MAI. Photomicrograph of a lymph node containing MAI showing histocytes filled with thousands of microorganisms (Fite stain, ×240).

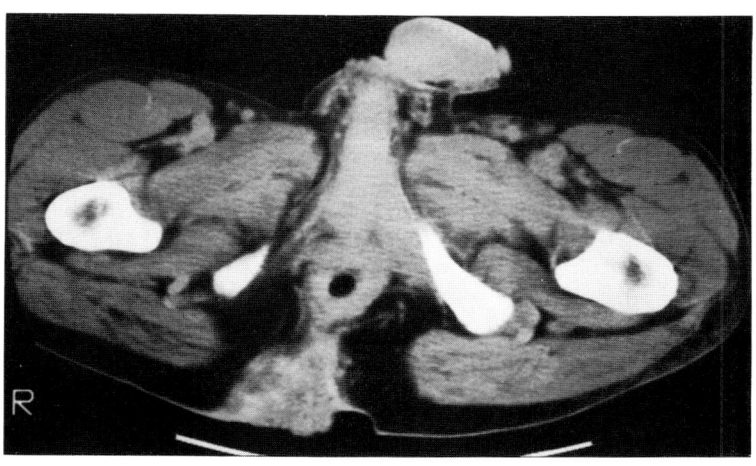

FIG. 40. Cloacogenic carcinoma. Extensive anorectal tumor invading buttocks and base of penis.

have an increased risk of carcinoma of the anorectum ("cloacogenic carcinoma") that may not be associated with AIDS per se (Fig. 40). As with KS and lymphoma, there is evidence of viral induction of squamous cell carcinoma, specifically by the papilloma virus. Other AIDS authorities, however, question whether neoplasms other than KS and NHL have an increased incidence in AIDS or just exhibit different biological behavior due to preexisting compromise of the immune system.

## INDICATIONS FOR ABDOMINAL CT IN AIDS

Indications for abdominal CT in AIDS patients include evaluation for suspected visceral or nodal infection with MAI, abdominal or pelvic abscesses, and diagnosis and staging of abdominal neoplasms such as KS and lymphoma. In patients with localized symptoms such as right upper quadrant pain, sonography often is a useful initial screening method. On occasion, sonography may reveal subtle hepatic lesions difficult to image by CT. Because of the frequency of mesenteric and retroperitoneal nodal disease in AIDS, CT remains the primary method for evaluation in most patients. Although chemotherapy for AIDS-related neoplasms often is limited in its effectiveness, repeat abdominal CT may be useful to assess the course of therapy.

## REFERENCES

1. Centers for Disease Control (1982): Epidemiologic aspects of the current outbreak of Kaposi's sarcoma and opportunistic infections. *N. Engl. J. Med.*, 306:248–252.
2. Friedman-Kein, A. E., Laubenstein, L. J., Rubinstein, P., et al. (1982): Disseminated Kaposi's sarcoma in homosexual men. *Ann. Intern. Med.*, 96:693–700.
3. Ziegler, J. L., Drew, W. L., Miner, R. C., et al. (1982): Outbreak of Burkitt's-like lymphoma in homosexual men. *Lancet*, 2:631–633.
4. Centers for Disease Control (1982): Diffuse, undifferentiated non-Hodgkin's lymphoma among homosexual males. United States. *M.M.W.R.*, 31:277–279.
5. Ziegler, J. L., Beckstead, J. A., Volberding, P. A., et al. (1984): Non-Hodgkin's lymphoma in 90 homosexual men: Relation to generalized lymphadenopathy and the acquired immunodeficiency syndrome. *N. Engl. J. Med.*, 311:565–570.
6. Levin, A. M., Meyer, P. M., Begandy, M. K., et al. (1984): Development of a B-cell lymphoma in homosexual men: Clinical and immunologic findings. *Ann. Intern. Med.*, 100:7–13.
7. Kalter, S. P., Riggs, S. A., Cabanillas, F., et al. (1985): Aggressive non-Hodgkin's lymphomas in immunocompromised homosexual males. *Blood*, 66:655–659.
8. Ioachim, H. L., Cooper, M. C., and Hellman, G. C. (1985): Lymphomas in men at high risk for acquired immunodeficiency syndrome (AIDS). *Cancer*, 56:2831–2842.
9. Centers for Disease Control Update (1985): Acquired immunodeficiency syndrome. United States. *M.M.W.R.*, 34:245–248.
10. Urba, W. S., and Longo, D. L. (1985): Clinical spectrum of human retroviral induced diseases. *Cancer Res.*, 45(*Suppl*):4637s–4643s.
11. Landesman, S. H., Ginzburg, H. M., and Weiss, S. H. (1985): Special report: The AIDS epidemic. *N. Engl. J. Med.*, 312:521–524.
12. Lozada, F., Silverman, S., and Conent, M. (1982): New outbreak of oral tumors. Malignancies and infectious disease strikes young male homosexuals. *C.D.A.J.* 19:39–42.
13. Cooper, H. S., Patchefsky, A. J., and Marks, G. (1979): Cloacogenic carcinoma of the anorectum in homosexual men: An observation of four cases. *Dis. Colon Rectum*, 22:557–558.
14. Gallo, R. C., Salahuddin, S. Z., Popovic, M., et al. (1984): Frequent detection and isolation of cytopathic retroviruses (HTLV-III) from patients with AIDS and pre-AIDS. *Science*, 224:500–503.
15. Buldgogh, I., Beth, E., Haang, E. S., et al. (1981): Kaposi's sarcoma: IV Detection of CMV, DNA, CMV RNA, and CMV NA in tumor biopsies. *Int. J. Cancer*, 28:469–474.
16. Drew, W. L., Miner, R. C., Ziegler, J. L., et al. (1982): Cytomegalovirus and Kaposi's sarcoma in young homosexual men. *Lancet*, 1:125.
17. Klein, G. (1981): The role of gene dosage and genetic transpositions in carcinogenesis. *Nature*, 294:313–318.
18. Hanto, W. H., Frizzera, G., Purtillo, D. T., et al. (1981): Clinical spectrum of lymphoproliferative disorders in renal transplant recipients and evidence for the role of Epstein-Barr virus. *Cancer Res.*, 141:4253–4261.
19. Oettle, A. G. (1962): Geographical and racial differences in the frequency of Kaposi's sarcoma as evidence of environmental or genetic causes. *Acta Un Int. Cancrum*, 18:330–363.
20. Safai, B., Mike, V., Giraldo, G., et al. (1980): Association of Kaposi's sarcoma with second primary malignancies. Possible etiopathogenic implications. *Cancer*, 45:1472–1479.
21. Reynolds, W. A., Winkelmann, R. K., and Soule, E. H. (1965): Kaposi's sarcoma: A clinicopathological study with particular reference to its relationship to the reticuloendothelial system. *Medicine*, 44:419–434.
22. Penn, I., Hammond, A., Brett-Scheider, L., et al. (1969): Malignant lymphomas in transplantation patients. *Transplant. Proc.*, 1:106–112.
23. Frizzera, G., Rosai, J., Dehner, L. P., et al. (1980): Lymphoreticular disorders in primary immunodeficiencies: New findings based on an up-to-date histologic classification of 35 cases. *Cancer*, 46:692–699.
24. Filipovich, A. H., Spector, B. D., and Kersey, J. H. (1980): Immunodeficiency in humans as a risk factor in the development of malignancy. *Prev. Med.*, 9:252–259.
25. Cox, F. H., and Helwig, E. G. (1959): Kaposi's sarcoma. *Cancer*, 12:289–298.
26. Taylor, J. P., Templeton, A. C., Vogel, C. L., et al. (1971): Kaposi's sarcoma in Uganda: A clinico-pathological study. *Int. J. Cancer*, 8:125–135.
27. Templeton, A. C. (1972): Studies in Kaposi's sarcoma. Post mortem findings and disease patterns in women. *Cancer*, 30:854–867.
28. Davies, J. N. P., and Lothe, F. (1962): Kaposi's sarcoma in African children. *Acta Un Int. Cancrum*, 18:394–399.
29. Satai, B., Sarngadharan, M. G., Koziner, B., et al. (1985): Spectrum of Kaposi's sarcoma in the epidemic of AIDS. *Cancer Res.*, 45(*Suppl*):4646–4648.
30. Centers for Disease Control Update (1983): Acquired immunodeficiency syndrome (AIDS). United States. *M.M.W.R.*, 32:389–391.
31. Drew, W. L., Mintz, L., Miner, R. C., et al. (1981): Prevalence of cytomegalovirus infection in homosexual men. *J. Infect. Dis.*, 143:180–191.
32. Giraldi, G., Beth, E., and Huang, E.-S. (1980): Kaposi's sarcoma and its relationship to human cytomegalovirus (CMV). CMV DNA and CMV early antigens in Kaposi's sarcoma. *Int. J. Cancer*, 26:23–27.
33. Longo, D. L. (1984): Kaposi's sarcoma and other neoplasms. *Ann. Intern. Med.*, 100:92–106.
34. Reichert, C. M., O'Leary, T. J., Lewens, D. L., et al. (1983): Autopsy pathology in the acquired immune deficiency syndrome. *Am. J. Pathol.*, 112:357–382.
35. Hui, A. N., Koss, M. N., and Meyer, P. R. (1984): Necropsy findings in acquired immunodeficiency syndrome: A comparison of pre-mortem diagnoses with post mortem findings. *Hum. Pathol.*, 15:670–676.
36. Welch, K., Finkbeiner, W., Alpers, C. E., et al. (1984): Autopsy findings in the acquired immune deficiency syndrome. *J.A.M.A.*, 252:1152–1159.
37. Niedt, G. W., and Schinella, R. A. (1985): Acquired immunodefi-

ciency syndrome. Clinicopathologic study of 56 autopsies. *Arch. Pathol. Lab. Med.,* 109:727–734.
38. Kelly, W. M., and Brant-Zawadski, M. (1983): Acquired immunodeficiency syndrome: Neuroradiologic findings. *Radiology,* 149:485–491.
39. Post, M. J. D., Kursunoglu, S. J., Hensley, G. T., et al. (1985): Cranial CT of the acquired immunodeficiency syndrome (AIDS): Spectrum of diseases and optimal contrast enhancement technique. *A.J.N.R.,* 6:743–754.
40. Post, M. J. D., Sheldon, J. J., Hensley, G. T., et al. (1986): Central nervous system in acquired immunodeficiency syndrome: Prospective correlation using CT, MR, imaging, and pathologic studies. *Radiology,* 158:141–148.
41. Murray, J. F., Felton, C. P., Gavay, S. M., et al. (1984): Special report: Pulmonary complications of the acquired immunodeficiency syndrome. *N. Engl. J. Med.,* 310:1682–1688.
42. Brown, R. K. J., Huberman, R. P., and Vanley, G. (1982): Pulmonary features of Kaposi's sarcoma. *A.J.R.,* 139:659–660.
43. Kornfield, H., and Axelrod, J. L. (1983): Pulmonary presentation of Kaposi's sarcoma in a homosexual patient. *Am. Rev. Respir. Dis.,* 127:248–249.
44. Ahmed, N., Nelson, R. S., Golstein, H. M., et al. (1975): Kaposi's sarcoma of the stomach and duodenum. Endoscopic and roentgenologic correlations. *Gastrointest. Endosc.,* 21:149–152.
45. Weprin, L., Zollinger, R., Clausen, K. M., et al. (1982): Kaposi's sarcoma: Endoscopic observations of gastric and colon involvement. *J. Clin. Gastroenterol.,* 4:357–600.
46. Friedman, S. L., Wright, T. L., and Altman, D. F. (1985): Gastrointestinal Kaposi's sarcoma in patients with acquired immunodeficiency syndrome: Endoscopic and autopsy findings: *Gastroenterology,* 89:102–108.
47. Lozada, F., Silverman, S., Migliorati, C. A., et al. (1983): Oral manifestations of tumor and opportunistic infections in the acquired immunodeficiency syndrome (AIDS). Findings in 53 homosexual men with Kaposi's sarcoma. *Oral Surg.,* 56:491–494.
48. Rose, H. S., Balthazar, E. J., Megibow, A. J., et al. (1982): Alimentary tract involvement in Kaposi's sarcoma: Radiographic and endoscopic findings in 25 homosexual men. *A.J.R.,* 139:661–666.
49. Hill, C. A., Harle, T. S., Mansell, P. W. A. (1983): The prodrome. Kaposi's sarcoma and infections associated with acquired immunodeficiency syndrome. Radiologic findings in 39 patients. *Radiology,* 149:393–399.
50. Frager, D. H., Frager, J. D., Brandt, L. J., et al. (1986): Gastrointestinal complications of AIDS: Radiologic features. *Radiology,* 158:597–603.
51. Jeffrey, R. B., Jr., Nyberg, D. A., Bottles, W., et al. (1986): Review: Abdominal CT in acquired immunodeficiency syndrome. *A.J.R.,* 146:7–14.
52. Wall, S. D., Ominsky, S., Altman, D. F., et al. (1986): Multifocal abnormalities of the gastrointestinal tract in AIDS. *A.J.R.,* 146:1–5.
53. Moon, K. L., Federle, M. P., Abrams, D. I., et al. (1984): Kaposi's sarcoma and lymphadenopathy syndrome: Limitations of abdominal CT in acquired immunodeficiency syndrome. *Radiology,* 150:479–483.
54. Nyberg, D. A., Jeffrey, R. B., Jr., Federle, M. P., et al. (1986): AIDS-related lymphomas: Evaluation by abdominal CT. *Radiology,* 159:59–63.
55. Shaw, G. M., Harper, M. E., Hahn, B. H., et al. (1985): HTLV-III infection in brains of children and adults with AIDS encephalopathy. *Science,* 227:177–182.
56. Levy, R. M., Bredesen, D. E., and Rosenblum, M. L. (1985): Neurological manifestations of the acquired immunodeficiency syndrome (AIDS): Experience at UCSF and review of the literature. *J. Neurosurg.,* 62:475–495.
57. Abrams, D. I., Lewis, B. J., Beckstead, J. H., et al. (1984): Persistent diffuse lymphadenopathy in homosexual men: Endpoint or prodrome? *Ann. Intern. Med.,* 100:801–808.
58. Centers for Disease Control, Department of Health and Human Services (1985): Revision of the case definition of acquired immunodeficiency syndrome for national reporting. United States. *Ann. Intern. Med.,* 103:402–403.
59. Schoeppel, S. L., Hoppe, R. T., Dorfman, R. F., et al. (1985): Hodgkin's disease in homosexual men with generalized lymphadenopathy. *Ann. Intern. Med.,* 102:68–70.
60. Bragg, D. G., Colby, T. V., and Ward, J. H. (1986): New concepts in the non-Hodgkin's lymphomas: Radiologic implications. *Radiology,* 1159:289–304.
61. Gill, P. S., Levin, A. M., Meyer, P. R., et al. (1985): Primary central nervous system lymphoma in homosexual men: Clinical, immunologic, and pathologic features. *Am. J. Med.,* 78:742–748.
62. Snider, W. D., Simpson, D. M., Nielson, S., et al. (1983): Neurological complications of acquired immune deficiency syndrome: Analysis of 50 patients. *Ann. Neurol.,* 14:403–418.
63. Schneck, S. A., and Penn, I. (1971): *De novo* brain tumors in renal transplant recipients. *Lancet,* 1:983–986.
64. Cohen, B. A., Pomeranz, S., Rabinowitz, J. G., et al. (1984): Pulmonary complications of AIDS: Radiologic features. *A.J.R.,* 143:115–122.
65. Stern, R. G., Gamsu, G., Golden, J. A., et al. (1984): Intrathoracic adenopathy: Differential feature of AIDS and diffuse lymphadenopathy syndrome. *A.J.R.,* 142:689–692.
66. Nyberg, D. A., Federle, M. P., Jeffrey, R. B., et al. (1985): Abdominal CT findings of disseminated Mycobacterium avium intracellulare. *A.J.R.,* 45:297–299.
67. Bottles, K., Cohen, M. B., Brodie, H., et al. (1986): Fine needle aspiration cytology and the differential diagnosis of lymphadenopathy in homosexual males. *Diagn. Cytopathol.,* 2:31–35.
68. Guillaumin, E., Jeffrey, R. B., Jr., Shea, W. J., et al. (1986): Perirectal inflammatory disease: CT findings. *Radiology,* 161:153–157.

# CHAPTER 6

# Pediatric AIDS

Nancy Branom Genieser, Marta Hernanz-Schulman, Keith Krasinski, M. Alba Greco, and William Borkowsky

Soon after the recognition of acquired immune deficiency syndrome (AIDS) in adults, it became apparent that children, without recognized immunosuppressive disorders, also were subject to opportunistic infections. The awareness of disease in children younger than 2 years of age who did not have the typical adult risk factors was an early clue to the viral etiology of AIDS. Children infected with the human immunodeficiency virus (HIV) display a wide range of abnormalities that are due to the direct effects of the virus on various organ systems, as well as those related to immunosuppression (14,32,36,38,39). Why disease should be different in children is partially explained by the time of infection, which occurs primarily by the transplacental route or by exposure to maternal blood at the time of delivery, during a period when the fetus or newborn is immunologically immature. A second important difference is the fact that children are antigenically naive. In the toddler age range, they have had insufficient opportunity to develop antibodies to the usual encapsulated bacterial pathogens of childhood, and consequently suffer from recurrent bacterial infections with typical pediatric pathogens (36).

By early 1987 there had been at least 450 children younger than 13 years of age ("Pediatric AIDS" applies to children under 13) reported to the Centers for Disease Control (CDC) as having AIDS. This figure probably represents only 20% of children with symptomatic HIV infection. The number of children with asymptomatic infection is not known. Pediatric AIDS accounts for 1.5% of total AIDS cases (2).

## PEDIATRIC AIDS

For the limited purposes of epidemiologic surveillance, in order to maintain the integrity and comparability of preexisting data, the CDC defined disease in a child as AIDS only if it met the following four criteria (10,33,42):

1. Disease must be reliably diagnosed and moderately indicative of underlying cellular immunodeficiency. Reliable diagnosis usually demands tissue biopsy with histologic confirmation of the suspected pathogen. Sentinel diseases that are sufficiently indicative of underlying cellular immunity include Pneumocystis carinii pneumonia (PCP), lymphoid interstitial pneumonitis atypical mycobacteria, esophageal or bronchopulmonary candidiasis, persistent diarrhea due to cryptosporidia, cryptococcal infections (excluding pulmonary cryptococcosis), toxoplasma pneumonia, or encephalitis beyond 28 days of age, disseminated cytomegalovirus (CMV) infection beyond 6 months of age, chronic ulceration due to herpes simplex virus (HSV) beyond 28 days of age, progressive multifocal leukoencephalopathy (PML), primary lymphoma of the brain, and Kaposi's sarcoma (KS). In order to use candidiasis as a criterion, serologic tests for HTLV-III must be positive. Although mothers at risk for AIDS may transmit a number of agents of congenital infection to their infants either antepartum or intrapartum, congenital infections are excluded from these sentinel diseases.

2. Known causes of underlying cellular immunodeficiency or reduced resistance that are associated with the sentinel disease must be excluded.

3. Primary immunodeficiency diseases of children must be excluded. These include severe combined immunodeficiency, DiGeorge syndrome, Wiskott-Aldrich syndrome, ataxia-telangectasia, graft-versus-host disease, neutropenia, neutrophil functional abnormality, agammaglobulinemia, and hypogammaglobulinemia with increased immunoglobulin M. (IgM).

4. Secondary immunodeficiency, associated with im-

munosuppressive therapy, lymphoreticular malignancy, or starvation also must be excluded.

## AIDS-RELATED COMPLEX

To be classified as having AIDS-related complex (ARC), the patient should have any two of the following clinical features: fever greater than 100° F for 3 months, weight loss of 10% total body weight or 15 pounds, lymphadenopathy for more than 3 months, diarrhea, fatigue, or night sweats. In addition, any two of the following laboratory tests should show an abnormality: helper T-cells less than $400/\mu L$, helper-suppressor ratio less than 1.0, leukothrombocytopenia, anemia, elevated serum globulins, depressed blastogenesis, or anergy to skin tests.

With the identification of the etiologic agent of AIDS, it has become possible to attribute recurrent bacterial infections and other clinical presentations to HIV. Recently the CDC have published a classification system that more closely parallels the clinical problem of HIV infection as it applies to children (10). HIV infection is considered established in children under 15 months of age if HIV is present in blood or tissue, or the case definition of AIDS (above) is met, or the child has antibody to HIV and evidence of humoral and cellular immunity and clinically apparent disease. Older children infected through any route are considered infected if virus or antiHIV antibody can be detected, or if they meet the case definition of AIDS (11) (see Appendix A).

The clinical appearance of children is divided into indeterminate status (P-0), and asymptomatic infection (P-1) with normal immune function (P-1-A), abnormal immune function (P-1-B), or immune function not tested (P-1-C). Symptomatic infection (P-2) is similarly divided into subclasses: nonspecific findings (P-2-A), progressive neurologic disease (P-2-B), lymphoid interstitial pneumonitis (P-2-C), secondary infectious diseases (P-2-D), secondary cancers (P-2-E), and other diseases possibly due to HIV infection (P-2-F). The subclass of secondary infectious diseases is subdivided further into those listed in the CDC surveillance definition for AIDS (D-1), recurrent serious bacterial infections (D-2), and other specified infectious diseases (D-3), such as persistent oral candidiasis or disseminated herpes zoster infection (10).

## PEDIATRIC RISK FACTORS

The principal risk for HIV infection in children is having a parent in a risk group: usually a drug-addicted mother or a mother who is a consort of a drug-addicted or bisexual father (15,34,35). Approximately 70% of cases are derived from this population (26). As in adults, children who require blood products also have developed AIDS (9,16,19,24,25,27,39); this risk factor accounts for approximately 20% of infected children. Adolescents account for the remaining 10% of infected children and appear to acquire HIV infection as a result of adult types of behavior, including sexual activity and i.v. drug use (14,36). One infant acquired AIDS from his mother while breast feeding (13), because the mother had been transfused with blood from an AIDS patient after the baby's delivery. Sexual abuse also has been responsible for transmission of HIV to children. The average incubation period for children with paternal risk factors only, from birth until presentation with symptomatic disease, is 1.7 years; however, we have seen infants of drug-addicted mothers with autoimmune thrombocytopenia in the newborn period, and children with latent infection for up to 7 years. Others have reported a mean of 29 months from birth to the development of AIDS (38). The incubation for symptomatic disease that results from postnatal exposure is difficult to assess because knowledge of contact with the virus is limited. In adults and children who have received transfusions, the incubation period appears to be approximately 2 years. However, an incubation period of 5 to 6 years following transfusions in patients under 6 years of age has been reported (25).

## CLINICAL FEATURES

The typical presentation of children with HIV-related disease includes, in the order of their frequency of occurrence, unexplained lymphadenopathy, hepatomegaly, splenomegaly, interstitial pneumonia, failure to thrive and/or weight loss, immune-mediated thrombocytopenia, chronic diarrhea, bacteremia, developmental delay or progressive neurologic deterioration, unexplained fever, low birthweight (in those with prenatal exposure), eczema, and parotitis. Many of these findings occur together. Others have reported similar findings although not necessarily in the same order (32,36,39). In older children, acquisition of HIV may be followed in approximately 6 weeks by a syndrome clinically resembling mononucleosis. In young infants, a nonspecific viral illness may occur in the first six weeks after exposure to the virus. KS, not uncommon in the adult, is very rare in children (7,30,38).

## LABORATORY DATA

Common abnormalities in laboratory parameters include unexplained anemias, hypergammaglobulinemia, or hypogammaglobulinemia, abnormal mononuclear cell functions, and an altered T lymphocyte subset ratio. Some children also are neutropenic. Ninety percent of HIV-infected children will have antiHIV antibody detectable by ELISA. Using a combination of serologic assays (including antigen determination) this can be raised to almost 100% (6).

## RADIOLOGIC MANIFESTATIONS

### Pulmonary

The majority of symptomatic pediatric patients recognized as having HIV infection suffer from acute or chronic chest disease, which causes a high morbidity and mortality. Acute lobar pneumonias due to encapsulated bacteria (such as the pneumococcus) are a common and recurring finding in those patients with lymphadenopathy. However, unlike adults (31), two very distinct clinical and radiographic entities of pulmonary infection are seen.

#### Pneumocystis Carinii Pneumonia

P. carinii pneumonia (PCP) tends to occur in children younger than 1 year of age, and rarely in the presence of other types of interstitial pneumonitis. The symptoms of PCP (cough and dyspnea) develop insidiously. In infants, this lung infection usually is associated with severe respiratory distress manifested by hypoxia and wheezing. Radiographically, early chest roentgenograms frequently are normal. Later in the course of the illness there is a fine interstitial perihilar infiltrate that progresses to a homogeneous granular pattern throughout the entire lung parenchyma. No hilar adenopathy or significant pleural effusions are observed. The infants who respond poorly to therapy develop respiratory distress syndrome (RDS) pattern with interstitial emphysematous changes, frequently complicated by pneumothorax and pneumomediastinum (Fig. 1). Because of the marked interstitial emphysema, the stiff lungs do not collapse in the presence of a pneumothorax. The disease responds slowly to therapy (trimethoprim—sulfameth-

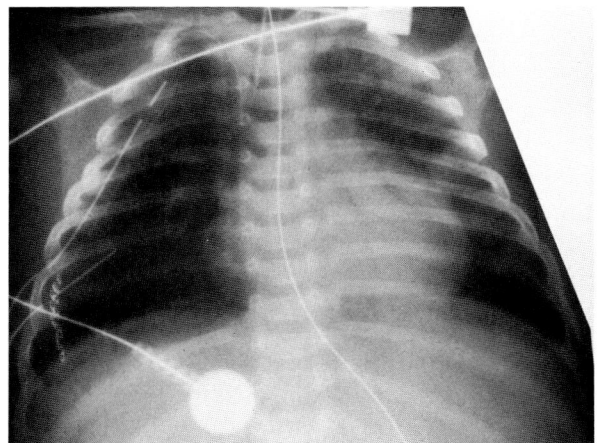
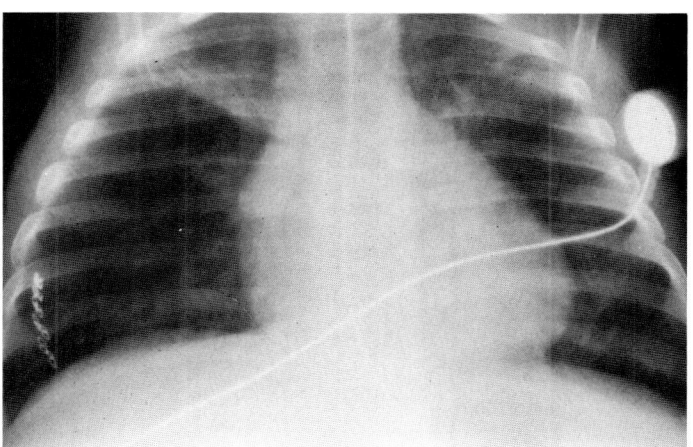
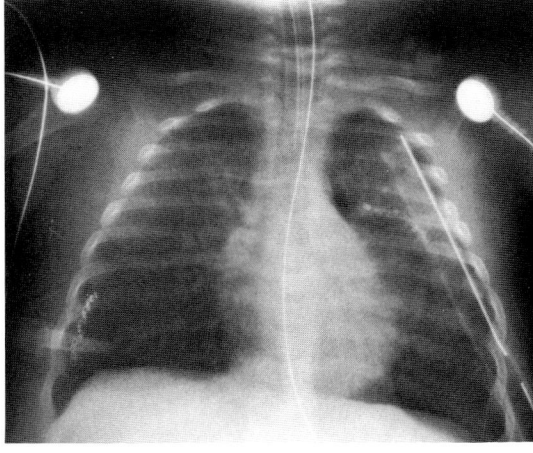
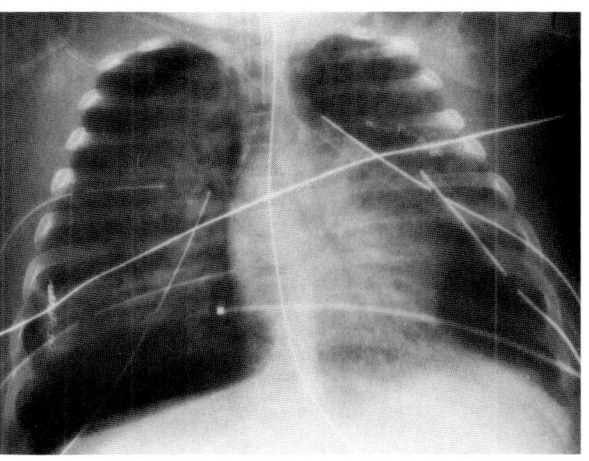

**FIG. 1.** Progression of PCP. **A:** Age 3 months. Chest film of a male infant, born of heterosexual parents, who experienced sudden onset of respiratory failure requiring high ventilatory pressure. Radiograph shows fine interstitial and alveolar densities. Air bronchogram in left lower lobe. Note two thoracotomy tubes *in situ* and biopsy clips at right base. **B:** Age 7 months. There are patchy alveolar infiltrates in both upper lobes with atelectasis on the right. Fine interstitial opacities persist. **C:** Age 8 months. Note progression of the interstitial and alveolar densities. A second lung biopsy (left-sided clips) was performed because of deteriorating respiratory status. The results were consistent with reinfection with P. carinii. A left-sided pneumothorax is evident, as is the thoracotomy tube. **D:** Age 9 months. Chest radiograph demonstrates stiff lungs and air block phenomena. Note five chest tubes *in situ*. Infant expired shortly thereafter.

oxazole or pentamidine). Clinical resolution requires 1 to 2 weeks while the roentgenographic changes remain for a much longer duration.

PCP is the most frequently encountered opportunistic pneumonia in pediatric AIDS. Approximately two thirds of the children who meet the CDC's case definition for AIDS do so as a result of biopsy-proven PCP. In PCP the number of organisms and inflammatory cells is variable, although in most cases the inflammation is minimal and consists of lymphocytes and plasma cells (21,22,37; see Figure 2, Chapter 3). In infants, infection with P. carinii carries a high mortality.

### Lymphocytic Interstitial Pneumonitis

In lymphocytic interstitial pneumonitis (LIP), the radiographs often are more impressive than the clinical signs and symptoms. The chest roentgenogram shows a diffuse reticulonodular infiltrate that usually becomes accentuated over time as the pneumonitis progresses; although this is not invariable, the findings may remain unchanged for long periods (Fig. 2). The mediastinum is widened and hilar adenopathy is present. The radiographic pattern resembles that seen in miliary tuberculosis, chronic interstitial pneumonitis, desquamative interstitial pneumonia (DIP), immunoblastic sarcoma, and bronchiolar-associated lymphoid tissue (BALT) (44). Opportunistic infections such as PCP do not develop in these patients.

This pneumonitis is chronic in nature and can significantly impair oxygen exchange, leading to chronic hypoxia and clubbing of the nail beds. Histologically, lymphocytes, plasma cells, and immunoblasts diffusely infiltrate the alveolar septa and peribronchiolar areas (Fig. 2F). Lymphoid nodules with and without germinal centers, and granulomalike collections of mononuclear and multinucleated giant cells may be present (21,22,37). Positive serologic testing for Epstein-Barr virus infection is a frequent concomitant finding in patients with LIP (37). Some investigators believe that LIP is secondary to a local response to antigenic stimulation (13).

In addition to these two clinical and radiologic entities the following pneumonias are seen.

### Cytomegalovirus Pneumonia

CMV pneumonia is an opportunistic infection in pediatric patients with AIDS. It can present insidiously or with the acute onset of respiratory failure. The radiographic pattern correlates with the clinical course (Fig. 3). An interstitial pattern is present in those patients with a more insidious onset, while a miliary pattern predominates in the acutely ill patients (5). These findings, however, are not specific and biopsy is required for diagnosis. Histologically, there is alveolar cell hyperplasia, interstitial edema, and inflammation (Fig. 3E). Large cells containing intranuclear and intracytoplasmic CMV inclusions are present (21,22).

### Mycobacterium Avium-Intracellulare

In the adult, infection with nontuberculous mycobacteria (NTMB), especially Mycobacterium avium-intracellulare (MAI), is a common complication of AIDS. MAI is found less frequently in children. The radiographic findings of alveolar or nodular infiltrates accompanied by adenopathy are nonspecific. Areas of collapse may be present (Fig. 4). Biopsy, bronchoscopic washings, or sputum are required for diagnosis. A positive culture may be obtained from the lung, even if the chest radiograph is negative; in such a case, the disease is assumed to be disseminated (28).

## Cardiac

Cardiac disease in children infected with HIV consists of cardiomyopathy and is estimated to occur in as many as 15% of these patients (20,41). Some of these children present with congestive heart failure amenable to the usual therapy. The etiology is not yet entirely clear, but it could be the direct result of the virus or of an opportunistic pathogen such as CMV. The cardiac complications also might result from the proliferation of lymphoid tissue in the pulmonary tree leading to increased pulmonary artery pressure and increased pulmonary vascular resistance. There is no distinctive roentgen constellation of findings: congestive heart failure and cardiomegaly are the most common abnormalities on chest radiographs. Echocardiograms reveal left ventricular hypertrophy with a decreased shortening fraction and an increased left ventricular diastolic volume. Occasionally a pericardial effusion is detected.

## Lymph Nodes

Due to the paucity of retroperitoneal fat in children, sonography is the preferred imaging method for assessing lymph node enlargement. The involved nodes usually are found in the periaortic, caval, mesenteric, and porta hepatis regions (Fig. 5). The nodes we have encountered have been uniformly hyperechoic, although hypoechoic nodes have been reported (3). This discrepancy may lie in the histological or infectious composition of the nodes (that is, lymphocytic proliferation, lymphoid depletion, or MAI).

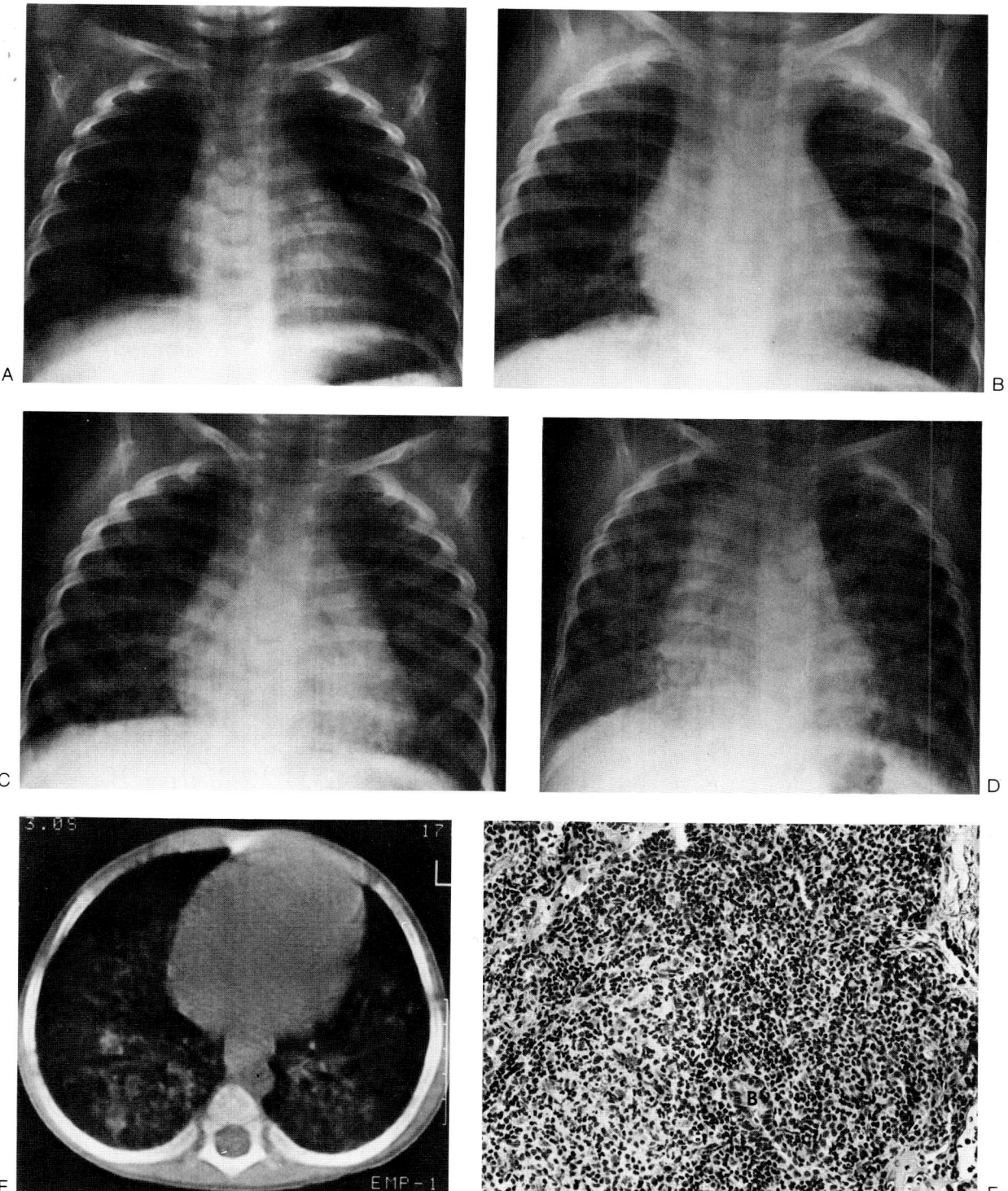

**FIG. 2.** Typical course of LIP. **A:** Age 7 months. Chest radiograph of an infant whose mother had several risk factors for HIV. The patient had unexplained fever; this initial roentgenogram is negative. **B:** Age 15 months. Generalized bilateral reticulonodular infiltrates are now present. **C:** Age 20 months. There is progression of the interstitial densities. **D:** Age 24 months. Chest roentgenogram demonstrates further progression of the interstitial findings. Chain lung sutures at right base indicate the site of lung biopsy. **E:** CT at age 24 months. A 10-mm section through the pulmonary bases depicts the interstitial nodular shadows well. **F:** Histologic section taken from the lung biopsy demonstrates a lymphoid interstitial infiltrate of the alveolar septa and peribronchiolar areas. B, bronchiole. (Hematoxylin and eosin stain, × 215.)

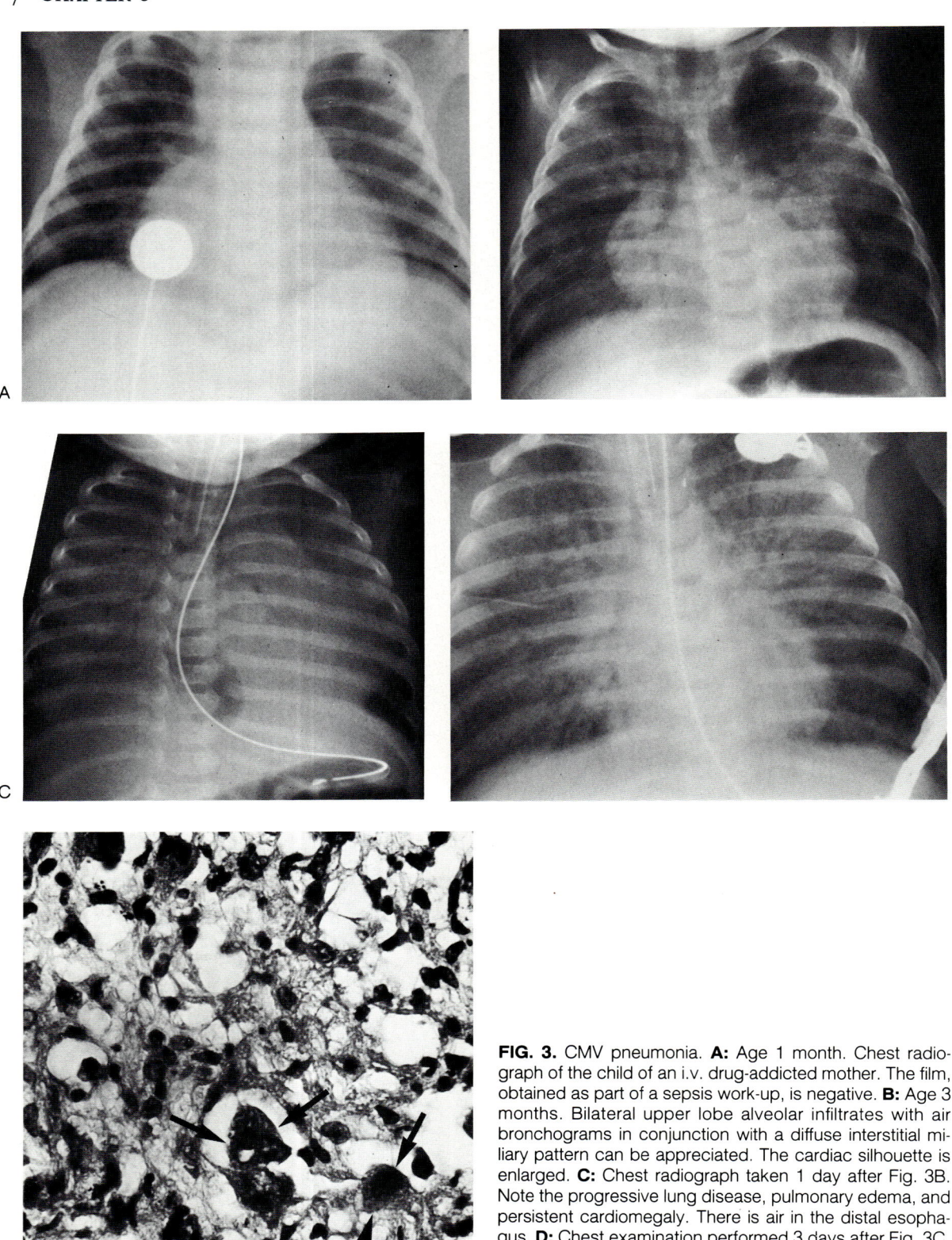

**FIG. 3.** CMV pneumonia. **A:** Age 1 month. Chest radiograph of the child of an i.v. drug-addicted mother. The film, obtained as part of a sepsis work-up, is negative. **B:** Age 3 months. Bilateral upper lobe alveolar infiltrates with air bronchograms in conjunction with a diffuse interstitial miliary pattern can be appreciated. The cardiac silhouette is enlarged. **C:** Chest radiograph taken 1 day after Fig. 3B. Note the progressive lung disease, pulmonary edema, and persistent cardiomegaly. There is air in the distal esophagus. **D:** Chest examination performed 3 days after Fig. 3C. Although better aeration has been achieved, there is persistent pulmonary edema and air bronchograms. **E:** Histologic section from postmortem lung specimen. The alveolar lining cells are enlarged and contain large intranuclear CMV inclusions (arrows). A concurrent bacterial pneumonia (P. aeruginosa) was also present. (Hematoxylin and eosin, × 672.)

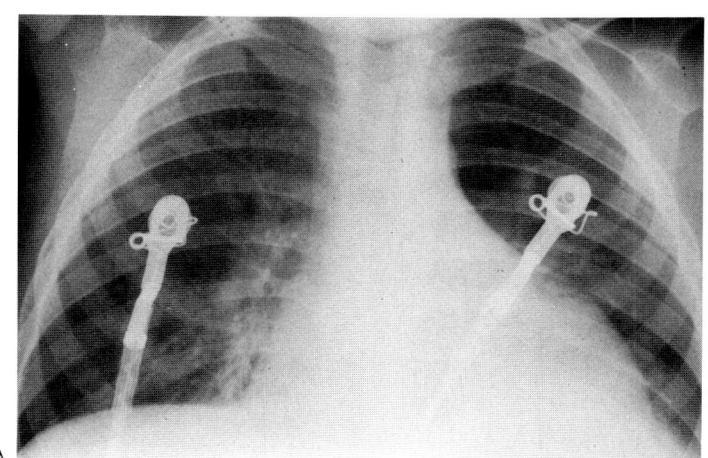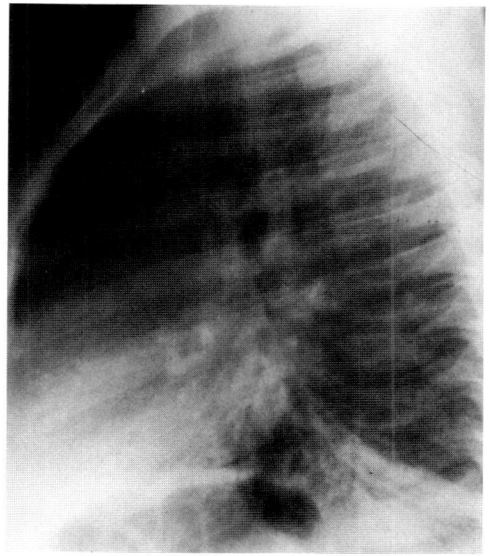

FIG. 4. MAI. **A, B:** Chest film of a 4-year-old boy demonstrates bilateral streaky densities with areas of atelectasis and air bronchograms at the lung bases. The diagnosis of MAI was made on positive blood cultures and confirmed at postmortem.

Lymphatic involvement in pediatric AIDS usually is generalized and on occasion may be the only manifestation of the disease, but is often accompanied by splenomegaly or other constitutional symptoms (1). To be indicative of HIV infection, lymphadenopathy must not be explainable by a coexisting infection and should be demonstrated in at least two noncontiguous sites for at least three months. Histologic examination of the nodes may show follicular hyperplasia with a normocellular or depleted paracortical zone or follicular atrophy with absence of germinal centers and lymphocytic depletion of the paracortical zone (Fig. 5B,C). Some degree of overlapping of these patterns may be seen. Additional findings are hyalinization of follicles and sinus histiocytosis. The germinal centers show transformed lymphoid cells, mitotic activity, macrophages, nuclear debris, and occasionally multinucleated giant cells. Around follicles, plasma cells and immunoblasts may be seen (21). Electron microscopic studies may show cylindrical-confronting cisternae and tuboloreticular inclusions in lymphocytes and endothelial cells (23) (Fig. 5D,E). MAI may be responsible for lymph node enlargement in pediatric AIDS, with microscopic examination revealing poorly formed granulomas or sheets of histocytes packed with mycobacteria.

### Hepatic

Chronic liver inflammation has occurred in 10% of pediatric AIDS patients. It is most common in the younger children and may be due to HIV, CMV, or MIA, or may include CMV as a cofactor. Chronic hepatic inflammation can lead to progressive liver failure with abnormal coagulation parameters resulting in bleeding abnormalities. Histologically, lymphocytes, plasma cells, immunoblasts, and histiocytes are seen in portal triads (21) (Fig. 6).

To date, sonography and computed tomography (CT) have not been helpful in detecting liver disease except for hepatic enlargement.

### Gastrointestinal

Although longstanding and debilitating diarrheal disease in children with HIV infection can result from the more typical bacterial gastrointestinal (GI) pathogens of childhood, opportunistic infections with coccidian parasites such as cryptosporidia and isospora, as well as mycobacterial infections with MAI, are characteristic (4). The course and pathogenesis of all diarrheal illness in this patient population have not been explained. The frequent histologic association of CMV suggests that this virus is also a cause of protracted diarrhea. One of our patients with severe diarrhea had an accompanying abdominal Burkitt's lymphoma (Fig. 7). The morphology of the GI mucosa usually is not diagnostic, although loss of mucosal integrity is common. Possibly this loss, coupled with deficient coagulation parameters, could be responsible for the massive upper and lower GI hemorrhages we have observed in some children. One of our patients showed multiple chronic ulcers in the segment of small bowel resected at the time of bleeding (Fig. 8). Electron microscopic studies of the intestinal epithelial cells showed viruslike particles as previously described (12) (Fig. 8D).

Fungal disease frequently presents as thrush; however,

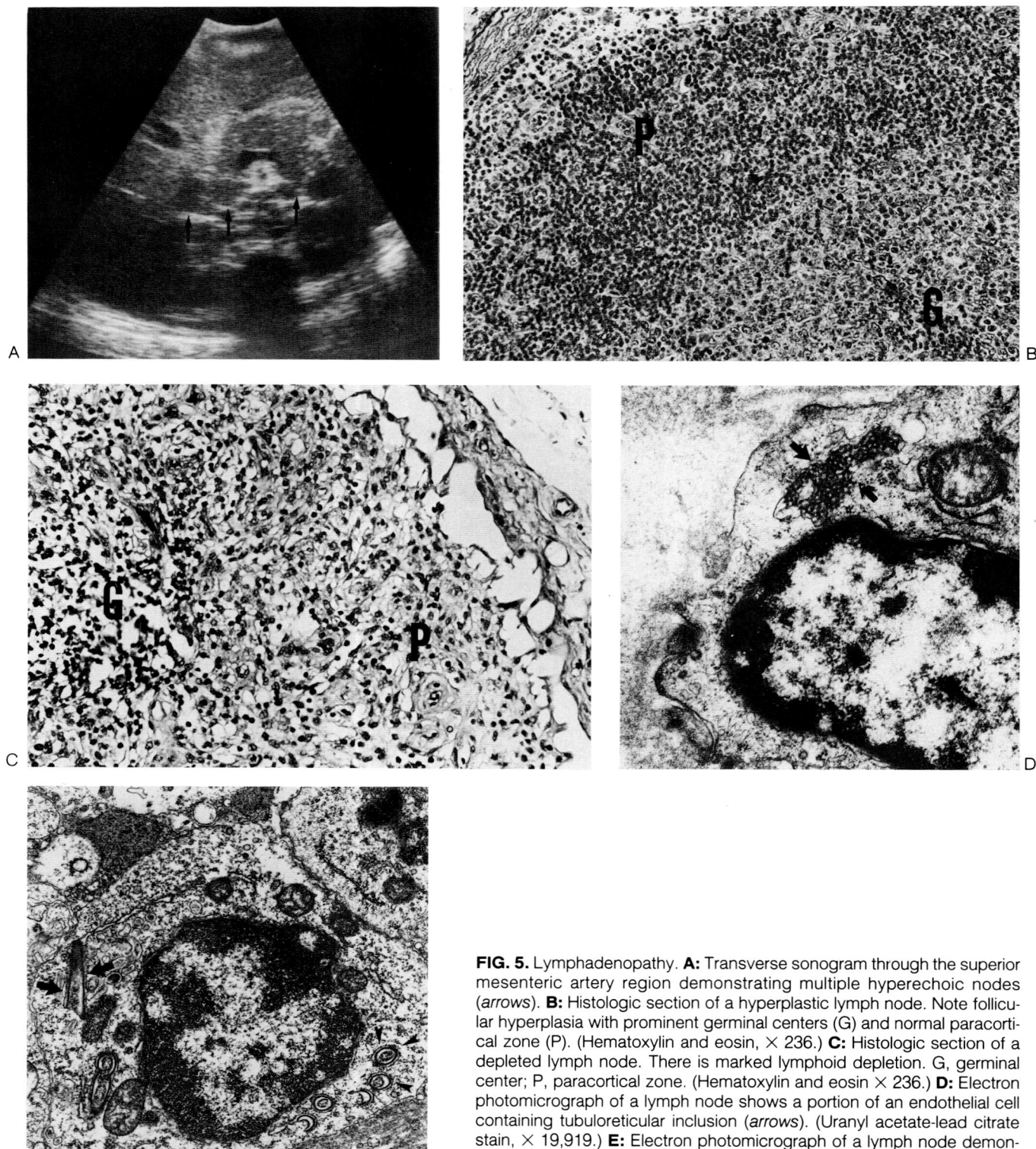

**FIG. 5.** Lymphadenopathy. **A:** Transverse sonogram through the superior mesenteric artery region demonstrating multiple hyperechoic nodes (*arrows*). **B:** Histologic section of a hyperplastic lymph node. Note follicular hyperplasia with prominent germinal centers (G) and normal paracortical zone (P). (Hematoxylin and eosin, × 236.) **C:** Histologic section of a depleted lymph node. There is marked lymphoid depletion. G, germinal center; P, paracortical zone. (Hematoxylin and eosin × 236.) **D:** Electron photomicrograph of a lymph node shows a portion of an endothelial cell containing tubuloreticular inclusion (*arrows*). (Uranyl acetate-lead citrate stain, × 19,919.) **E:** Electron photomicrograph of a lymph node demonstrates confronting cisternae. Note portion of a lymphocyte containing several longitudinal (*arrows*) and cross sections (*arrowheads*) of cylindrical confronting cisternae. (Uranyl acetate-lead citrate stain, × 11,344.)

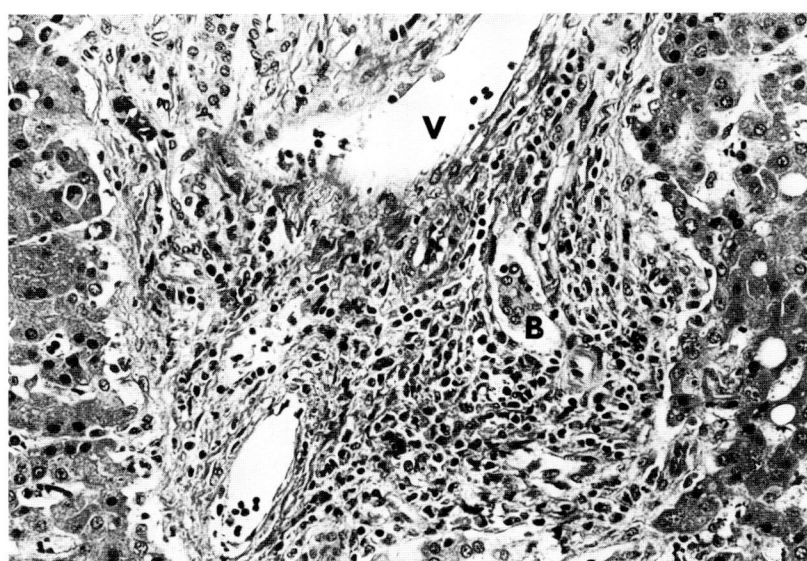

FIG. 6. Hepatic micropathology. Histologic specimen shows mild lymphohistiocytic cellular infiltrate in the portal triad. V, portal vein; B, bile duct. (Hematoxylin and eosin, × 258.)

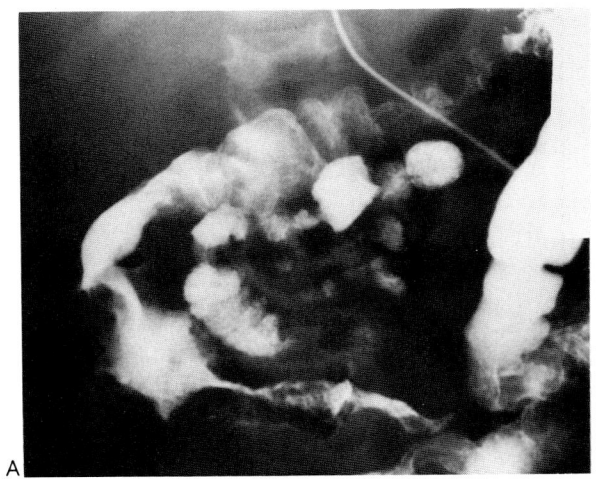
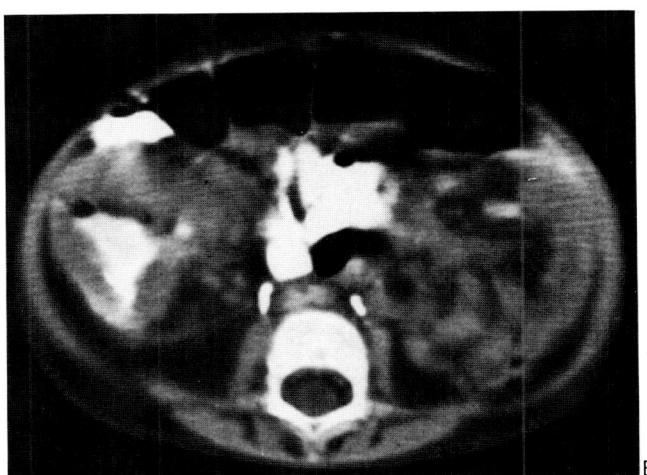
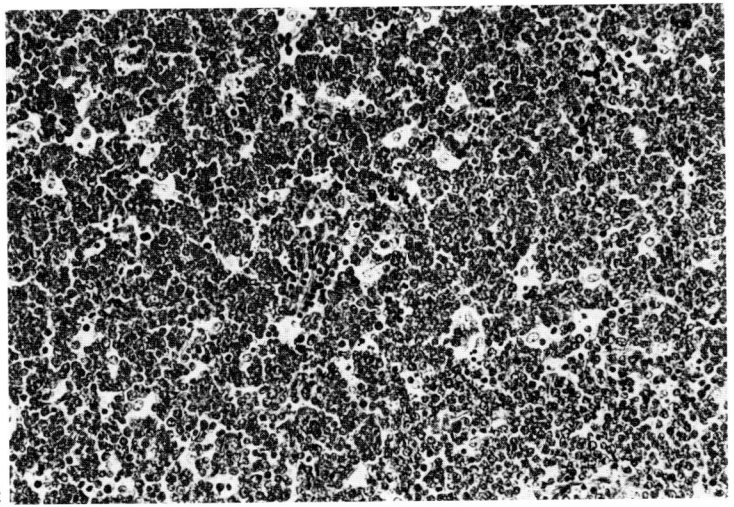

FIG. 7. Burkitt's lymphoma. A: Small bowel study of a 2-year-old boy with positive HIV serology, whose mother was addicted to i.v. drugs. There is destruction of the mucosa in the region of the terminal ileum and cecum, with associated ulceration (arrow) and mass effect. B: CT demonstrates thickening of the cecal wall and infiltration of the mesentery. C: Histologic section from surgical specimen of the terminal ileum. The lymphocytic infiltrates shows a typical "starry-sky" pattern seen in Burkitt's lymphoma. Hematoxylin and eosin, ×236.)

persistent candidal infection also results in esophagitis and enteritis. Among our patients, the diagnosis of candidal esophagitis has been an ominous finding, frequently heralding overwhelming disease due to opportunistic agents. A barium esophagram will demonstrate ulceration, fold thickening, and mucosal plaques (Fig. 9). Disseminated histoplasmosis has been reported in children although we have not observed any cases in our pediatric AIDS population. Cryptococcus, a frequent pathogen in adults, only rarely occurs in children.

Viral infections, especially herpes simplex virus (HSV) and CMV, can produce esophagitis but more commonly cause oral mucosal ulcerations. Herpes simplex stomatitis may recur with great frequency but rarely produces significant disease. In contrast, CMV is responsible for significant morbidity and mortality. In addition to its association with pneumonitis and hepatitis, it is also implicated in colitis. Severe or fatal varicella infection and recurrent zoster also have been documented in children.

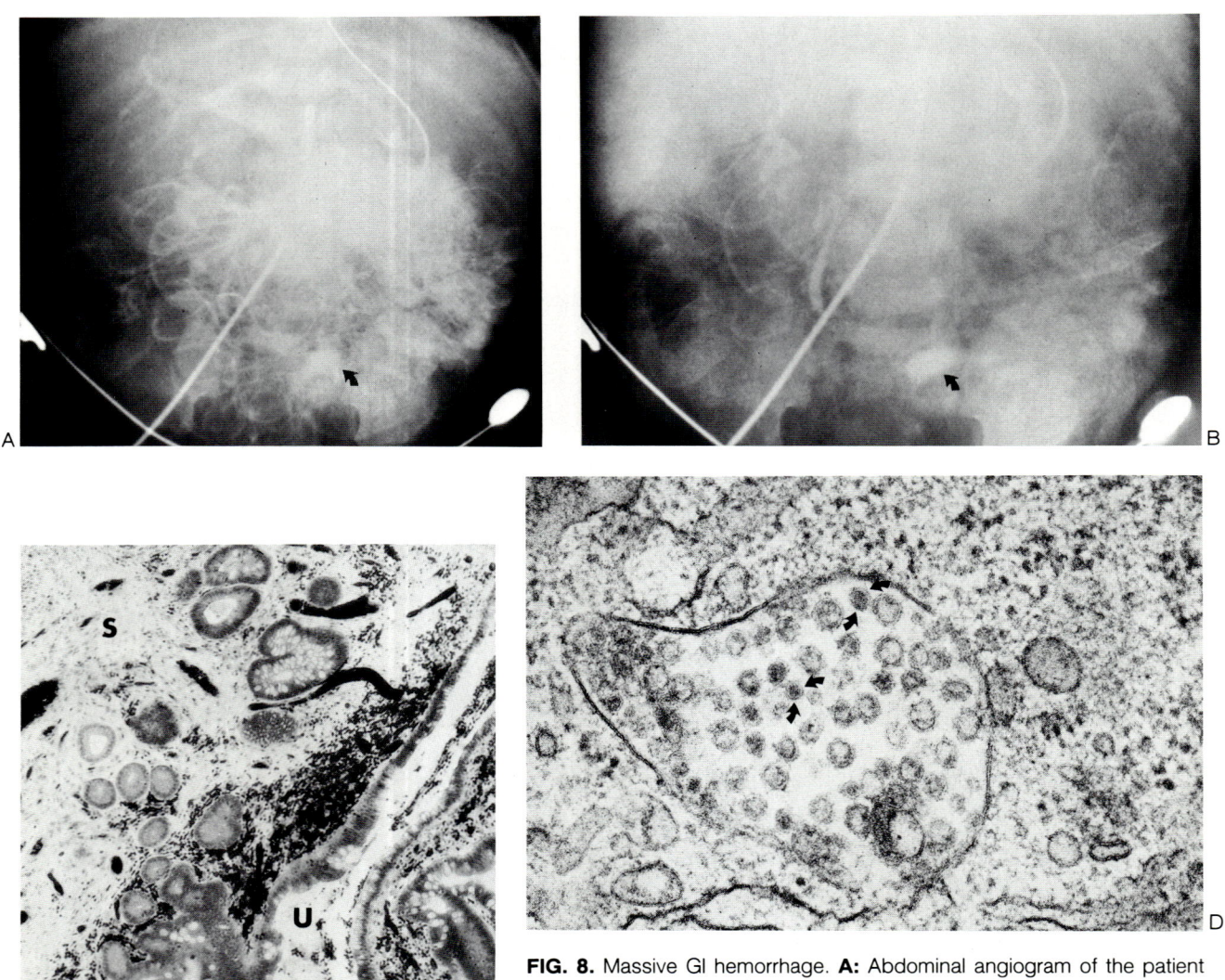

**FIG. 8.** Massive GI hemorrhage. **A:** Abdominal angiogram of the patient presented in Fig. 1, performed at a time when he had massive bright red blood per rectum. The study demonstrates pooling of contrast (*arrow*) overlying S1 in the region of the distal ileum. **B:** Delayed film from the same angiogram as shown in Fig. 7A. There is persistence of extravasated contrast in the same area (*arrow*). **C:** Histologic section from resected small bowel specimen shows a chronic ulcer (U) with reepithelialization. S, submucosa; B, ulcer bottom. (Hematoxylin and eosin, × 96.) **D:** Electron photomicrograph from the same surgical specimen demonstrates viruslike particles (*arrows*) contained within a portion of an intestinal epithelial cell (Uranyl acetate lead-citrate stain, × 70,125.)

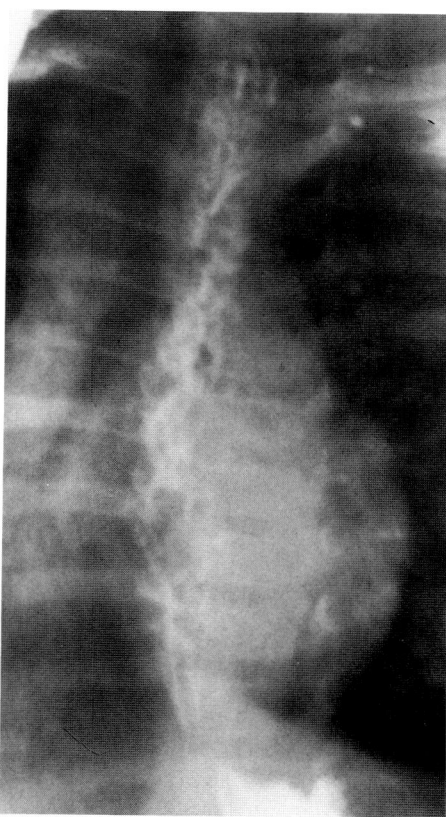

**FIG. 9.** Candidiasis. Esophagram of a 4-month-old infant with AIDS. There is marked mucosal fold thickening and ulceration.

### Recurrent Infections

More than 60% of children with symptomatic HIV infection suffer from recurring and/or chronic infections. Bacterial disease is common and presents as sepsis, pneumonia, urinary tract infection, meningitis, bone and joint infection, sinusitis, and otitis media. The organisms causing disease are commonly the pneumococcus, Haemophilus influenzae type B, enterococcus, both typical and atypical mycobacterial species, and gram-negative enteric bacilli, such as E. coli, Klebsiella, and Salmonella species. Pseudomonas auruginosa has complicated the terminal stages of illness in some of our patients. Nearly all our patients had otitis media and a large number had clinically significant sinusitis. In our experience, CT has been helpful in assessment of chronic sinusitis in young infants.

### Neurologic

Unlike adult patients with AIDS who frequently become superinfected with opportunistic pathogens such as toxoplasma, central nervous system disease in children with AIDS is often protracted and related to direct invasion of neural tissue by the HIV virus (8,43). HIV appears to have an extraordinary tropism for neural tissue (17,18). This tissue tropism results in encephalopathy in at least 10% of patients with clinical illness, and may occur in as many as 50%. HIV has been isolated from cerebrospinal fluid (CSF), and local production of antibody has been demonstrated. The virus appears to be located predominantly in multinucleated giant cells that are composed of macrophages (23). Common clinical features include arrest in or loss of developmental milestones, and generalized weakness, with lower extremities more commonly involved than upper extremities, truncal ataxia, pyramidal signs, secondary microcephaly, and rarely generalized seizures. The encephalopathy is progressive and may precede other manifestations of the disease. Routine CSF examination usually is normal or shows only mild elevations of protein. Other invasive viral infections also have been described, for example the progressive multifocal leukoencephalopathy, a slow viral subacute demyelinating disease, that is due to the SV 40-polyoma subgroup of slow viruses. CT scans may show cortical atrophy and occasionally, calcifications in the basal ganglia. Magnetic resonance imaging may identify alterations in basal ganglia relaxation parameters prior to the process of calcification. These findings are discussed in greater detail in Chapter 2.

### Dysmorphic Features

A characteristic pattern of dysmorphic features has been described in children affected with HIV (29). In addition to growth retardation, these include craniofacial abnormalities consisting of microcephaly, hypertelorism, high forehead, flattened nasal bridge, patulous lips, and a triangular philtrum. It has been suggested by Marion et al. that there is an inverse correlation between the severity of dysmorphia and the length of the incubation period. Other investigators have been unable to support this observation (40).

### REFERENCES

1. Abiri, M., Kirpekar, M., and Abiri, S. (1986): Role of ultrasound in detection of extrapulmonary TB in patients with AIDS. *J. Ultrasound Med.*, 4:471–473.
2. American Academy of Pediatrics Newsletter, May 1986.
3. Amodio, J., Abramson, S., Berdon, W., and Levy, J. (1987): Pediatric AIDS. *Semin. Roentgenol.*, 22:66–76.
4. Berkowitz, C. D., and Seidell, J. S. (1985): Spontaneous resolution of cryptosporidiosis in children with acquired immunodeficiency syndrome. *Am. J. Dis. Child.*, 139:967–969.
5. Beschorner, W., Hutchins, G., Burns, W., Saral, R., Tutschka, P., and Santos, G. (1980): Cytomegalovirus pneumonia in bone marrow transplant recipients: Miliary and diffuse patterns. *Am. Rev. Respir. Dis.*, 122:107–114.
6. Borkowsky, W., Krasinski, K., Paul, C., Moore, T., Beneroth, D., and Chandwani, S. (1988): Human immunodeficiency virus infections in infants negative for anti-HIV G enzyme linked immunoassay. *Lancet* (in press).
7. Buck, B. E., Scott, G. B., Valdes-Dapena, M., and Parks, W. P.

(1983): Kaposi sarcoma in two infants with acquired immune deficiency syndrome. *J. Pediatr.,* 103:911–913.
8. Bursztyn, E., Lee, B., and Bauman, J. (1984): CT of acquired immune deficiency syndrome. *Am. J. Neuroradiol.,* 5:711–714.
9. Centers for Disease Control (1983): Acquired immune deficiency syndrome in patients with hemophilia. *M.M.W.R.,* 32:613–616.
10. Centers for Disease Control (1987): Classification system for human immunodeficiency virus (HIV) infection in children under 13 years of age. *M.M.W.R.,* 36:225–235.
11. Center for Infectious Diseases: Revision of the CDC surveillance case definition for acquired immunodeficiency syndrome. *M.M.W.R.,* 36:35–145.
12. Chandler, F. W., White, E. H., Callaway, C. S., Spira, T. J., and Ewing, E. P., Jr. (1984): Unidentified virus-like particles in the intestine of patients with the acquired immune deficiency syndrome. *Ann. Intern. Med.,* 100:851–853.
13. Church, J. A., Isaacs, H., Saxon, A., Keens, T., and Richards, W., (1981): Lymphoid interstitial pneumonitis and hypogammaglobulinemia in children. *Am. Rev. Respir. Dis.,* 124:491–496.
14. Church, J. A., Allen, J. R., and Stiehm, E. R. (1986): New scarlet letter(s). Pediatric AIDS. *Pediatrics,* 77:423–428.
15. Cowan, M. J., Hellman, D., Chudwin, D., Wara, D. W., Chang, R. S., and Ammann, A. J. (1984): Maternal transmission of acquired immune deficiency syndrome. *Pediatrics,* 73:382–386.
16. Curran, J. W., Lawrence D. N., Jaffee H., et al. (1984): Acquired immune deficiency syndrome (AIDS) associated with transfusions. *N. Engl. J. Med.,* 310:69–75.
17. Elkin, C. M., Leon, E., Grenell S. L., and Leeds, N. E. (1985): Intracranial lesions in the acquired immune deficiency syndrome. *J.A.M.A.,* 253:393–396.
18. Epstein, L., Sharer, L., Connor, E., Goudsmit, S., and Oleske J. (1986): Persistent LAV/HTLV-III infection of brain in children with AIDS and AIDS-Related Complex (ARC). International Conference on AIDS, June 23–25, 1986, Paris, France.
19. Gill, J. C., Menitove, J. E., Wheeler, D., Aster, R. H., and Montgomery, R. R. (1983): Generalized lymphadenopathy and T-cell abnormalities in hemophilia A. *J. Pediatr.,* 103:18–22.
20. Issenberg, H., Charytan, M., and Rubinstein, A. (1985): Cardiac involvement in children with acquired immune deficiency syndrome. *Am. Heart J.,* 110:710.
21. Joshi, V. V., Oleske, J. M., Minnefor, A. B., Singh, R., Bokhari, T., and Rapkin, R. H. (1984): Pathology of suspected acquired immune deficiency syndrome in children. *Pediatr. Pathol.,* 2:71–87.
22. Joshi, V. V., Oleske, J. M., Minnefor, A. B., et al. (1985): Pathologic pulmonary findings in children with the acquired immune deficiency syndrome: A study of ten cases. *Hum. Pathol.,* 16:241–246.
23. Kostianovsky, M., Orenstein, J. M., Schaff, Z. A., and Grimley, P. M. (1987): Cytomembranous inclusions observed in acquired immune deficiency syndrome. *Arch. Pathol. Lab. Med.,* 111:218–223.
24. Landay, A., Poon, M. C., Abo, T., Stagno, S., Lurie, A., and Cooper, M. D. (1983): Immunologic studies in asymptomatic hemophilia patients: Relationship to acquired immune deficiency syndrome (AIDS). *J. Clin. Invest.,* 71:1500–1515.
25. Lawrence, D. N., Lui, K. J., Peterman, T. A., Jaffee, H. W., Jason, J. M., and Allen, J. R. (1986): Characteristics of incubation periods (IP) in pediatric cases of transfusion-associated acquired immune deficiency syndrome (TA-AIDS). Second International Conference on AIDS, 20;58A:33.
26. Lawrence, R., Krasinski, K., LaRussa, P., Flug, F., and Borkowsky, W. (1986): Presentations of HTLV-III infections in children. *Pediatr. Res.,* 20;937(Abstr.):314A.
27. Lederman, M. M., Ratnoff, O. D., Scillian, J. J., Jones, P. K., and Schacter, B. (1983): Impaired cell-mediated immunity in patients with classic hemophilia. *N. Engl. J. Med.,* 308:79–80.
28. Marinelli, D., Albeda, S., Williams, T., Kern, J., Iozzo, R., and Miller, W. (1986): Nontuberculous mycobacterial infection in AIDS: Clinical, pathologic, and radiographic features. *Radiology,* 160:77–82.
29. Marion, R., Wiznia, A., Hutcheon, G., and Rubinstein, A. (1987): Fetal AIDS syndrome score. *Am. J. Dis. Child.,* 141:429–431.
30. McCauley, D., Naidich, D., Leitman, B., Reede, D., and Laubenstein, L. (1982): Radiographic patterns of opportunistic lung infections and Kaposi sarcoma in homosexual men. *Am. J. Roentgenol.,* 139:653–658.
31. Naidich D., Garay S., Leitman B., and McCauley D. (1987): Radiographic manifestations of pulmonary disease in the acquired immune deficiency syndrome (AIDS). *Semin. Roentgenol.,* 22:14–30.
32. Oleske, J., Minnefor, A., Cooper, R., Jr., et al. (1983): Immune deficiency syndrome in children. *J.A.M.A.,* 249:2345–2349.
33. Centers for Disease Control (1985): Revision of the case definition of AIDS for national reporting. United States. *M.M.W.R.,* 32:691.
34. Rubinstein, A., Sicklick, M., Gupta, A., et al. (1983): Acquired immunodeficiency with reversed T4/T8 ratios in infants born to promiscuous and drug-addicted mothers. *J.A.M.A.,* 249:2350–2356.
35. Rubinstein, A. (1983): Acquired immunodeficiency syndrome in infants. *Am. J. Dis. Child.,* 137:825–827.
36. Rubinstein, A. (1986): Pediatric AIDS. *Curr. Prob. Pediatr.,* 7:361–409.
37. Rubinstein, A., Morecki, R., Silverman, B., et al. (1986): Pulmonary disease in children with acquired immune deficiency syndrome and AIDS-related complex. *J. Pediatr.,* 108:498–503.
38. Scott, G. B., Buck, B. E., Letterman, J. G., Bloom, F. L., and Parks, W. P. (1984): Acquired immunodeficiency syndrome in infants. *N. Engl. J. Med.,* 310:76–81.
39. Shannon, K. M., and Ammann, A. J. (1985): Acquired immune deficiency syndrome in childhood. *J. Pediatr.,* 106:332–341.
40. Sheikh, T. M., Qazi, Q. H., Fikrig, S., and Menikoff, H. (1987): Lack of evidence for cranial facial dysmorphism in children with AIDS. *Pediatr. Res.,* 21(Abstr.):230A.
41. Sherron, P., Pickoff, A. S., Ferrer, P. L., and Scott, G. B. (1985): Echocardiographic evaluation of myocardial function in pediatric AIDS patients. *Am. Heart J.,* 110:710.
42. Centers for Disease Control Update (1984): Acquired immunodeficiency syndrome. United States. *M.M.W.R.,* 32:691.
43. Whelan, M., Kricheff, I. I., Handler, M., et al. (1983): Acquired immunodeficiency syndrome: Computed tomographic manifestations. *Radiology,* 149:477–484.
44. Zimmerman, B. L., Haller, J. O., Price, A. P., Thelmo, W. L., and Fikrig, S. (1987): Children with AIDS—Is pathologic diagnosis possible based on chest radiographs? *Pediatr. Radiol.,* 17:303–307.

CHAPTER 7

# Handling AIDS Patients in the Radiology Department

Mary Anne G. Johnson

The high mortality of acquired immunodeficiency syndrome (AIDS) and its potential for transmission within the health care setting have precipitated a close reevaluation of infection control practices. Precautions for use with AIDS patients are precisely those precautions that should be practiced in all clinical situations (1,2); however, until the AIDS epidemic, adherence to good infection control practices frequently was lacking. In the Radiology Department, as throughout the hospital, infection control education about modes of disease transmission and means of preventing such transmission are of utmost importance.

## RISK IN THE HEALTH CARE SYSTEM

The human immunodeficiency virus (HIV) has been isolated from most body fluids. Semen, blood, cervical secretions, and, possibly, breast milk have all been implicated in disease transmission (3–7). Urine, tears, saliva, sweat, and cerebrospinal fluid (CSF), although found to contain HIV, have never been clearly linked to disease transmission (4,8–10); this lack of transmission may be related to the low concentrations of virus in most of these fluids (CSF concentrations are high but exposure to CSF is unlikely to occur in most settings).

Like hepatitis B infections, HIV infection is transmitted in three ways: parenterally, sexually, and perinatally (3). Multiple studies of close, nonsexual contacts of patients with AIDS have failed to show transmission of the disease in the home or institutional setting (11–14). In the health care setting, transmission of HIV potentially can occur from needlestick injuries or contamination of mucous membranes or open skin lesions by HIV-infected body fluids (15–17). Several large studies of health care workers have documented only rare transmission of HIV by these routes. The results of these studies indicate that the risk of acquiring HIV infection is less than 1% following a percutaneous exposure (18–23). This is in contrast to the risk of acquiring hepatitis B infection, which may be as high as 20%, following a needlestick injury from a patient with hepatitis B (24), and probably relates to the lower concentrations of HIV as compared with hepatitis B virus in the serum of infected individuals.

## BODY FLUID PRECAUTIONS

Not all patients with HIV infection, AIDS, or other blood-borne diseases are diagnosed before radiologic examination; therefore, all patients seen in the department should be assumed to have an infectious agent in their body fluids (2,18). Using special precautions for known AIDS patients or for those patients who are perceived to be in high-risk groups, and not using precautions for those perceived to be in low-risk groups is potentially dangerous and may be perceived as discriminatory. On the other hand, using body fluid precautions for all patients eliminates the need for judgment about whether patients are in high-risk groups, ensures confidentiality of patient diagnosis, and provides protection against all blood-borne infections that may be present in the general hospital population. In addition, a uniform application of infection control precautions for all patients is easier for staff to remember and to follow than an isolation system (disease-specific) that varies depending on patient diagnosis.

The intact skin of the health care worker provides the best defense against infection with nosocomial pathogens. If the skin unexpectedly becomes exposed to any patient's body fluid, the skin should be washed immediately with soap and water. Gloves should be worn for touching blood and body fluids, mucous membranes, or nonintact skin of all patients, and for performing venipuncture and other vascular access procedures. Gloves may not provide complete protection because of tears or defects; therefore, even if gloves have been worn, hands should be thoroughly washed after gloves are removed. Nonintact skin of health care workers may serve as a portal for the entrance of infectious agents. Any health care worker with nonintact skin should wear gloves when providing direct patient care.

When procedures are being done where splatter of body fluids is expected (e.g., invasive procedures or angiography) the mucous membranes, hands, and clothing of the health care worker should be protected by the use of masks, goggles, water-impermeable gowns, and gloves (25). For the protection of patients, staff with exudative skin lesions should not perform invasive procedures.

Needles and other sharp instruments should be disposed of close to the area of use; puncture-resistant needle boxes must be replaced frequently so that injuries from overfilling are avoided. Needles should not be left on guerneys or tables or placed in waste containers. To prevent needlestick injuries, needles should not be recapped, purposely bent or broken by hand, removed from disposable syringes, or otherwise manipulated by hand. Reusable procedure needles must be placed in puncture-resistant containers for transport for cleaning and sterilization. Such large needles should not be wrapped in the procedure tray, since cleaning personnel may suffer injuries while unwrapping the tray.

## HANDLING OF SPECIMENS

Fluids or biopsy specimens obtained from all patients in the Radiology Department should be handled as potentially infectious materials. Such specimens and their containers should be placed in impervious plastic bags for transport to the laboratory (18). Laboratory requisitions should be attached to the outside of the plastic bag.

## ENVIRONMENTAL CLEANING

Thorough cleaning of procedure rooms should occur after any procedures where splatter of body substances may have occurred. Adequate cleaning techniques after each patient eliminates the need to perform special cleaning after procedures on AIDS patients or to schedule AIDS patients at the end of the day.

Surfaces that become contaminated with body substances from any patient should be thoroughly cleaned with a detergent solution and then disinfected. Large spills of body fluids should first be mopped up by a gloved employee using disposable towels; the contaminated area should then be disinfected. Any disinfectant used on surfaces should be an approved mycobactericidal product. Since mycobacteria are quite resistant to chemicals, agents that are capable of killing mycobacteria will also inactivate most other organisms, including viruses (1,18). A freshly prepared 1:10 dilution of household bleach (sodium hypochlorite) is an effective disinfectant. Other routinely used hospital disinfectants such as phenolic compounds also are effective in inactivating HIV and other organisms (27,28). Commercially available chemical germicides may be more compatible with certain medical devices, such as the stainless steel components of x-ray equipment, that might be corroded by repeated exposure to bleach (25).

## WASTE, LINENS, MATERIALS, AND EQUIPMENT

All infectious waste (e.g., paper towels used to clean up a spill or drapes used during invasive procedures) should be disposed of in infectious waste containers. Linens that become contaminated with body fluids from any patient should be treated as infectious; transporting and laundering should follow hospital procedure for infectious linen, including the use of a hot water-soluble bag. Soiled linen should be handled as little as possible and should be bagged at the location where it was used; it should not be sorted or rinsed in patient care areas.

All reusable instruments must be cleaned and sterilized in the same way after use on any patient (18). Physical cleaning with detergent and water, using a brush if necessary, is extremely important in removing body fluids. Sterilization may be ineffective if large amounts of organic materials are present. Any employee who is cleaning instruments should wear heavy gloves and provide protection for mucous membranes and clothing. After cleaning, instruments that are used to enter normally sterile body spaces, such as the vascular system or internal organs, must be sterilized. Heat, steam, ethylene oxide, or 10 hours of immersion in activated glutaraldehyde are all effective sterilants. Instruments that enter nonsterile areas, such as the gastrointestinal tract, should be sterilized if possible or should receive high-level disinfection with an agent such as activated glutaraldehyde for 45 minutes (29).

## SPECIAL INFECTION CONTROL PROCEDURES

There are no data to suggest the transmission of HIV itself by the respiratory route. Therefore, masks are not routinely needed when patients with AIDS or HIV positivity are seen in the department. However, some patients with AIDS are infected with other agents such as Mycobacterium tuberculosis or varicella zoster, for which mask precautions are indicated.

Patients with diagnosed or suspected tuberculosis (TB) should be on respiratory precautions. Such patients should not be transported to the Radiology Department unless absolutely indicated. When such patients require procedures in the department, the patients must wear masks during transport and during all procedures. It is not necessary for transport personnel or radiology personnel to wear masks when the patient is masked.

For patients with disseminated varicella zoster infections, the risk of exposing nonimmune hospital staff, visitors, and other patients is significant if the infected patient is transported. Therefore, every effort should be made to avoid procedures that must be done in the department. If transport to the department is required, the patient must wear a mask at all times. Gowns and gloves must be worn by all staff who have direct contact with the patient. Staff with no history of chicken pox should not perform procedures on patients with varicella zoster infections.

## PORTABLE RADIOLOGIC PROCEDURES

When portable x-rays are taken of a patient, the radiology technician should follow standard procedures for prevention of exposure to body fluids. This includes wearing gloves if exposure to body fluids or skin lesions is likely and handwashing after patient contact, even when gloves have been worn. When contact with open skin lesions or body fluids is expected, the x-ray cassette should be covered with a sheet or pillowcase that should be placed in the infectious linen hamper after use. A nonpermeable plastic disposable cover for the cassette would be preferred, but is not yet commercially available. Masks should be worn when the patient is on respiratory precautions and indicated by a sign outside the patient's door. Masks are required if the patient has active pulmonary TB or if TB has not yet been excluded in a patient with pulmonary symptoms. If a patient has varicella zoster infection, radiology staff with no history of chicken pox should not enter the patient's room.

### Special Concerns

1. Needlestick injuries and mucous membrane splashes from body fluids are potential risks to the radiology staff. The major risk from such exposures is hepatitis B. Staff who suffer exposures should receive appropriate prophylaxis against hepatitis B. There is no risk of acquiring HIV infection from the immunoglobulins or hepatitis B vaccine that are used for postexposure prophylaxis (30,31).

Although the Centers for Disease Control (CDC; 18,25) recommend routine serial HIV antibody testing for health care workers with parenteral exposures to HIV-infected substances, such an approach overemphasizes the risk, which is extremely low. Health care workers who have experienced significant exposures to HIV should receive support and counseling, including a discussion of the actual risk involved. Serial HIV antibody testing can be offered to the exposed individual on a voluntary basis.

2. Cardiopulmonary resuscitation (CPR) may be required in the Radiology Department. Because mouth-to-mouth resuscitation in hospital patients potentially exposes the rescuer to a variety of pathogens, ventilation devices should be available in all rooms where cardiac or respiratory arrest could occur. Staff should receive training in the use of such devices as part of their annual CPR training (18,32).

3. Some authorities, including the CDC, feel that pregnant women can provide direct care to AIDS patients as long as appropriate precautions are followed (18,25). However, because of the potential risk from cytomegalovirus (which is common in AIDS patients) and HIV infection (which may be more virulent during pregnancy), pregnant employees in the Radiology Department may be excused from performing procedures on patients with AIDS or AIDS-related conditions when exposure to body fluids may occur (29,33). Because many patients who are HIV-seropositive will not be identified at the time of their radiology procedures, pregnant women should be particularly careful to follow body fluid precautions for all patients.

4. There are no documented cases of HIV transmission from a health care worker to a patient. Radiology employees who have AIDS but are asymptomatic, or who are HIV-seropositive can continue to perform their regular duties. If symptoms are present, HIV-positive employees should refrain from direct patient contact until a potentially transmissible infection has been excluded.

## SUMMARY

Using standard infection precautions in all situations where exposure to body substances may occur will protect health care workers from HIV as well as other agents commonly found in body fluids (Table 1). The CDC's recommended (25) "universal blood and body fluid precautions" should be used in the care of all patients, especially including those in emergency care settings in which the risk of blood exposure is increased and the infection status of the patient is usually unknown.

Handwashing remains the most effective protective mechanism and should be used routinely after contact with any patient or body substance. Gloves should be worn for any anticipated exposure to body fluids. Gloves, gowns, goggles, and masks should be used to protect skin, clothing, and mucous membranes when splatter of body fluids is expected, as during invasive procedures. Masks are indicated when a patient has TB or an undiagnosed pulmonary process where TB is a possibility. Extreme care should be used in the handling of needles and other sharp instruments. All patient specimens should be placed in plastic bags for transport.

**TABLE 1.** *Summary of precautions for all patient contact*

1. Use body fluid precautions
   Handwashing
   Gloves, if body fluid contact likely
   Masks, goggles if splatter expected
   Gowns, if splatter expected
   Additional precautions if indicated
2. Avoid needlestick injuries and mucous membrane splashes
3. Contain all patient specimens in plastic bags for transport
4. Physically clean all instruments before sterilizing
5. Sterilize all instruments between patients
6. Use approved hospital disinfectants for environmental surfaces
7. Handle as infectious waste all disposables that are contaminated with body fluids
8. Handle as infectious linen all linen that is contaminated with body fluids

Usual hospital disinfection and sterilization procedures are effective in inactivating HIV as well as other infectious agents.

## REFERENCES

1. Garner, J. S., and Favero, M. S. (1985): *Guideline For Handwashing and Hospital Environmental Control.* Centers for Disease Control. Publication no. PB85-923404, Atlanta, Georgia.
2. Gerberding, J. L., and the University of California, San Francisco Task Force on AIDS. (1986): Recommended infection control policies for patients with human immunodeficiency virus infection: An update. *N. Engl. J. Med.,* 315:1562–1564.
3. Centers for Disease Control. Update (1986): Acquired immunodeficiency syndrome. United States. *M.M.W.R.,* 35:757–766.
4. Levy, J. A., Kaminsky, L. S., Morrow, W. J. W., et al. (1987): Infection by the retrovirus associated with the acquired immunodeficiency syndrome: Clinical, biological, and molecular features. *Ann. Intern. Med.,* 155:54–63.
5. Redfield, R. R., Markham, P. D., Salahuddin, S. Z., et al. (1985): Heterosexually acquired HTLV III/LAV disease (AIDS-related complex and AIDS). *J.A.M.A.,* 254:2094–2096.
6. Vogt, M. W., Witt, D. J., Craven, D. E., et al. (1987): Isolation patterns of the human immunodeficiency virus from cervical secretions during the menstrual cycle of women at risk for the acquired immunodeficiency syndrome. *Ann. Intern. Med.,* 106:380–382.
7. Ziegler, J. B., Cooper, D. A., Johnson, R. O., and Gold, J. (1985): Postnatal transmission of AIDS-associated retrovirus from mother to infant. *Lancet,* 1:896–897.
8. Fujikawa, L. S., Salahuddin, S. Z., Palestine, et al. (1985): Isolation of human T-lymphotropic virus type III from the tears of a patient with the acquired immunodeficiency syndrome. *Lancet,* 2:529–530.
9. Groopman, J. E., Salahuddin, S. Z., Sarngadharan, M. G., et al. (1984): HTLV-III in saliva of people with AIDS-related complex and healthy homosexual men at risk for AIDS. *Science,* 226:447–449.
10. Ho, D. D., Rota, T. R., Schooley, R. T., et al. (1985): Isolation of HTLV-III from cerebrospinal fluid and neural tissues of patients with neurologic syndromes related to the acquired immunodeficiency syndrome. *N. Engl. J. Med.,* 313:1493–1497.
11. Friedland, G. H., Saltzman, B. R., Rogers, M. F., et al. (1986): Lack of transmission of HTLV-III/LAV infection to household contacts of patients with AIDS or AIDS-related complex with oral candidiasis. *N. Engl. J. Med.,* 314:344–349.
12. Kaplan, J. E., Oleske, J. M., Getchell, J. P., et al. (1985): Evidence against transmission of human T-lymphotropic virus/lymphadenopathy-associated virus (HTLV-III/LAV) in families of children with the acquired immunodeficiency syndrome. *Pediatr. Infect. Dis.,* 4:468–471.
13. Lawrence, D. N., Jason, J. M., Bouhasin, J. D., et al. (1985): HTLV-III/LAV antibody status of spouses and household contacts assisting in home infusion of hemophilia patients. *Blood,* 66:703–705.
14. Martin, K., Katz, B. Z., and Miller, G. (1987): AIDS and antibodies to human immunodeficiency virus (HIV) in children and their families. *J. Infect. Dis.,* 155:54–63.
15. Anonymous (1984): Needlestick transmission of HTLV-III from a patient infected in Africa. *Lancet,* 2:1376–1377.
16. Oksenhendler, E., Harzic, M., LeRoux, J. M., et al. (1986): Letter: HIV infection with seroconversion after a superficial needlestick injury to the finger. *N. Engl. J. Med.,* 315:582.
17. Stricoff, R. L., and Morse, D. L. (1986): Letter: HTLV-III/LAV seroconversion following a deep intramuscular needlestick injury. *N. Engl. J. Med.,* 314:115.
18. Centers for Disease Control (1985): Recommendations for preventing transmission of infection with human T-lymphotropic virus type III/lymphadenopathy-associated virus in the workplace. *M.M.W.R.,* 34:682–695.
19. Henderson, D. K., Saah, A. J., Zak, B. J., et al. (1986): Risk of nosocomial infection with human T-cell lymphotropic virus type III/lymphadenopathy-associated virus in a large cohort of intensively exposed health care workers. *Ann. Intern. Med.,* 104:644–647.
20. Hirsch, M. S., Wormser, G. P., Schooley, R. T., et al. (1985): Risk of nosocomial infection with human T-cell lymphotropic virus III (HTLV-III). *N. Engl. J. Med.,* 313:1493–1497.
21. Kuhls, T. L., Viker, S., Parris, N. B., et al. (1986): A prospective cohort study of the occupational risk of AIDS and AIDS-related infections in health care personnel. *Clin. Res.,* 34:120A–124A.
22. McCray, E., and the Cooperative Needlestick Group (1986): Occupational risk of the acquired immunodeficiency syndrome among health care workers. *N. Engl. J. Med.,* 314:1127–1132.
23. Weiss, S. H., Saxinger, C., Rechtman, D., et al. (1985): HTLV-III infection among health care workers. Association with needlestick injuries. *J.A.M.A.,* 254:2089–2093.
24. Seef, L. B., Wright, E. C., Zimmerman, H. J., et al. (1978): Type B hepatitis after needlestick exposure: Prevention with hepatitis B immune globulin. *Ann. Intern. Med.,* 88:285–293.
25. Centers for Disease Control (1987): Recommendations for prevention of HIV transmission in health care settings. *M.M.W.R.,* 36 (Suppl.):2S–17S.
26. Wormser, G. P., Joline, C., Duncanson, F., et al. (1984): Letter: Needlestick injuries during the care of patients with AIDS. *N. Engl. J. Med.,* 310:1461–1462.
27. Martin, L. S., McDougal, J. S., and Loskoski, S. L. (1985): Disinfection and inactivation of the human T lymphotropic virus type III/lymphadenopathy-associated virus. *J. Infect. Dis.,* 152:400–403.
28. St. Pierre, B., Barre-Sinoussi, F., Montagnier, L., et al. (1984): Inactivation of lymphadenopathy associated virus by chemical disinfectants. *Lancet,* 2:899–901.
29. Conte, J. E. (1986): Infection with human immunodeficiency virus in the hospital. *Ann. Intern. Med.,* 105:730–736.
30. Centers for Disease Control (1986): Safety of therapeutic immune globulin preparations with respect to transmission of human T-lymphotropic virus type III/lymphadenopathy-associated virus infection. *M.M.W.R.,* 35:231–233.
31. Wood, C. C., Williams, A. E., McNamara, J. G., et al. (1986): Antibody against the human immunodeficiency virus in commercial intravenous gammaglobulin preparations. *Ann. Intern. Med.,* 105:536–538.
32. Conte, J. E., Hadley, W. K., Sande, M., and the University of California Task Force on the Acquired Immunodeficiency Syndrome (1983): Infection control guidelines for patients with the acquired immunodeficiency syndrome (AIDS). *N. Engl. J. Med.,* 309:740–744.
33. Ziegler, J. B., Cooper, D. A., Johnson, R. O., et al. (1985): Postnatal transmission of AIDS-associated retrovirus from mother to infant. *Lancet,* 1:896–897.

# APPENDIX A

# Revision of the CDC Surveillance Case Definition for Acquired Immunodeficiency Syndrome

Council of State and Territorial Epidemiologists, AIDS Program, Center for Infectious Diseases, CDC

The following revised case definition for surveillance of acquired immunodeficiency syndrome (AIDS) was developed by the Centers for Disease Control (CDC) in collaboration with public health and clinical specialists. The Council of State and Territorial Epidemiologists (CSTE) has officially recommended adoption of the revised definition for national reporting of AIDS. The objectives of the revision are a) to track more effectively the severe disabling morbidity associated with infection with human immunodeficiency virus (HIV) (including HIV-1 and HIV-2); b) to simplify reporting of AIDS cases; c) to increase the sensitivity and specificity of the definition through greater diagnostic application of laboratory evidence for HIV infection; and d) to be consistent with current diagnostic practice, which in some cases includes presumptive, i.e., without confirmatory laboratory evidence, diagnosis of AIDS-indicative diseases (e.g., Pneumocystis carinii pneumonia, Kaposi's sarcoma).

The definition is organized into three sections that depend on the status of laboratory evidence of HIV infection (e.g., HIV antibody). The major proposed changes apply to patients with laboratory evidence for HIV infection: a) inclusion of HIV encephalopathy, HIV wasting syndrome, and a broader range of specific AIDS-indicative diseases (Section II.A); b) inclusion of AIDS patients whose indicator diseases are diagnosed presumptively (Section II.B); and c) elimination of exclusions due to other causes of immunodeficiency (Section I.A).

Application of the definition for children differs from that for adults in two ways. First, multiple or recurrent serious bacterial infections and lymphoid interstitial pneumonia/pulmonary lymphoid hyperplasia are accepted as indicative of AIDS among children but not among adults. Second, for children <15 months of age whose mothers are thought to have had HIV infection during the child's perinatal period, the laboratory criteria for HIV infection are more stringent, since the presence of HIV antibody in the child is, by itself, insufficient evidence for HIV infection because of the persistence of passively acquired maternal antibodies <15 months after birth.

The new definition is effective immediately. State and local health departments are requested to apply the new definition henceforth to patients reported to them. The initiation of the actual reporting of cases that meet the new definition is targeted for September 1, 1987, when modified computer software and report forms should be in place to accommodate the changes. CSTE has recommended retrospective application of the revised definition to patients already reported to health departments. The new definition follows:

## 1987 REVISION OF CASE DEFINITION FOR AIDS FOR SURVEILLANCE PURPOSES

For national reporting, a case of AIDS is defined as an illness characterized by one or more of the following "indicator" diseases, depending on the status of laboratory evidence of HIV infection, as shown below.

### I. Without Laboratory Evidence Regarding HIV Infection

If laboratory tests for HIV were not performed or gave inconclusive results (see Appendix I) and the patient had no other cause of immunodeficiency listed in Section I.A below, then any disease listed in Section I.B indicates AIDS if it was diagnosed by a definitive method (see Appendix II).

- A. **Causes of immunodeficiency that disqualify diseases as indicators of AIDS in the absence of laboratory evidence for HIV infection**
    1. high-dose or long-term systemic corticosteroid therapy or other immunosuppressive/cytotoxic therapy ≤3 months before the onset of the indicator disease
    2. any of the following diseases diagnosed ≤3 months after diagnosis of the indicator disease: Hodgkin's disease, nonHodgkin's lymphoma (other than primary brain lymphoma), lymphocytic leukemia, multiple myeloma, any other cancer of lymphoreticular or histiocytic tissue, or angioimmunoblastic lymphadenopathy
    3. a genetic (congenital) immunodeficiency syndrome or an acquired immunodeficiency syndrome atypical of HIV infection, such as one involving hypogammaglobulinemia
- B. **Indicator diseases diagnosed definitively (see Appendix II)**
    1. candidiasis of the esophagus, trachea, bronchi, or lungs
    2. cryptococcosis, extrapulmonary
    3. cryptosporidiosis with diarrhea persisting >1 month
    4. cytomegalovirus disease of an organ other than liver, spleen, or lymph nodes in a patient >1 month of age
    5. herpes simplex virus infection causing a mucocutaneous ulcer that persists longer than one month; or bronchitis, pneumonitis, or esophagitis for any duration affecting a patient >1 month of age
    6. Kaposi's sarcoma affecting a patient <60 years of age
    7. lymphoma of the brain (primary) affecting a patient <60 years of age
    8. lymphoid interstitial pneumonia and/or pulmonary lymphoid hyperplasia (LIP/PLH complex) affecting a child <13 years of age
    9. Mycobacterium avium complex or M. kansasii disease, disseminated (at a site other than or in addition to lungs, skin, or cervical or hilar lymph nodes)
    10. Pneumocystis carinii pneumonia
    11. progressive multifocal leukoencephalopathy
    12. toxoplasmosis of the brain affecting a patient >1 month of age

### II. With Laboratory Evidence for HIV Infection

Regardless of the presence of other causes of immunodeficiency (I.A), in the presence of laboratory evidence for HIV infection (see Appendix I), any disease listed above (I.B) or below (II.A or II.B) indicates a diagnosis of AIDS.

- A. **Indicator diseases diagnosed definitively (see Appendix II)**
    1. bacterial infections, multiple or recurrent (any combination of at least two within a two-year period), of the following types affecting a child <13 years of age: septicemia, pneumonia, meningitis, bone or joint infection, or abscess of an internal organ or body cavity (excluding otitis media or superficial skin or mucosal abscesses), caused by Haemophilus, Streptococcus (including pneumococcus), or other pyogenic bacteria
    2. coccidioidomycosis, disseminated (at a site other than or in addition to lungs or cervical or hilar lymph nodes)
    3. HIV encephalopathy (also called "HIV dementia," "AIDS dementia," or "subacute encephalitis due to HIV") (see Appendix II)

4. histoplasmosis, disseminated (at a site other than or in addition to lungs or cervical or hilar lymph nodes)
5. isosporiasis with diarrhea persisting >1 month
6. Kaposi's sarcoma at any age
7. lymphoma of the brain (primary) at any age
8. other non-Hodgkin's lymphoma of B-cell or unknown immunologic phenotype and the following histologic types:
    a. small noncleaved lymphoma (either Burkitt or nonBurkitt type) (*see Appendix IV for equivalent terms and numeric codes used in the International Classification of Diseases, Ninth Revision, Clinical Modification*)
    b. immunoblastic sarcoma (equivalent to any of the following, although not necessarily all in combination: immunoblastic lymphoma, largecell lymphoma, diffuse histiocytic lymphoma, diffuse undifferentiated lymphoma, or high-grade lymphoma) (*see Appendix IV for equivalent terms and numeric codes used in the International Classification of Diseases, Ninth Revision, Clinical Modification*)
    Note: Lymphomas are not included here if they are of T-cell immunologic phenotype or their histologic type is not described or is described as "lymphocytic," "lymphoblastic," "small cleaved," or "plasmacytoid lymphocytic"
9. any mycobacterial disease caused by mycobacteria other than M. tuberculosis, disseminated (at a site other than or in addition to lungs, skin, or cervical or hilar lymph nodes)
10. disease caused by M. tuberculosis, extrapulmonary (involving at least one site outside the lungs, regardless of whether there is concurrent pulmonary involvement)
11. Salmonella (nontyphoid) septicemia, recurrent
12. HIV wasting syndrome (emaciation, "slim disease") (*see Appendix II for description*)

B. **Indicator diseases diagnosed presumptively (by a method other than those in Appendix II)**
Note: Given the seriousness of diseases indicative of AIDS, it is generally important to diagnose them definitively, especially when therapy that would be used may have serious side-effects or when definitive diagnosis is needed for eligibility for antiretroviral therapy. Nonetheless, in some situations a patient's condition will not permit the performance of definitive tests. In other situations, accepted clinical practice may be to diagnose presumptively based on the presence of characteristic clinical and laboratory abnormalities. Guidelines for presumptive diagnoses are suggested in Appendix III.
1. candidiasis of the esophagus
2. cytomegalovirus retinitis with loss of vision
3. Kaposi's sarcoma
4. lymphoid interstitial pneumonia and/or pulmonary lymphoid hyperplasia (LIP/PLH complex) affecting a child <13 years of age
5. mycobacterial disease (acid-fast bacilli with species not identified by culture), disseminated (involving at least one site other than or in addition to lungs, skin, or cervical or hilar lymph nodes)
6. Pneumocystis carinii pneumonia
7. toxoplasmosis of the brain affecting a patient >1 month of age

### III. With Laboratory Evidence Against HIV Infection

With laboratory test results negative for HIV infection (*see Appendix I*), a diagnosis of AIDS for surveillance purposes is ruled out *unless:*
A. all the other causes of imunodeficiency listed above in Section I.A are excluded; and
B. the patient has had either:
   1. Pneumocystis carinii pneumonia diagnosed by a definitive method (*See Appendix II*); or
   2. a. any of the other diseases indicative of AIDS listed above in Section I.B diagnosed by a definitive method (*See Appendix II*); and
      b. a T-helper/inducer (CD4) lymphocyte count $< 400/mm^3$.

## COMMENTARY

The surveillance of severe disease associated with HIV infection remains an essential, though not the only, indicator of the course of the HIV epidemic. The number of AIDS cases and the relative distribution of cases by demographic, geographic, and behavioral risk variables are the oldest indices of the epidemic, which began in 1981 and for which data are available retrospectively back to 1978. The original surveillance case definition, based on then-available knowledge, provided useful epidemiologic data on severe HIV disease (1). To ensure a reasonable predictive value for underlying immunodeficiency caused by what was then an unknown agent, the indicators of AIDS in the old case definition were restricted to particular opportunisitic diseases diagnosed by reliable methods in patients without specific known causes of immunodeficiency. After HIV was discovered to be the cause of AIDS, however, and highly sensitive and specific HIV-antibody tests became available, the spectrum of manifestations of HIV infection became better defined, and classification systems for HIV infection were developed (2–5). It became apparent that some progressive, seriously disabling, and even fatal conditions (e.g., encephalopathy, wasting syndrome) affecting a substantial number of HIV-infected patients were not subject to epidemiologic surveillance, as they were not included in the AIDS case definition. For reporting purposes, the revision adds to the definition most of those severe noninfectious, noncancerous HIV-associated conditions that are categorized in the CDC clinical classification systems for HIV infection among adults and children (4, 5).

Another limitation of the old definition was that AIDS-indicative diseases are diagnosed presumptively (i.e., without confirmation by methods required by the old definition) in 10% to 15% of patients diagnosed with such diseases; thus, an appreciable proportion of AIDS cases were missed for reporting purposes (6, 7). This proportion may be increasing, which would compromise the old case definition's usefulness as a tool for monitoring trends. The revised case definition permits the reporting of these clinically diagnosed cases as long as there is laboratory evidence of HIV infection.

The effectiveness of the revision will depend on how extensively HIV-antibody tests are used. Approximately one-third of AIDS patients in the United States have been from New York City and San Francisco, where, since 1985, <7% have been reported with HIV-antibody test results, compared with > 60% in other areas. The impact of the revision on the reported numbers of AIDS cases also will depend on the proportion of AIDS patients in whom indicator diseases are diagnosed presumptively rather than definitively. The use of presumptive diagnostic criteria varies geographically, being more common in certain rural areas and in urban areas with many indigent AIDS patients.

To avoid confusion about what should be reported to health departments, the term "AIDS" should refer only to conditions meeting the surveillance definition. This definition is intended only to provide consistent statistical data for public health purposes. Clinicians will not rely on this definition alone to diagnose serious disease caused by HIV infection in individual patients because there may be additional information that would lead to a more accurate diagnosis. For example, patients who are not reportable under the definition because they have either a negative HIV-antibody test or, in the presence of HIV antibody, an opportunistic disease not listed in the definition as an indicator of AIDS, nonetheless may be diagnosed as having serious HIV disease on consideration of other clinical or laboratory characteristics of HIV infection or a history of exposure to HIV.

Conversely, the AIDS surveillance definition may rarely misclassify other patients as having serious HIV disease if they have no HIV-antibody test but have an AIDS-indicative disease with a background incidence unrelated to HIV infection, such as cryptococcal meningitis.

The diagnostic criteria accepted by the AIDS surveillance case definition should not be interpreted as the standard of good medical practice. Presumptive diagnoses are accepted in the definition because not to count them would be to ignore substantial morbidity resulting from HIV infection. Likewise, the definition accepts a reactive screening test for HIV antibody without confirmation by a supplemental test because a repeatedly reactive screening test result, in combination with an indicator disease, is highly indicative of true HIV disease. For national surveillance purposes, the tiny proportion of possibly false-positive screening tests in persons with AIDS-indicative diseases is of little consequence. For the individual patient, however, a correct diagnosis is critically important. The use of supplemental tests therefore, is, strongly endorsed. An increase in the diagnostic use of HIV-antibody tests could improve both the quality of medical care and the function of the new case definition, as well as assist in providing counseling to prevent transmission of HIV.

*References*

1. World Health Organization. Acquired immunodeficiency syndrome (AIDS) (1986); WHO/CDC case definition for AIDS. *WHO Wkly. Epidemiol Rec.,* 61:69–72.
2. Haverkos, H. W., Gottlieb, M. S., Killen, J. Y., and Edelman, R. (1985): Letter: Classification of HTLV-III/LAV-related diseases. *J. Infect. Dis.,* 152:1095.
3. Redfield, R. R., Wright, D. C., and Tramont, E. C. (1986): The Walter Reed staging classification of HTLV-III infection. *N. Engl. J. Med.,* 314:131–132.
4. Centers for Disease Control. (1986): Classification system for human T-lymphotropic virus type III/lymphadenopathy-associated virus infections. *M. M. W. R.,* 35:334–339.
5. Centers for Disease Control. (1987): Classification system for human immunodeficiency virus (HIV) infection in children under 13 years of age. *M. M. W. R.,* 36:225–30, 235.
6. Hardy, A. M. Starcher, E. T., Morgan, W. M., et al. (1987): Review of death certificates to assess completeness of AIDS case reporting. *Pub. Hlth. Rep.* 102:386–391.
7. Starcher, E. T., Biel, J. K., Rivera-Castano, R, Day, J. M., Hopkins, S. G., and Miller, J. W. (1987): The impact of presumptively diagnosed opportunistic infections and cancers on national reporting of AIDS. Washington, DC: Third International Conference on AIDS, June 1–5, 1987 (*Abstr.*).

# APPENDIX I
## Laboratory evidence for or against HIV infection

1. **For infection:**
   When a patient has disease consistent with AIDS:
   a. a serum specimen from a patient ≥15 months of age, or from a child <15 months of age whose mother is not thought to have had HIV infection during the child's perinatal period, that is repeatedly reactive for HIV antibody by a screening test (e.g., enzyme-linked immunosorbent assay [ELISA]) as long as subsequent HIV-antibody tests (e.g., Western blot, immunofluorescence assay), if done, are positive; OR
   b. a serum specimen from a child < 15 months of age, whose mother is thought to have had HIV infection during the child's perinatal period, that is repeatedly reactive for HIV antibody by a screening test (e.g., ELISA), plus increased serum immunoglobulin levels and at least one of the following abnormal immunologic test results: reduced absolute lymphocyte count, depressed CD4 (T-helper) lymphocyte count, or decreased CD4/CD8 (helper/suppressor) ratio, as long as subsequent antibody tests (e.g., Western blot, immunofluorescence assay), if done, are positive; OR
   c. a positive test for HIV serum antigen; OR
   d. a positive HIV culture confirmed by both reverse transcriptase detection and a specific HIV-antigen test or *in situ* hybridization using a nucleic acid probe; or
   e. a positive result on any other highly specific test for HIV (e.g., nucleic acid probe of peripheral blood lymphocytes).

2. **Against infection:**
   A nonreactive screening test for serum antibody to HIV (e.g., ELISA) without a reactive or positive result on any other test for HIV infection (e.g., antibody, antigen, culture), if done.

3. **Inconclusive (neither for nor against infection):**
   a. a repeatedly reactive screening test for serum antibody to HIV (e.g., ELISA) followed by a negative or inconclusive supplemental test (e.g., Western blot, immunofluorescence assay) without a positive HIV culture or serum antigen test, if done; OR
   b. a serum specimen from a child < 15 months of age, whose mother is thought to have had HIV infection during the child's perinatal period, that is repeatedly reactive for HIV antibody by a screening test, even if positive by a supplemental test, without additional evidence for immunodeficiency as described above (in 1.b) and without a positive HIV culture or serum antigen test, if done.

## APPENDIX II
## Definitive diagnostic methods for diseases indicative of AIDS

| Diseases | Definitive diagnostic methods |
|---|---|
| Cryptosporidiosis<br>Cytomegalovirus<br>Isosporiasis<br>Kaposi's sarcoma<br>Lymphoma<br>Lymphoid pneumonia or hyperplasia<br>Pneumocystis carinii pneumonia<br>Progressive multifocal leukoencephalopathy<br>Toxoplasmosis | Microscopy (histology or cytology) |
| Candidiasis | Gross inspection by endoscopy or autopsy or by microscopy (histology or cytology) on a specimen obtained directly from the tissues affected (including scrapings from the mucosal surface), not from a culture |
| Coccidioidomycosis<br>Cryptococcosis<br>Herpes simplex virus<br>Histoplasmosis | Microscopy (histology or cytology), culture, or detection of antigen in a specimen obtained directly from the tissues affected or a fluid from those tissues |
| Tuberculosis<br>Other mycobacteriosis<br>Salmonellosis<br>Other bacterial infection | Culture |
| HIV encephalopathy* (dementia) | Clinical findings of disabling cognitive and/or motor dysfunction interfering with occupation or activities of daily living, or loss of behavioral developmental milestones affecting a child, progressing over weeks to months, in the absence of a concurrent illness or condition other than HIV infection that could explain the findings. Methods to rule out such concurrent illnesses and conditions must include cerebrospinal fluid examination and either brain imaging (computed tomography or magnetic resonance) or autopsy |
| HIV wasting syndrome* | Findings of profound involuntary weight loss >10% of baseline body weight plus either chronic diarrhea (at least two loose stools per day for $\geq$ 30 days) or chronic weakness and documented fever (for $\geq$ 30 days, intermittent or constant) in the absence of a concurrent illness or condition other than HIV infection that could explain the findings (e.g., cancer, tuberculosis, cryptosporidiosis, or other specific enteritis) |

* For HIV encephalopathy and HIV wasting syndrome, the methods of diagnosis described here are not truly definitive, but are sufficiently rigorous for surveillance purposes.

## APPENDIX III
## Suggested guidelines for presumptive diagnosis of diseases indicative of AIDS

| Diseases | Presumptive Diagnostic Criteria |
|---|---|
| Candidiasis of esophagus | a. Recent onset of retrosternal pain on swallowing; and<br>b. Oral candidiasis diagnosed by the gross appearance of white patches or plaques on an erythematous base or by the microscopic appearance of fungal mycelial filaments in an uncultured specimen scraped from the oral mucosa. |
| cytomegalovirus retinitis | A characteristic appearance on serial ophthalmoscopic examinations (e.g., discrete patches of retinal whitening with distinct borders, spreading in a centrifugal manner, following blood vessels, progressing over several months, frequently associated with retinal vasculitis, hemorrhage, and necrosis). Resolution of active disease leaves retinal scarring and atrophy with retinal pigment epithelial mottling. |
| Mycobacteriosis | Microscopy of a specimen from stool or normally sterile body fluids or tissue from a site other than lungs, skin, or cervical or hilar lymph nodes, showing acid-fast bacilli of a species not identified by culture. |
| Kaposi's sarcoma | A characteristic gross appearance of an erythematous or violaceous plaque-like lesion on skin or mucous membrane. (Note: Presumptive diagnosis of Kaposi's sarcoma should not be made by clinicians who have seen few cases of it.) |
| Lymphoid interstitial pneumonia | Bilateral reticulonodular interstitial pulmonary infiltrates present on chest x-ray for $\geq$ 2 months with no pathogen identified and no response to antibiotic treatment. |
| Pneumocystis carinii pneumonia | a. a history of dyspnea on exertion or nonproductive cough of recent onset (within the past 3 months); and<br>b. chest x-ray evidence of diffuse bilateral interstitial infiltrates or gallium scan evidence of diffuse bilateral pulmonary disease; and<br>c. arterial blood gas analysis showing an arterial $pO_2$ of <70 mm Hg or a low respiratory diffusing capacity (<80% of predicted values) or an increase in the alveolar-arterial oxygen tension gradient; and<br>d. no evidence of a bacterial pneumonia. |
| Toxoplasmosis of the brain | a. Recent onset of a focal neurologic abnormality consistent with intracranial disease or a reduced level of consciousness; and<br>b. Brain imaging evidence of a lesion having a mass effect (on computed tomography or nuclear magnetic resonance) or the radiographic appearance of which is enhanced by injection of contrast medium; and<br>c. Serum antibody to toxoplasmosis or successful response to therapy for toxoplasmosis. |

# Subject Index

**A**
Abdominal lymph nodes, 115–119
Abdominal lymphoma, 112
Abdominal opportunistic infections, 125, 128
Absolute lymphopenia, 3
Acquired immune deficiency syndrome (AIDS)
 case definitions of, 5
  CDC revised, 147–151
 casual transmission of, 2–3
 classification of, 5
 definitive diagnosis methods for diseases indicative of, 155
 diagnosis of, 1
 epidemiology of, 1–3
 etiologic agents of, 4–5
 immune abnormalities and immunopathogenesis of, 3–4
 incidence of, 1
 occupational exposure to, 2–3
 suggested guidelines for presumptive diagnosis of diseases indicative of, 157
Actinomycosis, 80
Acute appendicitis, causes by KS, 98
Acyclovir, 14, 34
ADC, see Diffuse cerebral atrophy
Adenopathy, 73
Africa, AIDS in, 2
AIDS, see Acquired immune deficiency syndrome
AIDS-associated neoplasms, 9–11
AIDS-related complex (ARC), 13–15, 123, 124
 adrenal insufficiency in, 15
 bacterial infections of skin in, 14
 in children, 132
 constitutional symptoms of, 13
 dermatophytic infections in, 14
 hematologic manifestations of, 15
 manifestations of, 14
 mucotaneous manifestations of, 13
 neurologic manifestations of, 15
 ophthalmologic changes due to, 15
 oral manifestations of, 14
 reticuloendothelial system as affected by, 13
 viral infections of skin in, 14

AIDS-related lymphomas (ARLs), 11–13, 62–68
 in alimentary tract, 122
 clinical manifestations of, 107
 mortality in, 113
 multiple abdominal sites in, 115
 pathologic findings in, 113–114
 spinal involvement in, 114
 thoracic involvement in, 114, 116
Air-space disease, in PCP, 47
AL-721, 16
Alimentary tract, ARLs in, 11–13, 62–68
Alpha-interferon, 11, 16
Amitriptylline, 15
Amphotericin-B, 7, 58, 59
Anemia, 15
Angular stomatitis (cheilitis), 14
Ansamycin, 9
Antibody-dependent cytotoxic cellular response (ADCC), 3
Antimoniotungstate (HPA-23), 15, 16
Antiretroviral agents, 16
ARC, see AIDS-related complex
ARLS, see AIDS-related lymphomas
Aseptic meningitis, 34
Aspergillosis, 59, 61
Atrophy, see Diffuse cerebral atrophy
AZT, 9, 15–17

**B**
B-cell immunoglobulin production, 3
B-lymphocyte defects, 3
Bacterial infections, 59
BAL, see Bronchoalveolar lavage
Benign adenoidal enlargement, 44, 45
Beta-interferon, 16
Biliary disease, 102–104
BK, see Burkitt's lymphoma
Body fluids, precautions regarding, 143–144
Bovine transfer factor, 8, 87
Bowel lymphoma, 122
Brain, see also Toxoplasmosis
 KS and, 110
 lymphoma of, 114
 mass lesions in, 29–31
Bronchoalveolar lavage (BAL), 57, 71–72

Bulky abdominal lymphadenopathy, 115–119
Burkitt's lymphoma (BK), 11, 68, 99, 102, 114, 121, 122, 139

**C**
Candida
 of esophagus, 78, 79, 82
  in children, 140
 of stomach, 82
Candidal esophagitis, in children, 140
Candidiasis, 78, 141
 definitive diagnostic methods for, 155
 presumptive diagnosis of, 157
Cardiac disease, 69–71
 in children, 134
 gallium scintigraphy for, 69–71
 incidence of, 69
Cardiomyopathy, 134
$CD_4/CD_8$ ratio, 3, 11
$CD_4$ lymphocytes, 11
 in binding and penetration of HIV, 16
CDC, see Centers for Disease Control
Cell-mediated immunity (CMI), 2
Centers for Disease Control (CDC)
 classification of HIV infection by, 2
 surveillance case definition for, revised, 147–151
Central Africa, AIDS in, 2
Central nervous system (CNS), 21
Central nervous system (CNS) disease, in children, 141
Central nervous system (CNS) lymphoma, 112
Cerebral toxoplasmosis, see Toxoplasma gondii
Children, see also Pediatric AIDS
 ARC in, 132
 candidal esophagitis in, 140
 cardiac disease in, 134
 CDC revised surveillance case definition for AIDS in, 147
 central nervous system disease in, 141
 disseminated histoplasmosis in, 58
 dysmorphia in, 141
 gastrointestinal disease in, 137–140
 herpes simplex virus (HSV) in, 140
 histoplasmosis in, 140

Children, *(contd.)*
  laboratory evidence for or against HIV infection in, 153
  LIP in, 134, 135
  liver disease in, 137
  lymph nodes in, 134–137
  MAI in, 134, 137
  PCP in, 133–134
  recurrent infections in, 141
Cholangitis, 102–104
Clindamycin, 7
Clofazamine, 9, 55
Clotrimazole, 13
CMI, *see* Cell-mediated immunity
CMV, *see* Cytomegalovirus
CMV colitis, *see* Colitis
CMV esophagitis, 79–81
CNS, *see* Central nervous system
Coccidiomycosis, 58–59, 60
  definitive diagnostic methods for, 155
Cofactors
  for AIDS, 5
  for KS, 9
Colitis, 92–99
  barium enema in, 92–97
  clinical presentation, 97–98
  CMV in, 8
Colon, 92–101
  KS in, 98–100
  lymphoma of, 99–101, 102
  neoplasms in, 98–102
Colonic lymphoma, *see* Lymphoma, of colon
Computed tomography (CT), 73–74
  of abdominal opportunistic infections in AIDS, 125, 128
  double dose compared with single dose contrast, 25
  MR compared with, 28
  of neurological manifestations in AIDS, 22–24
Condyloma cauminata, in ARC, 15
Cryptococcal meningitis, 5, 27, 29, 36
Cryptococcosis, definitive diagnostic methods for, 155
Cryptococcus, in children, 140
Cryptococcus immitis, 58–59
Cryptococcus neoformans, 6, 7, 57–58
Cryptosporidial enteritis, 87
Cryptosporidiosis, 8, 84–87, 90, 91, 92
Cryptosporidium, 102
CT, *see* Computed tomography
Cutaneous lesions, 10
Cytomegalovirus (CMV), 4, 55–57, 79
  bronchoalveolar lavage (BAL) for, 57
  in children, 140
  in colitis, 92–98
  diffuse cerebral atrophy and, 24
  in ependymal disease, 34–36
  general information on, 8
  in leptomeningeal disease, 34–36
  of small bowel, 89–90
  treatment of, 8
  in white matter disease, 33
Cytomegalovirus (CMV) gastritis, 81–82, 86, 87
Cytomegalovirus (CMV) pneumonia, in children, 134, 136
Cytomegalovirus (CMV) retinitis, 157
Cytosine arabinoside, 32

## D

Danazol, 15
Dapsone, 7
Delayed-type hypersensitivity (DTH) reaction, 3
Deoxyfluoromethoxyornithine, 7
Dermatophytic infections, in ARC, 14
DHPG, 8
Diffuse cerebral atrophy (ADC), 24, 26, 40
Diffuse encephalitis, 6
Diffuse enteritis, 89
Disseminated histoplasmosis, 58, 59
  in children, 140
Disseminated mycobacteriosis, 5
Distal sensory polyneuropathy, 15
Duodenum, 83–89, 92
Dysmorphia, in children, 141
Dysphagia, 78

## E

EKS (epidemic Kaposi's sarcoma), *see* Kaposi's sarcoma
Endobronchial tumors, 60
Enteroclysis, 90–92
Ependymal disease, 34–36
Epidural lymphoma, 114
Epstein-Barr virus, 14, 43, 134
Esophageal candida infection, 78
Esophagitis, 78–80, 82
Esophagography, 78–79
Esophagus
  candida of, 78, 79, 82, 140
  candidiasis of, 157
  gastrointestinal radiology of, 78–81
  KS of, 80–81
  MAI of, 80
  neoplasms of, 80–81
Ethambutol, 9
Etoposide (VP-16), 11
Europe, AIDS in, 2

## F

Fansidar, 7
Fiberoptic bronchoscopy (FOB), 71–72
Fluconazole, 7
5-Fluorocytosine, 7
FOB, *see* Fiberoptic bronchoscopy
Focal parenchymal disease, 59
Fungal infections, 27–29
Fungi, 57–59

## G

Gallium scintigraphy, 69–73
Gamma-interferon, 16
Gammaglobulin, 15
Ganciclovir, 8
Gastric lesions, 81
Gastric neoplasms, 82–83
Gastric tuberculosis (TB), 82
Gastrointestinal disease, in children, 137–140
Gastrointestinal KS, 82–83
Gastrointestinal radiology, 77–104, 110–111
  biliary disease, 102–104
  colon, 92–101
  duodenum, 83–89, 92
  esophagus, 78–81
  radiographic technique, 77–78
  small bowel, 83–91
  stomach, 81–83

## H

Hairy leukoplakia, 13–14
Handling AIDS patients, 143–146
  body fluid precautions, 143–144
  environmental cleaning, 144
  handling of specimens, 144
  portable radiologic procedures, 145
  risk in health care system, 143
  special infection control procedures, 144–145
  summary of precautions for all patient contact, 146
  waste, linens, materials, and equipment, 144
HD, *see* Hodgkin's disease
Head and neck, 40–45
  benign adenoidal enlargement of, 45
  Kaposi's sarcoma of, 42–43
  lymph node enlargement of, 45
  mycobacterial infections of, 42
  non-Hodgkin's lymphoma of, 42, 43, 44
  sinus disease of, 45
  squamous cell carcinoma of, 43
  tumors of, 42–43
Health care workers, and risk of HIV infection, 3; *see also* Handling AIDS patients
Hematologic manifestations, of ARC, 15
Hemophilus influenza, 59
Hepatic disease, in children, 137
Herpes simplex encephalitis, 33–34
Herpes simplex esophagitis, 80
Herpes simplex stomatitis, 14
Herpes simplex virus (HSV; I and II), 33–34
  in children, 140
Hilar adenopathy, 73
Hilar lymphadenopathy, 114–115

Histoplasmosis, in children, 140
HIV, see Human immunodeficiency virus
HIV-$CD_4$ antigen binding, 16
HIV-dementia, 9
HIV encephalitis, 32, 35, 36
HIV encephalopathy, definitive diagnostic methods for, 155
HIV-induced subacute encephalitis, 6
HIV-infected individuals, immune abnormalities and immunopathogenesis in, 3–4
HIV infection
  cases of, by risk group, 2
  CDC classification of, 2
  epidemiology of, 1–3
  health care workers and risk of, 3
  laboratory evidence for or against, 153
  natural history of, 2
  therapeutic approach to, 15–17
HIV seropositivity, rate of, 2
HIV wasting syndrome, definitive diagnostic methods for, 155
Hodgkin's disease (HD), 11–13, 115, 117, 122
  atypical manifestation of, in AIDS, 114
  clinical hallmark of, 12
  incidence of, 11
  as indicator of AIDS, 114
  presentation of, 12
  treatment of, 12
  in visceral organs, 119
Homosexuals, AIDS in, 108–109
HPA-23, see Antimoniotungstate
HSV; I and II, see Herpes simplex virus
HTLV-III, see Human T-lymphotropic virus-III
Human T-lymphotropic virus-III (HTLV-III), 4
Human immunodeficiency virus (HIV)
  as causes of AIDS, body of evidence for, 4
  composition of, 4
  immunopathogenesis of, 4
  naming of, 4
  vaccine for, 17
Hydrocephalus, 34
Hypopharynx, Kaposi's sarcoma of, 80–81

I
Ileo colitis, 89
Immune thrombocytopenia (ITP), 15
Immune thrombocytopenia purpura, 4
Immunorestorative agents, 16
Imreg-1, 16
Infarcts, 34
Interferons, 16
Interleukin-2 (IL-2), 16
Intracranial mass lesions, 29–31

Intracranial tuberculosis, 29
Isoniazid, 9
Isoprinosine (Insiplex), 16
ITP, see Immune thrombocytopenia

J
J-C virus, see Papova virus

K
Kaposi's sarcoma, 1, 9–11, 59–60, 64–66, 73, 83, 84, 108–114
  acute appendicitis caused by, 98
  brain involvement with, 110
  $CD_4/CD_8$ ratio and, 11
  $CD_4$ lymphocytes and, 11
  classic form of, 9
  clinical course of, in AIDS, 108–109
  clinical manifestations of, 107
  clinical subtypes of, 108
  cofactors for development of, 9
  in colon, 98–100
  cutaneous lesions of, 10
  endobronchial tumors, 60
  of esophagus, 80–81, 110
  gastrointestinal lesions of, 10
  in gastrointestinal tract, 110–111
  of head and neck, 42–43
  in homosexuals versus other AIDS patients, 108–109
  of hypopharynx, 80–81
  incidence of, 9, 59, 107–109
  lymph nodes as site of, 111–112
  lymphadenopathy and, 10
  lymphoma and, 107
  origin of malignant cell in, 10
  pleural effusion secondary to, 10
  premortem diagnosis of, 59–60
  presumptive diagnosis of, 157
  prognosis following, 109
  pulmonary involvement in, 10, 59–60
  radiographic descriptions of, 60
  in renal transplants, 107
  of small bowel, 90–92, 96, 97
  staging system for, 10, 11
  in stomach, 82
  survival rate of patients with, 10
  treatment for, 11
Ketoconazole, 13
KS, see Kaposi's sarcoma

L
LAS, see Lymphadenopathy syndrome
LAV, see Lymphadenopathy virus
LDH, see Serum lactate dehydrogenase
Legionella pneumonia, 59, 62
Leptomeningeal disease, 34–36
LIP, see Lymphocytic interstitial pneumonitis
Liver disease, see Hepatic disease, in children

Lymph nodes
  in children, 134–137
  enlargement of, 45
  as site of KS, 111–112
Lymphadenopathy, 10, 111, 138
Lymphadenopathy syndrome (LAS), see Persistent generalized lymphadenopathy
Lymphadenopathy virus (LAV), 4
Lymphocytic interstitial pneumonitis (LIP), 60–62, 67
  in children, 134, 135
  diagnosis of, 60–61
Lymphoid interstitial pneumonia, 157
Lymphoma, 112–122
  bulky abdominal lymphadenopathy due to, 115–119
  in colon, 99, 101,
  of gastrointestinal tract, 83
  as indicator of AIDS, 112
  Kaposi's sarcoma and, 107
  of small bowel, 90–91, 97

M
Magnetic resonance imaging (MR), in neurological manifestations of AIDS, 22–24
MAI, see Mycobacterium avium-intracellulare
Malignant neoplasms, 107–128; see also Kaposi's sarcoma, Lymphoma
  differential diagnosis, 122–125
  other malignancies, 125–128
Mass lesions, 24–31; see also specific lesions
  biopsy for, 26
  in brain, 29–31
  incidence of, 24
  presentation, 24
Mediastinal adenopathy, 73
Mediastinal lymphadenopathy, 114–115
Meningeal disease, 34
Meningitis, 6
Metastatic Kaposi's sarcoma, 29
Metastatic non-Hodgkin's lymphoma, 39, 42
Monocytes, 3–4
Mucotaneous manifestations, of ARC, 13
MTB, see Mycobacterial tuberculosis
Mycobacterial infections, 36, 52–55
  of GI tract, 87–89
Mycobacterial meningitis, 38
Mycobacterial tuberculosis (MTB), 53–56
  diagnosis of, 54
  incidence of, 53
  therapy for, 54–55
Mycobacteriosis, presumptive diagnosis of, 157

Mycobacterium avium-intracellulare
    (MAI), 5, 6, 43, 72, 93, 94, 124–127
  bulky abdominal lymphadenopathy
      due to, 115–119
  in children, 134, 137
  CT in, 125
  of esophagus, 80
  general information on, 8–9
  granuloma formation in, 88
  presentation, 55
  "pseudo-Whipple" appearance of,
      88–89
  treatment of, 9, 55
Myelopathy, 38–40, 41
Myocarditis, 69

## N

Naltrexone (Trexan), 16
Neck, see Head and neck disease
Neoplasms
  of colon, 98–102
  of esophagus, 80–81
  of small bowel, 90–92
  of stomach, 82–83
Neuroimaging, 22
Neurologic manifestations
  of ARC, 15
  of AIDS, 21
Neurologic syndromes, 6
Neuroradiology of AIDS, 21–45
  atrophy, 24–31
  neurologic manifestations, 21
  radiologic manifestations, 22–24
New York City, AIDS in, 2, 3
NHL, see Non-Hodgkin's lymphoma
Nocardia, 59, 61
Non-Hodgkin's lymphoma (NHL),
    11–13, 67, 68, 69, 115, 118–123
  clinical hallmark of, 12
  grading of, 11
  of head and neck, 42, 43, 44, 45
  incidence of, 11
  presentation, 12
  treatment of, 12
  in visceral organs, 119–122
Nonviral infections, caused by AIDS,
    21–22
Nystatin, 13

## O

OI, see Opportunistic infections
Open-lung biopsy, 72
Ophthalmologic changes, due to ARC,
    15
Opportunistic infections (OI), 5–11; see
    also specific infections
  presentations of, 5
  symptom complexes caused by, 5
Oral candidiasis (thrush), 13
Oral manifestations, of ARC, 14

## P

Papova virus (J-C virus), 31, 32
PCP, see Pneumocystis carinii pneumonia
Pediatric AIDS, 36–38, 131–141; see
    also Children
  clinical features of, 132
  criteria for, 131–132
  incidence of, 131
  laboratory data on, 132
  radiologic manifestations, 133–141
  risk factors, 132
Pentamidine, 6–7, 134
Peptide-T, 16
Peripheral lymph nodes, biopsy of, 119
Peripheral neuropathy, 39
Persistent generalized lymphadenopathy (PGL), 113
  diagnostic criteria for, 123
  mortality in, 113
  node size in, 119, 123–125
PGL, see Persistent generalized lymphadenopathy
Phosphonoformate (Foscarnet), 16
PML, see Progressive multifocal leukoencephalopathy
Pleural effusion, secondary to KS, 10
Pneumocystis carinii pneumonia
    (PCP), 47–55, 60, 61, 63, 71
  air-space disease in, 47
  atypical radiographic findings in, 49
  BAL in, 72
  in children, 133–134
  cystic changes in, 49–50
  diagnosis of, 6
  gallium scintigraphy for, 70–71
  general information, 6–7
  incidence of, 6, 47
  presentation, 47
  presumptive diagnosis of, 157
  pulmonary fibrosis in, 52
  pulmonary symptoms of, 5–6
  radiographic resolution of, 50–52
  relapse and/or recurrence of, 52–53
  residual or recurrent infection, 50–51
  symptoms of, 6
  TBB in, 72
  treatment of, 6–7
Primary CNS lymphoma, 26–27, 31,
    32, 33
  as indicator of AIDS, 114
Progressive generalized lymphadenopathy (PGL), 10, 13
Progressive multifocal lymphadenopathy (PML), 32–33, 37
Pulmonary fibrosis, 52
Pulmonary KS, 110
Pulmonary lymphoma, 67
Pulmonary manifestations of AIDS, 5,
    6, 47–74; see also specific diseases
  diagnosis of, 71–74
  incidence of, 47
  types and frequency of, 73

## R

Radiography, guidelines for, 73–74
Radiological manifestations of AIDS,
    22–24
  in children, 133–141
  indications, 22
  technique, 22–24
Rectum, squamous cell carcinoma of,
    39
Recurrent aseptic meningitis, 15
Renal transplants, KS in, 107
Respiratory distress syndrome (RDS),
    133
Reticuloendothelial system, ARC and,
    13
Retrovir, 9, 15–17
Reverse transcriptase, 15–16
Ribavirin (Virazole), 16
Rifabutine (ansamycin), 55

## S

Sclerosing cholangitis, 102
Seborrheic dermatitis, in ARC, 14
Serum lactate dehydrogenase (LDH), 6
Simian T-lymphotropic virus (STIV-III), 4
Sinus disease, 45
Skin, ARC and infections of, 14
Small bowel, 83–92
  CMV of, 89–90
  cryptosporidiosis, 84–87
  gastrointestinal radiology of, 83–91
  KS of, 90–92, 96, 97
  lymphoma of, 90–92, 97
  mycobacterial infections of, 87–89,
      93, 94
  neoplasms of, 90–92
Sonography, for lymph nodes, 134
Spine, in ARLs, 114
Spiramycin, 8, 87
Splenomegaly, 13, 111
Spontaneous pneumotosis coli, 97
Squamous cell carcinoma, 61
  of anorectal region, 12
  of head and neck, 43
  of rectum, 39
Stenosing papillitis, 102, 103
STIV-III, see Simian T-lymphotropic
    virus
Stomach, 81–83
  candida of, 82
  gastric lesions, 81
  gastric neoplasms, 82–83
  gastrointestinal radiology of, 81–83
  KS of, 82
  nonneoplastic lesions, 81–82

Streptococcus pneumonia, 59
Sulfamethoxazole, 133–134
Suramin, 15, 16

**T**
T-helper cells, 4
T-helper lymphocytes ($CD_{4+}$), 3
T-suppressor cells ($CD_{+8}$), 3
TBB, 71–72
Testicular carcinoma, 12
Thorax, in ARC, 114
Thrush, see Oral candidiasis

Tmp/smx, see Trimethoprim/sulfamethoxazole
Toxoplasmic gondii, 5–7
Toxoplasmosis, 23, 24–30, 36, 39
   incidence of, 24
   presumptive diagnosis of, 157
   treatment for, 26
TP-5 (Thymopentane), 16
Transbronchial lung biopsy, 6
Trimerexate, 7
Trimethoprim, 133
Trimethoprim/sulfamethoxazole (Tmp/smx), 6–7
Tuberculoma, 34

**V**
Varicella zoster virus (VZV), 14, 33, 34
Vidarabine, 33
Vinblastine, 11
Vincristine, 11, 15
Viral messenger RNA, 16
Viral syndromes, caused by AIDS, 21
VZV, see Varicella zoster virus

**W**
White matter disease, 31–34

**Z**
Zodivudine, 9, 15–17

RC 607.A26R23 1988

circ — Radiology of AIDS / Bergen Community College Library

3 5936 000 121 834

**DATE DUE**
Student

MAY 0 5 2008

AUG 0 7 2008

AUG 1 4 2008

SEP 1 6 2008

Nov. 21

Dec 3, 08

MAR 3 1 2009

**Library and Learning
Resources Center
Bergen Community College**
400 Paramus Road
Paramus, N.J. 07652-1595

Return Postage Guaranteed